Core Concepts in Hypertension in Kidney Disease

Ajay K. Singh • Rajiv Agarwal

Editors

Core Concepts in Hypertension in Kidney Disease

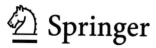 Springer

Editors
Ajay K. Singh
Global and Continuing Education
Harvard Medical School
Boston, MA, USA

Rajiv Agarwal
VA Medical Center
Indiana University School of Medicine
Indianapolis, IN, USA

ISBN 978-1-4939-8199-1   ISBN 978-1-4939-6436-9   (eBook)
DOI 10.1007/978-1-4939-6436-9

Printed on acid-free paper

This Springer imprint is published by Springer Nature
The registered company is Springer Science+Business Media LLC New York

Preface

Hypertension is ubiquitous in chronic kidney disease (CKD); textbooks on hypertension in CKD are not. The specialist wants to master the art of managing hypertension in CKD, yet there are few resources to go to. This book, we hope, fills the vacuum for the specialist who wants a comprehensive review of hypertension in CKD.

In approaching the difficult task to fill this void, we created topics that would have minimal overlap among them and asked each of the authors to provide a comprehensive, yet succinct, narrative on the subject. Authors need little introduction as they are respected authorities in the field from around the world; we are grateful for their efforts in creating this text. As editors, we did not try to change their opinions—even when our approach may have been different—because the evidence base for practice is often thin and opinion-based. We did ask our authors to rationalize their unique approach in the hopes that this would allow the readers to appreciate the variations in practice among authorities.

Books are old-fashioned and often have the quality of being outdated even before they are published. So we may ask: why do we still read books? There is something real about holding a book; the smell of paper, turning the pages, highlighting, and making notes allow us to develop a GPS image in our brains; it provides a connection with the material that we feel is not possible with electronic texts. We are decidedly old-fashioned when it comes to touching real paper and learning by reading books on paper.

This book is written with primarily the renal fellow or a practicing nephrologist in mind. The renal fellow may want to master the subject and read the book cover to cover in bite-sized chapters. The practicing nephrologist may simply want to review a few areas of interest to her. Each chapter stands on its own, and the book, in order to be understood, does not need to be read from the first page to the last.

We owe a debt of gratitude to our wives, Anuja and Ritu, while we took time to edit this work. The editorial team at Springer, in particular Barbara Lopez-Lucio, gets a big thank you from us for keeping us on track; without the editorial team (and Barbara in particular), there was little hope of creating this textbook.

Lastly, we hope that our daughters, Radhika and Anika, both medical students, and Vikrum and Nikki, will join them in reading this text (and approve of it).

Boston, MA, USA   Ajay K. Singh
Indianapolis, IN, USA   Rajiv Agarwal

Contents

Contributors

Anil K. Bidani, MD Edward Hines Jr. VA Hospital and Loyola University Medical Center, Maywood, IL, USA

Jordana B. Cohen, MD Renal, Electrolyte, Hypertension Division, Department of Medicine, University of Pennsylvania, Philadelphia, PA, USA

Joseph T. Flynn, MD, MS Department of Pediatrics, University of Washington, Seattle Children's Hospital, Seattle, WA, USA

Division of Nephrology, Seattle Children's Hospital, Seattle, WA, USA

Panagiotis I. Georgianos, MD, PhD AHEPA Hospital, Aristotle University of Thessaloniki, Thessaloniki, Greece

Karen A. Griffin, MD Edward Hines Jr. VA Hospital and Loyola University Medical Center, Maywood, IL, USA

Susan M. Halbach, MD, MPH Department of Pediatrics, University of Washington, Seattle Children's Hospital, Seattle, WA, USA

Division of Nephrology, Seattle Children's Hospital, Seattle, WA, USA

Sandra M. Herrmann, MD Nephrology and Hypertension Division, Mayo Clinic, Rochester, MN, USA

Sharon Maynard, MD Associate Professor of Medicine, University of South Florida Morsani College of Medicine, Lehigh Valley Health Network, Allentown, PA, USA

Dipti Patel, MD Department of Nephrology, University of Maryland Medical Center, Baltimore, MD, USA

Aldo J. Peixoto, MD Department of Internal Medicine (Section of Nephrology), Yale University, New Haven, CT, USA

Mark A. Perazella, MD, MS Department of Medicine, Section of Nephrology, Yale University School of Medicine, Yale-New Haven Hospital, New Haven, CT, USA

Aaron J. Polichnowski, PhD Edward Hines Jr. VA Hospital and Loyola University Medical Center, Maywood, IL, USA

Pantelis A. Sarafidis, MD, MSc, PhD Hippokration Hospital, Aristotle University of Thessaloniki, Thessaloniki, Greece

Arjun D. Sinha, MD, MS Division of Nephrology, Richard L. Roudebush VA Medical Center, University of Indiana School of Medicine, Indianapolis, IN, USA

Stephen C. Textor, MD Nephrology and Hypertension Division, Mayo Clinic, Rochester, MN, USA

George Thomas, MD, FACP Department of Nephrology and Hypertension, Glickman Urological and Kidney Institute, Cleveland Clinic, Cleveland, OH, USA

Hakan R. Toka, MD, PhD Graduate Medical Education, Manatee Memorial Hospital, Bradenton, FL, USA

Raymond R. Townsend, MD Renal, Electrolyte, Hypertension Division, Department of Medicine, University of Pennsylvania, Philadelphia, PA, USA

Hina K. Trivedi, DO Department of Nephrology, University of Maryland Medical Center, Baltimore, MD, USA

Sebastian Varas, MD Division of Nephrology, Maine Medical Center, Portland, ME, USA

John Vella, MD, FRCP, FACP, FASN Maine Transplant Program, Maine Medical Center, Portland, ME, USA

Alfred A. Vichot, MD Department of Internal Medicine, Yale University, New Haven, CT, USA

Angela Yee-Moon Wang, MBBS, MD, PhD, FRCP Department of Medicine, Queen Mary Hospital, University of Hong Kong, Hong Kong, China

Matthew R. Weir, MD Department of Nephrology, University of Maryland School of Medicine, Baltimore, MD, USA

Chapter 1
Epidemiology of Hypertension in Chronic Kidney Disease

Angela Yee-Moon Wang

Prevalence of Chronic Kidney Disease and Its Determinants

Chronic kidney disease (CKD) is defined as persistent kidney damage, which is often reflected by either a reduction in glomerular filtration rate or increased urine albumin excretion, or both. CKD is now a worldwide public health challenge. According to the 2010 Global Burden of Disease study, CKD is ranked 18th in the list of causes of total number of global deaths with an estimated annual death rate of 16.3 per 100,000 [1]. The prevalence of CKD varies across different countries and regions and is estimated to range between 8 and 16 % of the adult population [2–9]. The prevalence of CKD has shown a steady global increase over the years. For example, in the USA, the prevalence of CKD was estimated to be around 10 % between 1988 and 1994 and it increased to 13.1 % between 1999 and 2004 [4]. The prevalence estimates of CKD differ slightly depending on the GFR estimating equations used [4, 10]. The rise in CKD prevalence and incidence has been attributed to an aging population as well as an increased prevalence of hypertension, diabetes, and obesity, all of which are recognized as important global health challenges [4, 11, 12].

According to the 2010 United States Renal Data System (USRDS) Annual Data Report, the leading causes of kidney failure in the USA are diabetes, hypertension, and glomerulonephritis. Hypertension and diabetes account for 99 and 153 per million population of incident cases of end-stage renal disease (ESRD), respectively [13]. The prevalence of stage 3 or higher CKD in diabetics in the USA exceeds 15 % [13]. Over 5 % of people with newly diagnosed type 2 diabetes already have CKD and an estimated 40 % of diabetics will develop CKD in their time course [14]. Data from World Health Organization showed that the number of individuals with diabetes is currently around 154 million globally and is projected to double within

A.Y.-M. Wang, MBBS, MD, PhD, FRCP (✉)
Department of Medicine, Queen Mary Hospital, University of Hong Kong,
102 Pok Fu Lam Road, Hong Kong, China
e-mail: aymwang@hku.hk

© Springer Science+Business Media New York 2016
A.K. Singh, R. Agarwal (eds.), *Core Concepts in Hypertension in Kidney Disease*, DOI 10.1007/978-1-4939-6436-9_1

the next 20 years. The increase is most notable in less developed countries, where the number of diabetic patients could rise from 99 million to 286 million by 2025 [15]. China and India are projected to have 139 million people with diabetes in 2025 [16]. A parallel increase in the global incidence and prevalence of CKD due to diabetic nephropathy is therefore anticipated. CKD in diabetes is associated with an increased risk of progression to ESRD [17].

The aging population also in part explains an increase in the incidence of hypertension, diabetes, and CKD worldwide. The prevalence of CKD was reported to be 7.4% among women aged 18–39 years and increased to 18.0 and 24.2% among those aged 60–69 and 70 years or above, respectively, in the Chinese general population [2]. Similar parallel increase in CKD prevalence with aging was observed across the USA, Canada, and Europe although the absolute prevalence differed across countries [4, 8, 18]. Cardiovascular disease is also an important cause of CKD.

Definition of Hypertension

The American Heart Association defines hypertension as a blood pressure of 140/90 mmHg or more, measured in clinic setting, based on two readings, 5 min apart and sitting in chair and confirmed with elevated reading in contralateral arm.

Prevalence of Hypertension in CKD

Hypertension is very common in CKD, with a prevalence estimated around 60–95% in CKD stage 3–5 [19–22]. Hypertension has a complex interrelationship with CKD. Hypertension is an important modifiable cause for CKD as well as a consequence of CKD. Nearly a billion of the adult population (around 26.4%) in 2000 had hypertension (defined as >140/90 mmHg) and this proportion is projected to increase by about 60% to 1.56 billion by 2025 (24% in developed countries and 80% in developing regions such as Africa and Latin America) [23]. A corresponding global increase in the prevalence of CKD is therefore anticipated. The Global Burden of Disease Study identified elevated blood pressure as the leading risk factor, among 67 studied, for death and disability-adjusted life years lost during 2010 [24]. According to the USRDS Annual Data report for 2014, up to 25% of CKD was attributed to hypertension. Of the 10.7% of Medicare patients diagnosed with CKD in 2013, nearly half also have diabetes, and over 92% also have hypertension [25]. The rate of ESRD caused by hypertension has grown 8.1% since 2000, to 99.1 per million population. In contrast, the incident rate of diabetic ESRD fell 1.5% between 2007 and 2008, to 153 per million population—a rate nearly unchanged from that of 2000 while that of ESRD due to glomerulonephritis has fallen 23.4%, to 23.7 per million population [25].

Fig. 1.1 Prevalence of
hypertension in different
CKD stages [27]

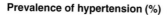

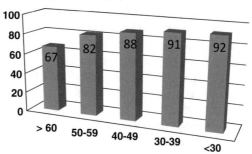

The prevalence of hypertension in CKD shows racial disparities in being higher among non-Hispanic blacks versus whites or Mexican Americans, as reported in several cohorts. In the Modification of Diet in Renal Disease (MDRD) study, the prevalence of hypertension was higher in blacks versus whites [93 % versus 81 %] [26]. Similarly, in Chronic Renal Insufficiency Cohort (CRIC) study, hypertension was reported in 93 % of African Americans versus 80 % of whites although Hispanics show a greater risk for CKD and ESRD compared to non-Hispanics [27]. Socioeconomic status and lifestyle also influence the prevalence of hypertension in CKD patients. Patients with poorer socioeconomic status, lower income, and education level showed a higher prevalence of hypertension [27].

The prevalence of hypertension increases with worsening estimated glomerular filtration rate (eGFR), as shown in CRIC study [27] (see Fig. 1.1). The prevalence of hypertension was 92 % for those with eGFR <30 ml/min per 1.73 m^2 and 67 % for those with eGFR >60ml/min per 1.73 m^2. The prevalence estimates for hypertension among CKD patients in China, India, and Mexico were similar to those reported in CRIC cohort [28–30].

The prevalence of hypertension varies by the etiology of CKD. CKD due to diabetic nephropathy showed the highest prevalence of hypertension independent of kidney function [27]. Hypertension was also more frequent among patients with polycystic kidney disease, renal artery stenosis when compared to glomerulonephritis, tubulointerstitial disease, or chronic pyelonephritis [31]. Albuminuria was an important, independent risk factor for hypertension as shown by pooled data from National Health and Nutrition Examination Survey (NHANES) III and NHANES 1999–2005 [32, 33]. In the United States National Kidney Foundation's Kidney Early Evaluation Program (KEEP), decreasing GFR by 10 ml/min/1.73 m^2, increasing age, obesity, African American race, and microalbuminuria were all associated with an increased prevalence of hypertension [22]. Urine albumin to creatinine ratio greater than 6.67 mg/g in men and above 15.24 mg/g in women resulted in doubling the risk of developing hypertension when accounting for baseline blood pressure, body mass index, and creatinine [34]. Higher albumin/creatinine ratios, even within the normal range, are independently associated with increased risk for development of hypertension in the general population [35]. Proteinuria was shown to be one of the most important correlates of systolic blood pressure in older men, especially with ambulatory and home systolic blood pressure [36]. The association between albuminuria and hypertension may be mediated via an increased inflammation, endothelial dysfunction, and renal sodium handling [37].

Obesity was an important predictor of hypertension among CKD patients. In the MDRD study, body mass index was a strong predictor of hypertension among patients with a GFR of 25–55 ml/min per 1.73 m² [26]. Likewise, both the KEEP (78.6% versus 60.3%) and NHANES study (52% versus 30.8%) showed a greater prevalence of hypertension among obese subjects as compared to non-obese subjects [22]. Obesity was also an independent risk factor for CKD [38].

Suboptimal blood pressure control was common in CKD, especially those at the highest risk of adverse outcomes due to diabetes or albuminuria [39]. The NHANES data showed that elevated serum creatinine level was strongly related to suboptimal treatment of high blood pressure [20]. Only 36% of subjects met the blood pressure target of <140/90 while only 14% of treated hypertensive individuals met the older blood pressure target of <130/85 proposed for individuals with kidney disease [20]. In the KEEP program for people at high risk for CKD, the prevalence (86%), awareness (80%), and treatment (70%) of hypertension were high but good blood control was achieved in only 13% [40]. Poor medication adherence was associated with 23% increased risk of uncontrolled hypertension [41]. These data suggest poorly controlled hypertension is associated with much of the high burden of CKD and there is a need to improve blood pressure control in CKD.

Clinic Blood Pressure and Ambulatory Blood Pressure

The diagnosis and control of hypertension critically depend on accuracy of blood pressure measurements. Clinic blood pressure frequently overestimates and underestimates true blood pressure in hypertensive general population and this is also observed in patients with CKD. Misclassification of blood pressure control at the office was observed in 1 of 3 hypertensive patients with CKD, suggesting that ambulatory-based control rates were far better than office-based rates [42]. Using ambulatory blood pressure monitoring as the reference standard, home blood pressure monitoring showed the best diagnostic performance for hypertension compared with routine or standardized clinic measurements in CKD. One week-averaged home blood pressure >140/80 mmHg was associated with awake ambulatory blood pressure >130/80, a threshold considered as hypertensive in the CKD population [43]. White coat hypertension is defined as an elevated clinic blood pressure but controlled blood pressure out of clinics. Masked hypertension is defined as controlled blood pressure in clinic setting with elevated blood pressure out of clinics. According to a systematic analysis including six studies with 980 CKD subjects, the overall prevalence of white coat hypertension was 18.3% (range, 10–28%) and masked hypertension 8.3% (range, 5–28%). Notably, 40.4% of subjects with CKD considered to have normal or controlled blood pressure in fact had masked uncontrolled hypertension (range, 26–54%) while 30% of subjects with CKD that were thought to have hypertension had normotension at home [44]. Similarly, a high rate of masked hypertension was observed in the follow-up study of the African American Study of Kidney Disease (AASK) cohort; of the 61% subjects with controlled clinic blood pressure, 70% had masked hypertension [45]. This location-dependent hypertension, namely masked hypertension and white coat hypertension, has been shown to predict prognosis in patients with hypertension. Masked hypertension carries a risk equivalent to sustained hypertension, whereas white coat hypertension carries a risk almost equivalent to normotension [46]. In the general population, the risk of CKD was significantly increased in sustained hypertension, masked hypertension, and white coat hypertension [47]. The AASK study showed that target organ damage was more common in subjects with sustained or masked hypertension [45]. CKD patients with masked hypertension were more likely to progress to end-stage renal disease [48]. The prevalence rates of masked hypertension depend very much on the definitions used to define masked hypertension. Conventionally, masked uncontrolled hypertension was defined as clinic blood pressure >140/90 mmHg or daytime ambulatory blood pressure ≥135/85 mmHg. In a recent study of 333 veterans with CKD, the prevalence of masked uncontrolled hypertension was 26.7% defined by daytime ambulatory blood pressure, 32.8% by 24-hour ambulatory blood pressure and more than doubled to 56.1% if defined by daytime or nighttime ambulatory blood pressure [49].

Ambulatory blood pressure was superior to clinic blood pressure measurements in correlating with end-organ damage [36]. Ambulatory blood pressure showed a stronger association with proteinuria [36] and echocardiographic left ventricular hypertrophy [50, 51] than clinic blood pressure in CKD population. In keeping with these observations, a prospective cohort study conducted in 217 veterans with CKD showed that 24 h ambulatory systolic blood pressure provided additional prognostic value for composite cardiovascular endpoint of myocardial infarction, stroke, and mortality beyond clinic blood pressure, indicating the importance of ambulatory blood pressure in predicting clinical outcomes in CKD (see Fig. 1.2) [48]. Clinic blood pressure above goal and ambulatory blood pressure at goal identify a low risk condition while clinic blood pressure at goal and ambulatory blood pressure above goal are both associated with higher cardio-renal risk similar to that observed in patients with both clinic and ambulatory blood pressure above goal [52]. Furthermore, the definitions used to classify patients as having hypertension or normotension can influence the risk for being classified as having masked hypertension in favor of white coat hypertension. A meta-analysis has shown that when the thresholds for classification of clinic and ambulatory blood pressure are equal, the risk for diagnosis of masked hypertension is less (risk ratio of 0.74). When the clinic blood pressure threshold is higher and home blood pressure threshold is lower, the risk (risk ratio of 1.36) for diagnosing masked hypertension is greater [44]. More recent analysis by Agarwal and co-workers showed that clinic blood pressure was a good determinant of masked uncontrolled hypertension with area under the receiver-operating characteristics curve of 0.82 (95% confidence intervals, 0.76–0.87). Home blood pressure was no better than clinic blood pressure in

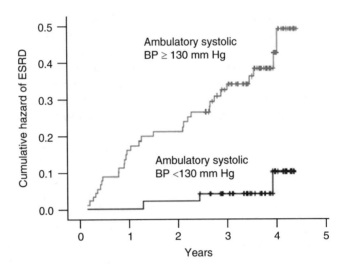

Fig. 1.2 Cumulative incidence of ESRD in patients with elevated systolic clinic blood pressure. Adapted from Agarwal R, et al. Prognostic importance of ambulatory blood pressure recordings in patients with chronic kidney disease. Kidney Int 2006;69:1175–80; used with permission

diagnosing masked uncontrolled hypertension in CKD. Thus, the use of home blood pressure to diagnose masked uncontrolled hypertension was not supported. Nevertheless, ambulatory blood pressure showed short-term reproducibility in diagnosing masked uncontrolled hypertension and may detect a phenotype with increased cardiovascular risk [49].

Hypertension and Kidney Outcomes in Chronic Kidney Disease

There are compelling data from observational studies that high blood pressure was associated with the development and progression of CKD [53–55]. Lowering blood pressure has also been a key treatment strategy in slowing the progression of CKD. However, the blood pressure threshold level of which this risk was increased remains controversial. The NHANES study showed an eightfold higher risk of an elevated serum creatinine among those with hypertension versus those with a normal blood pressure [20]. In the Multiple Risk Factor Intervention Trial, systolic and diastolic blood pressure was identified as strong risk factors for progression to ESRD, independent of age, race, income, use of medication for diabetes mellitus, history of myocardial infarction, serum cholesterol concentration, and cigarette smoking as well as baseline serum creatinine and proteinuria over an average follow-up duration of 16 years [53]. Those with blood pressure more than 210/120 mmHg showed at least a 20-fold increased risk of ESRD than those with blood pressure less than 120/80 mmHg. The estimated risk of ESRD associated with systolic blood pressure was also greater than that with diastolic blood pressure when both systolic and diastolic blood pressure were considered together. The risk appeared to start at systolic blood pressure of 140 mmHg rather than 130 mmHg and was the highest among those with systolic blood pressure of 150 mmHg or above [53].

The KEEP cohort showed that high systolic blood pressure accounted for most of the risk of progression to ESRD [56]. There is also evidence that the risk of ESRD appeared to increase even with modest elevation of blood pressure and the observed relationship did not appear to be due to confounding by clinically evident baseline kidney disease. Notably, among subjects with eGFR over 60 ml/min per 1.73 m^2, those with blood pressure of 12–129/80–84 mmHg were 62 % more likely to develop ESRD while those with blood pressure of 130–139/85–89 mmHg were 98 % more likely to develop ESRD compared to those with blood pressure below 120/80 mmHg [57]. Several earlier clinical trials also established that lower blood pressure levels were associated with slower progression of CKD among subjects with proteinuria [55, 58].

On the other hand, post-hoc analysis from the Homocysteinemia in Kidney and ESRD (HOST) study, a double-blind randomized controlled trial in 2056 subjects with advanced CKD (mean eGFR 18 ml/min per 1.73 m^2) showed no graded association between systolic blood pressure and cardiovascular events or ESRD. However, those with systolic blood pressure >157 mmHg were associated with an increased risk of ESRD [59]. A systematic analysis putting together 11 randomized controlled trials of 9287 patients with CKD concluded that a more intensive blood pressure lowering reduced the risk of composite kidney failure events by 17 % and the risk of ESRD alone by 18 %, especially those with proteinuria. However, intensive blood pressure lowering appeared to have no effect on kidney failure among those who did not have proteinuria [60]. Another systematic review of three large trials in this field, namely the MDRD study [58, 61, 62], Ramipril Efficacy in Nephropathy-2 (REIN-2) study [63], and the AASK study [64–66] including 2272 CKD subjects failed to show any significant benefit by lowering blood pressure to less than 125/75 to 130/80 as compared to 140/90 mmHg. However, subgroup analysis suggested that a lower target may benefit in subjects with proteinuria [67].

These observations are in contrast to the Systolic Blood Pressure Intervention Trial (SPRINT) which is a randomized controlled trial that examined >9000 hypertensive subjects with an increased cardiovascular risk but without diabetes. Among those with baseline CKD, the number of subjects showing ≥50 % decline in GFR or ESRD did not differ between intensive treatment (target 120 mmHg) versus standard treatment (target 140 mmHg). However, among those with no CKD at baseline, those randomized to intensive treatment showed more adverse renal outcomes compared to standard treatment [68]. This finding adds to the growing uncertainties of target blood pressure for kidney protection in high risk subjects with and without CKD. Although the JNC 7 recommended a target blood pressure of less than 130/80 mmHg for CKD subjects [69], more recent recommendations from JNC 8 acknowledged the limitations of available evidence and suggest a target of less than 140/90 mmHg be used [70]. The CRIC study showed that having longitudinal blood pressure values and time-updated systolic blood pressure greater than 130 mmHg may be more strongly associated with CKD progression than analyses based on a single baseline systolic blood pressure [71]. Given the clinical uncertainties and the potential for harm, it appears that a BP target of <140/90 mmHg in the clinic or <135/85 mmHg at home appears reasonable even among those with CKD.

Hypertension and Cardiovascular Outcomes in CKD

Blood pressure is an important determinant of cardiovascular risk in the general population [72] and lowering blood pressure reduces cardiovascular events in this population [73, 74]. A previous meta-analysis showed that lowering blood pressure was the main target to lower major cardiovascular event risk in hypertensive subjects [74]. Earlier study demonstrated the importance of blood pressure reduction in CKD. In the MDRD study, each 10 mmHg increase in follow-up systolic blood pressure increased the risk of hospitalization for cardiovascular and cerebrovascular disease by 35 % [61]. However, it remains controversial as to what ideal blood pressure target should be in terms of cardiovascular protection in CKD. A recent systematic analysis including 26 trials with 152,290 participants of which 30,295 subjects had CKD (defined as having eGFR <60 ml/min per 1.73 m^2) confirmed that blood pressure lowering significantly reduced the risk of major cardiovascular events by about one-sixth (for each 5 mmHg reduction in systolic blood pressure) in those with CKD (hazard ratio, 0.83, 95 % confidence intervals, 0.76–0.90) and the risk reduction was very comparable to those without CKD (hazard ratio, 0.83, 95 % confidence intervals, 0.79–0.88) [75]. Specifically, the systematic analysis showed that blood pressure lowering per se, rather than a particular anti-hypertensive drug class, was associated with cardiovascular risk reduction [75]. Notably, these observations are in keeping with the SPRINT trial showing that among adults with hypertension but without diabetes, lowering systolic blood pressure to a target goal of less than 120 mmHg significantly reduced the risk of fatal or non-fatal cardiovascular events and death from all causes as compared with the standard goal of less than 140 mmHg [68]. On the other hand, two retrospective cohort studies raised uncertainties with lower blood pressure targets [76, 77]. One study examined elderly veterans with CKD and initially uncontrolled hypertension and found higher mortality among subjects treated to a systolic blood pressure of less than 120 mmHg versus 120–139 mmHg (hazard ratio, 1.7, 95 % confidence intervals, 1.63–1.78) [77]. Another retrospective analysis of a large diverse cohort of hypertensive subjects observed a U-shaped curve for the risk associated with both achieved systolic and diastolic blood pressure in relation to a composite endpoint of all-cause mortality or ESRD [76]. Thus, while lowering blood pressure is recognized as one of the core strategies in reducing cardiovascular risk in CKD, the blood pressure target that confers the largest cardiovascular benefit has remained uncertain. Randomized trials rather than observational studies should inform clinical practice. Thus, guidelines such as the JNC 8 have taken the position that BP lowering to <140/90 mmHg measured in the clinic, even among those with CKD, appears reasonable.

Conclusions

Both hypertension and CKD are important global health problems and are strongly interrelated. Hypertension may cause CKD and modify the outcomes of CKD. On the other hand, hypertension may also result from CKD. High blood pressure increases the onset and progression of CKD and worsens the clinical outcomes of CKD patients. More attention is needed to raise awareness of hypertension and improve blood pressure control among CKD population.

References

1. Lozano R, Naghavi M, Foreman K, Lim S, Shibuya K, Aboyans V, et al. Global and regional mortality from 235 causes of death for 20 age groups in 1990 and 2010: a systematic analysis for the Global Burden of Disease Study 2010. Lancet. 2012;380(9859):2095–128.
2. Zhang L, Wang F, Wang L, Wang W, Liu B, Liu J, et al. Prevalence of chronic kidney disease in China: a cross-sectional survey. Lancet. 2012;379(9818):815–22.
3. Jha V, Wang AY, Wang H. The impact of CKD identification in large countries: the burden of illness. Nephrol Dial Transplant. 2012;27 (Suppl 3):iii32–8.
4. Coresh J, Selvin E, Stevens LA, Manzi J, Kusek JW, Eggers P, et al. Prevalence of chronic kidney disease in the United States. JAMA. 2007;298(17):2038–47.
5. Imai E, Horio M, Watanabe T, Iseki K, Yamagata K, Hara S, et al. Prevalence of chronic kidney disease in the Japanese general population. Clin Exp Nephrol. 2009;13(6):621–30.
6. Wen CP, Cheng TY, Tsai MK, Chang YC, Chan HT, Tsai SP, et al. All-cause mortality attributable to chronic kidney disease: a prospective cohort study based on 462 293 adults in Taiwan. Lancet. 2008;371(9631):2173–82.
7. Hallan SI, Coresh J, Astor BC, Asberg A, Powe NR, Romundstad S, et al. International comparison of the relationship of chronic kidney disease prevalence and ESRD risk. J Am Soc Nephrol. 2006;17(8):2275–84.
8. Zhang QL, Rothenbacher D. Prevalence of chronic kidney disease in population-based studies: systematic review. BMC Public Health. 2008;8:117.
9. Varma PP, Raman DK, Ramakrishnan TS, Singh P, Varma A. Prevalence of early stages of chronic kidney disease in apparently healthy central government employees in India. Nephrol Dial Transplant. 2010;25(9):3011–7.
10. Stevens LA, Schmid CH, Greene T, Zhang YL, Beck GJ, Froissart M, et al. Comparative performance of the CKD Epidemiology Collaboration (CKD-EPI) and the Modification of Diet in Renal Disease (MDRD) Study equations for estimating GFR levels above 60 mL/min/1.73 m2. Am J kidney Dis. 2010;56(3):486–95.
11. Jha V, Garcia-Garcia G, Iseki K, Li Z, Naicker S, Plattner B, et al. Chronic kidney disease: global dimension and perspectives. Lancet. 2013;382(9888):260–72.
12. Couser WG, Remuzzi G, Mendis S, Tonelli M. The contribution of chronic kidney disease to the global burden of major noncommunicable diseases. Kidney Int. 2011;80(12):1258–70.
13. Collins AJ, Foley RN, Herzog C, Chavers B, Gilbertson D, Ishani A, et al. United States Renal Data System 2008 Annual Data Report. Am J kidney Dis. 2009;53(1 Suppl):S1–374.
14. Huang ES, Basu A, O'Grady M, Capretta JC. Projecting the future diabetes population size and related costs for the U.S. Diabetes Care. 2009;32(12):2225–9.
15. King H, Aubert RE, Herman WH. Global burden of diabetes, 1995-2025: prevalence, numerical estimates, and projections. Diabetes Care. 1998;21(9):1414–31.
16. World Health Organization. Preventing chronic diseases: a vital investment. World Health Organization; 2005.

17. Jones CA, Krolewski AS, Rogus J, Xue JL, Collins A, Warram JH. Epidemic of end-stage renal disease in people with diabetes in the United States population: do we know the cause? Kidney Int. 2005;67(5):1684–91.
18. Arora P, Vasa P, Brenner D, Iglar K, McFarlane P, Morrison H, et al. Prevalence estimates of chronic kidney disease in Canada: results of a nationally representative survey. Can Med Assoc J. 2013;185(9):E417–23.
19. Kalaitzidis R, Li S, Wang C, Chen SC, McCullough PA, Bakris GL. Hypertension in early-stage kidney disease: an update from the Kidney Early Evaluation Program (KEEP). Am J kidney Dis. 2009;53(4 Suppl 4):S22–31.
20. Coresh J, Wei GL, McQuillan G, Brancati FL, Levey AS, Jones C, et al. Prevalence of high blood pressure and elevated serum creatinine level in the United States: findings from the third National Health and Nutrition Examination Survey (1988-1994). Arch Intern Med. 2001;161(9):1207–16.
21. Collins AJ, Foley RN, Herzog C, Chavers B, Gilbertson D, Ishani A, et al. US Renal Data System 2010 Annual Data Report. Am J kidney Dis. 2011;57(1 Suppl 1):A8. e1-526.
22. Rao MV, Qiu Y, Wang C, Bakris G. Hypertension and CKD: Kidney Early Evaluation Program (KEEP) and National Health and Nutrition Examination Survey (NHANES), 1999-2004. Am J kidney Dis. 2008;51(4 Suppl 2):S30–7.
23. Kearney PM, Whelton M, Reynolds K, Muntner P, Whelton PK, He J. Global burden of hypertension: analysis of worldwide data. Lancet. 2005;365(9455):217–23.
24. Lim SS, Vos T, Flaxman AD, Danaei G, Shibuya K, Adair-Rohani H, et al. A comparative risk assessment of burden of disease and injury attributable to 67 risk factors and risk factor clusters in 21 regions, 1990-2010: a systematic analysis for the Global Burden of Disease Study 2010. Lancet. 2012;380(9859):2224–60.
25. Saran R, Li Y, Robinson B, Ayanian J, Balkrishnan R, Bragg-Gresham J, et al. US Renal Data System 2014 Annual Data Report: Epidemiology of kidney disease in the United States. Am J Kidney Dis. 2015;66(1 Suppl 1):Svii, S1–305.
26. Buckalew Jr VM, Berg RL, Wang SR, Porush JG, Rauch S, Schulman G. Prevalence of hypertension in 1,795 subjects with chronic renal disease: the modification of diet in renal disease study baseline cohort. Modification of Diet in Renal Disease Study Group. Am J Kidney Dis. 1996;28(6):811–21.
27. Muntner P, Anderson A, Charleston J, Chen Z, Ford V, Makos G, et al. Hypertension awareness, treatment, and control in adults with CKD: results from the Chronic Renal Insufficiency Cohort (CRIC) Study. Am J kidney Dis. 2010;55(3):441–51.
28. Zheng Y, Cai GY, Chen XM, Fu P, Chen JH, Ding XQ, et al. Prevalence, awareness, treatment, and control of hypertension in the non-dialysis chronic kidney disease patients. Chin Med J. 2013;126(12):2276–80.
29. Obrador GT, Garcia-Garcia G, Villa AR, Rubilar X, Olvera N, Ferreira E, et al. Prevalence of chronic kidney disease in the Kidney Early Evaluation Program (KEEP) Mexico and comparison with KEEP US. Kidney Int Suppl. 2010;116:S2–8.
30. Singh AK, Farag YM, Mittal BV, Subramanian KK, Reddy SR, Acharya VN, et al. Epidemiology and risk factors of chronic kidney disease in India - results from the SEEK (Screening and Early Evaluation of Kidney Disease) study. BMC Nephrol. 2013;14:114.
31. Ridao N, Luno J, de Vinuesa SG, Gomez F, Tejedor A, Valderrabano F. Prevalence of hypertension in renal disease. Nephrol Dial Transplant. 2001;16 Suppl 1:70–3.
32. Peralta CA, Hicks LS, Chertow GM, Ayanian JZ, Vittinghoff E, Lin F, et al. Control of hypertension in adults with chronic kidney disease in the United States. Hypertension. 2005;45(6):1119–24.
33. Inker LA, Coresh J, Levey AS, Tonelli M, Muntner P. Estimated GFR, albuminuria, and complications of chronic kidney disease. J Am Soc Nephrol. 2011;22(12):2322–31.
34. Wang TJ, Evans JC, Meigs JB, Rifai N, Fox CS, D'Agostino RB, et al. Low-grade albuminuria and the risks of hypertension and blood pressure progression. Circulation. 2005;111(11):1370–6.

35. Takase H, Sugiura T, Ohte N, Dohi Y. Urinary albumin as a marker of future blood pressure and hypertension in the general population. Medicine (Baltimore). 2015;94(6), e511.
36. Agarwal R, Andersen MJ. Correlates of systolic hypertension in patients with chronic kidney disease. Hypertension. 2005;46(3):514–20.
37. Romero CA, Peixoto AJ, Orias M. Estimated GFR or albuminuria: which one is really associated with resistant hypertension? Semin Nephrol. 2014;34(5):492–7.
38. Gelber RP, Kurth T, Kausz AT, Manson JE, Buring JE, Levey AS, et al. Association between body mass index and CKD in apparently healthy men. Am J kidney Dis. 2005;46(5):871–80.
39. Fraser SD, Roderick PJ, McIntyre NJ, Harris S, McIntyre CW, Fluck RJ, et al. Suboptimal blood pressure control in chronic kidney disease stage 3: baseline data from a cohort study in primary care. BMC Fam Pract. 2013;14:88.
40. Sarafidis PA, Li S, Chen SC, Collins AJ, Brown WW, Klag MJ, et al. Hypertension awareness, treatment, and control in chronic kidney disease. Am J Med. 2008;121(4):332–40.
41. Schmitt KE, Edie CF, Laflam P, Simbartl LA, Thakar CV. Adherence to antihypertensive agents and blood pressure control in chronic kidney disease. Am J Nephrol. 2010;32(6):541–8.
42. Gorostidi M, Sarafidis PA, de la Sierra A, Segura J, de la Cruz JJ, Banegas JR, et al. Differences between office and 24-hour blood pressure control in hypertensive patients with CKD: A 5,693-patient cross-sectional analysis from Spain. Am J kidney Dis. 2013;62(2):285–94.
43. Andersen MJ, Khawandi W, Agarwal R. Home blood pressure monitoring in CKD. Am J kidney Dis. 2005;45(6):994–1001.
44. Bangash F, Agarwal R. Masked hypertension and white-coat hypertension in chronic kidney disease: a meta-analysis. Clin J Am Soc Nephrol. 2009;4(3):656–64.
45. Pogue V, Rahman M, Lipkowitz M, Toto R, Miller E, Faulkner M, et al. Disparate estimates of hypertension control from ambulatory and clinic blood pressure measurements in hypertensive kidney disease. Hypertension. 2009;53(1):20–7.
46. Hansen TW, Kikuya M, Thijs L, Bjorklund-Bodegard K, Kuznetsova T, Ohkubo T, et al. Prognostic superiority of daytime ambulatory over conventional blood pressure in four populations: a meta-analysis of 7,030 individuals. J Hypertens. 2007;25(8):1554–64.
47. Kanno A, Metoki H, Kikuya M, Terawaki H, Hara A, Hashimoto T, et al. Usefulness of assessing masked and white-coat hypertension by ambulatory blood pressure monitoring for determining prevalent risk of chronic kidney disease: the Ohasama study. Hypertens Res. 2010;33(11):1192–8.
48. Agarwal R, Andersen MJ. Prognostic importance of ambulatory blood pressure recordings in patients with chronic kidney disease. Kidney Int. 2006;69(7):1175–80.
49. Agarwal R, Pappas MK, Sinha AD. Masked Uncontrolled Hypertension in CKD. J Am Soc Nephrol. 2016;27:924–32.
50. Tucker B, Fabbian F, Giles M, Thuraisingham RC, Raine AE, Baker LR. Left ventricular hypertrophy and ambulatory blood pressure monitoring in chronic renal failure. Nephrol Dial Transplant. 1997;12(4):724–8.
51. Peterson GE, de Backer T, Gabriel A, Ilic V, Vagaonescu T, Appel LJ, et al. Prevalence and correlates of left ventricular hypertrophy in the African American Study of Kidney Disease Cohort Study. Hypertension. 2007;50(6):1033–9.
52. Minutolo R, Gabbai FB, Agarwal R, Chiodini P, Borrelli S, Bellizzi V, et al. Assessment of achieved clinic and ambulatory blood pressure recordings and outcomes during treatment in hypertensive patients with CKD: a multicenter prospective cohort study. Am J Kidney Dis. 2014;64(5):744–52.
53. Klag MJ, Whelton PK, Randall BL, Neaton JD, Brancati FL, Ford CE, et al. Blood pressure and end-stage renal disease in men. N Engl J Med. 1996;334(1):13–8.
54. Tozawa M, Iseki K, Iseki C, Kinjo K, Ikemiya Y, Takishita S. Blood pressure predicts risk of developing end-stage renal disease in men and women. Hypertension. 2003;41(6):1341–5.
55. Jafar TH, Stark PC, Schmid CH, Landa M, Maschio G, de Jong PE, et al. Progression of chronic kidney disease: the role of blood pressure control, proteinuria, and angiotensin-converting enzyme inhibition: a patient-level meta-analysis. Ann Intern Med. 2003;139(4):244–52.

56. Peralta CA, Norris KC, Li S, Chang TI, Tamura MK, Jolly SE, et al. Blood pressure components and end-stage renal disease in persons with chronic kidney disease: the Kidney Early Evaluation Program (KEEP). Arch Intern Med. 2012;172(1):41–7.

57. Hsu CY, McCulloch CE, Darbinian J, Go AS, Iribarren C. Elevated blood pressure and risk of end-stage renal disease in subjects without baseline kidney disease. Arch Intern Med. 2005;165(8):923–8.

58. Klahr S, Levey AS, Beck GJ, Caggiula AW, Hunsicker L, Kusek JW, et al. The effects of dietary protein restriction and blood-pressure control on the progression of chronic renal disease. Modification of Diet in Renal Disease Study Group. N Engl J Med. 1994;330(13):877–84.

59. Palit S, Chonchol M, Cheung AK, Kaufman J, Smits G, Kendrick J. Association of BP with death, cardiovascular events, and progression to chronic dialysis in patients with advanced kidney disease. Clin J Am Soc Nephrol. 2015;10(6):934–40.

60. Lv J, Ehteshami P, Sarnak MJ, Tighiouart H, Jun M, Ninomiya T, et al. Effects of intensive blood pressure lowering on the progression of chronic kidney disease: a systematic review and meta-analysis. CMAJ. 2013;185(11):949–57.

61. Lazarus JM, Bourgoignie JJ, Buckalew VM, Greene T, Levey AS, Milas NC, et al. Achievement and safety of a low blood pressure goal in chronic renal disease. The Modification of Diet in Renal Disease Study Group. Hypertension. 1997;29(2):641–50.

62. Peterson JC, Adler S, Burkart JM, Greene T, Hebert LA, Hunsicker LG, et al. Blood pressure control, proteinuria, and the progression of renal disease. The Modification of Diet in Renal Disease Study. Ann Intern Med. 1995;123(10):754–62.

63. Ruggenenti P, Perna A, Loriga G, Ganeva M, Ene-Iordache B, Turturro M, et al. Blood-pressure control for renoprotection in patients with non-diabetic chronic renal disease (REIN-2): multicentre, randomised controlled trial. Lancet. 2005;365(9463):939–46.

64. Norris K, Bourgoigne J, Gassman J, Hebert L, Middleton J, Phillips RA, et al. Cardiovascular outcomes in the African American Study of Kidney Disease and Hypertension (AASK) Trial. Am J Kidney Dis. 2006;48(5):739–51.

65. Appel LJ, Wright Jr JT, Greene T, Agodoa LY, Astor BC, Bakris GL, et al. Intensive blood-pressure control in hypertensive chronic kidney disease. N Engl J Med. 2010;363(10):918–29.

66. Wright Jr JT, Bakris G, Greene T, Agodoa LY, Appel LJ, Charleston J, et al. Effect of blood pressure lowering and antihypertensive drug class on progression of hypertensive kidney disease: results from the AASK trial. JAMA. 2002;288(19):2421–31.

67. Upadhyay A, Earley A, Haynes SM, Uhlig K. Systematic review: blood pressure target in chronic kidney disease and proteinuria as an effect modifier. Ann Intern Med. 2011;154(8):541–8.

68. Group SR, Wright Jr JT, Williamson JD, Whelton PK, Snyder JK, Sink KM, et al. A randomized trial of intensive versus standard blood-pressure control. N Engl J Med. 2015;373(22):2103–16.

69. Chobanian AV, Bakris GL, Black HR, Cushman WC, Green LA, Izzo Jr JL, et al. Seventh report of the Joint National Committee on Prevention, Detection, Evaluation, and Treatment of High Blood Pressure. Hypertension. 2003;42(6):1206–52.

70. James PA, Oparil S, Carter BL, Cushman WC, Dennison-Himmelfarb C, Handler J, et al. 2014 evidence-based guideline for the management of high blood pressure in adults: report from the panel members appointed to the Eighth Joint National Committee (JNC 8). JAMA. 2014;311(5):507–20.

71. Anderson AH, Yang W, Townsend RR, Pan Q, Chertow GM, Kusek JW, et al. Time-updated systolic blood pressure and the progression of chronic kidney disease: a cohort study. Ann Intern Med. 2015;162(4):258–65.

72. MacMahon S, Peto R, Cutler J, Collins R, Sorlie P, Neaton J, et al. Blood pressure, stroke, and coronary heart disease. Part 1, Prolonged differences in blood pressure: prospective observational studies corrected for the regression dilution bias. Lancet. 1990;335(8692):765–74.

73. Murray CJ, Lauer JA, Hutubessy RC, Niessen L, Tomijima N, Rodgers A, et al. Effectiveness and costs of interventions to lower systolic blood pressure and cholesterol: a global and regional analysis on reduction of cardiovascular-disease risk. Lancet. 2003;361(9359):717–25.

74. Turnbull F, Blood Pressure Lowering Treatment Trialists Collaboration. Effects of different blood-pressure-lowering regimens on major cardiovascular events: results of prospectively-designed overviews of randomised trials. Lancet. 2003;362(9395):1527–35.
75. Blood Pressure Lowering Treatment Trialists Collaboration, Ninomiya T, Perkovic V, Turnbull F, Neal B, Barzi F, et al. Blood pressure lowering and major cardiovascular events in people with and without chronic kidney disease: meta-analysis of randomised controlled trials. BMJ. 2013;347:f5680.
76. Sim JJ, Shi J, Kovesdy CP, Kalantar-Zadeh K, Jacobsen SJ. Impact of achieved blood pressures on mortality risk and end-stage renal disease among a large, diverse hypertension population. J Am Coll Cardiol. 2014;64(6):588–97.
77. Kovesdy CP, Lu JL, Molnar MZ, Ma JZ, Canada RB, Streja E, et al. Observational modeling of strict vs conventional blood pressure control in patients with chronic kidney disease. JAMA Intern Med. 2014;174(9):1442–9.

Chapter 2
Assessment of Hypertension in Chronic Kidney Disease

Aldo J. Peixoto

Hypertension is highly prevalent in chronic kidney disease (CKD). It is estimated that up to 80 % of patients have high blood pressure (BP) by the time they reach advanced stages of kidney disease (glomerular filtration rate <15 ml/min), and remains highly prevalent among dialysis [1] and kidney transplant [2] patients. Because of the importance of BP control to decrease cardiovascular risk and limit the progression of CKD, adequate assessment of hypertension is essential to the care of CKD patients. In this chapter, we review relevant aspects of the assessment of BP in the office and out-of-office environments in patients with CKD (not on dialysis) and with kidney transplants. Issues related to dialysis patients are discussed in Chap. 7.

General Elements of the Assessment of Hypertension Burden

Besides the careful measurement of BP, the evaluation of hypertension in patients with CKD should include the same general approach as used in any patient with hypertension. Other critical components of the clinical evaluation include the consideration of features that suggest secondary causes of hypertension other than CKD itself, the identification of comorbid conditions that may impact on treatment decisions, the discussion of lifestyle practices and preferences that may affect management, and the systematic evaluation of extra-renal target organ involvement, such as cerebrovascular disease, cognitive impairment, left ventricular hypertrophy, heart failure, coronary disease, and peripheral arterial disease.

A.J. Peixoto, MD (✉)
Department of Internal Medicine (Section of Nephrology), Yale University,
Boardman 114, 330 Cedar Street, New Haven, CT 06518, USA
e-mail: aldo.peixoto@yale.edu

© Springer Science+Business Media New York 2016
A.K. Singh, R. Agarwal (eds.), *Core Concepts in Hypertension
in Kidney Disease*, DOI 10.1007/978-1-4939-6436-9_2

Mounting evidence indicates that the objective assessment of extracellular fluid volume expansion and systemic hemodynamics can improve BP management. Such measurements can be obtained with different non-invasive technologies. Although it is cumbersome to directly measure extracellular fluid volume, various methods exist to estimate it indirectly and include bioimpedance, ultrasonographic measurement of inferior vena cava diameter and collapsibility with inspiration, estimation of right atrial pressure with hepatic vein flow patterns, or through thoracic ultrasound to estimate the amount of extravascular lung water. Systemic hemodynamics, on the other hand, can be easily determined non-invasively through echocardiography, impedance cardiography, bioreactance, and several oscillometric methods. Impedance cardiography can simultaneously measure volume (thoracic fluid content) and hemodynamic variables (cardiac output, systemic vascular resistance). In patients with resistant hypertension, use of this technology to guide treatment resulted in better BP control in two randomized trials [3, 4]. The experience in non-dialysis CKD is small, but some have called for more extensive use of formal volume assessment in the treatment of hypertension [5], particularly in the setting of kidney disease, where extracellular fluid volume expansion is common, and often covert.

Most relevant to the present discussion is the careful measurement of BP both in the office and in the home and ambulatory setting. The following sections will cover each of these elements in detail.

Principles of Blood Pressure Measurement

Adequate management decisions demand accurate BP measurement. Cuff-based brachial BP is the most commonly used method to measure BP, typically in the office setting. However, current evidence progressively points to the value of out-of-office BP methods, such as 24-hour BP monitoring (ABPM) and home BP monitoring, as superior methods to evaluate BP burden and BP-related risk in hypertensive patients [6–8].

Conventional Office Blood Pressure Measurement

BP measurement is traditionally made in the office using either the auscultatory technique or oscillometric method (manual or automated cuff following specific proprietary algorithms to impute systolic and diastolic BP). In some countries such as in the USA, mercury sphygmomanometers are now seldom available in clinical practice because of environmental concerns [9], so most measurements are made either with aneroid devices or electronic oscillometric manometers. Both types of manometers are accurate but should have periodic maintenance to ensure that they are properly calibrated. This is typically done every 12 months or anytime poor function is suspected or anticipated (such as following drop from height of the instrument).

Table 2.1 Technique of office blood pressure measurement

Patient rests quietly for at least 3–5 min prior to measurements.
Patient sits on a chair with arm and back support, with both legs on the floor.
The arm is the preferred site of measurement, using a well-fitting cuff based on arm circumference. The bladder length covers at least 80 % of the arm circumference. Recommended cuff sizes for adults are: • "Small adult" (12×22 cm): for arm circumferences between 22 and 26 cm. • "Adult" (16×30 cm): for arm circumferences between 27 and 34 cm. • "Large adult" (16×36 cm): for arm circumferences between 35 and 44 cm. • "Adult thigh" (16×42 cm): for arm circumferences between 45 and 52 cm
Lower end of the cuff rests 2–3 cm above the antecubital fossa.
Arm is positioned at the level of the heart.
At least two BP measurements are obtained and averaged. Obtain more measurements if there is disparity between the first two values. Allow at least 1 min between readings.
BP is checked in both arms to identify inter-arm differences. If different, report the values obtained on the arm with higher BP.
If using the auscultatory method with a stethoscope, first confirm the approximate systolic BP through palpation to avoid errors due to the auscultatory gap. Use Korotkoff phase I (appearance) and V (disappearance) to define systolic and diastolic BP, respectively. Record the value that is the nearest even number (nearest 2 mmHg).
If using an aneroid or mercury manometer, the cuff is deflated at 2–3 mmHg/s. (Deflation rates with oscillometric devices are defined by proprietary algorithms and usually not adjusted by the clinician.)

Most patients should have their BP measured in the arm in the seated position [10]. In selected situations, such as malformations, injuries or vascular disease of the upper extremities, or when comparisons of BP levels in the upper and lower extremities is warranted, it may be necessary to use thigh measurements with an appropriately sized thigh cuff, which should be obtained in the supine position to allow the cuff to be at the level of the heart. Thigh cuffs are most easily used with an oscillometric automated device, but can also be used with the auscultatory method (Korotkoff sounds are auscultated in the popliteal fossa). Table 2.1 provides the essential elements of proper BP measurement in the office.

Inter-Arm Blood Pressure Differences

As noted in Table 2.1, patients should have their BP measured in both arms at the time of their initial evaluation and periodically thereafter. Differences >10 mmHg between arms can occur in a variable proportion of hypertensive patients (average ~14%) [11]. Inter-arm BP differences had been thought to be due to occlusive arterial disease of the upper extremities, but this has not been confirmed by prospective imaging studies [11], and the underlying mechanisms remain uncertain, possibly related to vascular calcification and arterial stiffness. Regardless of this uncertainty there is general agreement that clinical decisions should be made based on BP levels from the arm with higher BP.

A recent meta-analysis indicates that the presence of an inter-arm SBP difference >10 mmHg is associated with a 2.7-fold increase in risk of fatal and non-fatal cardiovascular events in populations with increased vascular risk, including one with CKD [11]. Reproducibility of the difference, however, is limited. In one study of 443 patients with simultaneous bilateral measurements on two separate occasions, the reproducibility of an inter-arm difference >10 mmHg or >20 mmHg was only 27 % and 41 %, respectively [12]. Therefore, while recognizing inter-arm differences should be noted to optimize decisions on which BP level to use on a given visit, the limited reproducibility makes the prognostic implications of that difference still uncertain.

Pseudohypertension

Pseudohypertension is the detection of spuriously elevated BP due to poor compressibility of the brachial artery and its branches. In the past, the Osler maneuver, or palpation of the radial artery during cuff inflation above the systolic BP level, was purported to effectively diagnose pseudohypertension. However, several studies have repudiated this, and it is no longer considered to be a useful test [10]. Therefore, if pseudohypertension is being considered in a patient, the only definitive means of confirming it is through arterial cannulation and direct measurement of intra-arterial pressure.

The Auscultatory Gap

A common source of error when using the auscultatory method is the auscultatory gap, which consists of a prolonged period of disappearance of Korotkoff sounds after their initial appearance. Therefore, if the cuff is not inflated high enough, the observer may record an incorrectly low systolic BP. The auscultatory gap is most common in older patients with underlying vascular disease and systolic hypertension with wide pulse pressure [10]. It can be easily avoided by identification of the systolic BP through palpation of the radial or brachial artery so as to guarantee that the cuff is being inflated to a pressure that is above the systolic BP. The auscultatory gap does not occur with oscillometric BP measurements.

Orthostatic Blood Pressure Measurements

Orthostatic hypotension is common in patients treated for hypertension, especially in older patients (8–34 %) [13, 14]. It is recommended that standing BP be obtained as a screen for orthostatic hypotension in elderly patients with hypertension, as well as in patients at increased risk of autonomic dysfunction, such as those with diabetes and kidney disease [7, 15]. Orthostatic vital signs (heart rate and BP) should be obtained after at least 5 min in the supine position followed by immediate assumption of the standing position for up to 3 min [14]. The practical difficulties of following this method in a busy office cannot be ignored, so it is acceptable to compare values in the seated position with those after standing for 1 min. This method is less sensitive for the detection of orthostatic hypotension but is better than no measurement at all [14]. The definition of orthostatic hypotension is a drop in BP >20/10 mmHg after 3 min of standing [16]. Among patients with supine hypertension, the required systolic fall in BP for the diagnosis is >30 mmHg because the level of baseline supine BP is directly proportional to the orthostatic BP drop [14, 16]. Integration of the heart rate response to changes in BP with standing is important to guide the differential diagnosis and further evaluation of orthostatic hypotension. In the absence of medications that slow heart rate, the lack of a rise in heart rate by at least 20 bpm in response to hypotension suggests baroreflex or sympathetic autonomic dysfunction. Conversely, patients with an appropriate heart rate response likely have volume depletion or excessive vasodilatation.

Office BP Measurement During Exercise

BP measurement is necessary during exercise stress testing, which is commonly performed in the office setting. There are issues related to both the measurement and the interpretation of BP levels during exercise. BP measurement may be difficult during exercise; auscultatory measurements can be plagued by difficulties hearing Korotkoff sounds due to equipment noise, and many of the available automatic devices are inaccurate during exercise testing or have not been appropriately validated in this setting. As a general rule, the auscultatory method should be used preferentially, as it is less susceptible to systematic or random error during exercise. Oscillometric measurements are not recommended to assess BP response to exercise. Some automated devices are available that concurrently record Korotkoff sounds with EKG which enable better separation of signal from noise during exercise.

On average, systolic BP increases by ~10 mmHg per metabolic equivalent (MET) of exercise (~30 mmHg during the early stages of aerobic exercise and by 50–60 mmHg above baseline at peak exercise), with average increases higher in men than women [17]. Diastolic BP response is less adequately characterized; typically it stays the same or is slightly lower but may increase during exercise. Despite lack of formal guidelines, the generally accepted upper limit of BP during peak exercise is 210/110 mmHg for men and 190/110 mmHg for women [17].

Several studies suggest that the delayed rate of recovery of systolic BP after exercise has been associated with the presence of coronary artery disease.

Automated Office Blood Pressure Measurement

Multiple office BP measurements can now be performed automatically while the patient is alone in the room. The devices are programmed to perform several sequential readings (typically 6), discard the first reading, and provide an average that is used as the value for the visit. Using this method, the white coat effect is largely eliminated [18, 19]. In addition, this automated approach results in better correlations with ambulatory BP averages and left ventricular mass than routine office BP [19, 20]. Obviously, this may lead to significant slowing of patient flow in physician offices, but if planned appropriately, can be performed as the patient waits while the clinician see other patients. Using this technology is particularly relevant for patients who are being treated for hypertension and those who cannot or do not want to perform self-measured BP monitoring in the home environment (see below). This idea was initially launched by the BpTRU company (and the method is often referred to as "the BpTRU"), but others are now available on the market such as the Omron HEM-907 and the Welch-Allyn ProBP 2400.

Out-of-Office Blood Pressure Monitoring

Even though office BP has been the most commonly used measure to guide hypertension diagnosis and treatment, growing evidence indicates that out-of-office techniques (home BP and ABPM) are better markers of hypertension-related risk and as such, have been increasingly used in research and clinical practice. Indications for home BP and ABPM are listed in Table 2.2 and a summary of the advantages and shortcomings of these monitoring methods is presented in Table 2.3.

Home Blood Pressure Monitoring

Home BP monitoring is performed by the patient in the home and/or work environment and is increasingly used in practice; as many as 65 % of patients with hypertension own a home monitor [21], although accessibility to low-income patients is still a problem despite the availability of low cost devices ($40–50) and coverage by many healthcare insurance plans.

Just as with office BP, it is important that the equipment works properly and fits the patient well. Home BP measurements should be obtained using the same attention to technique as described for office BP (see Table 2.1). In general, it is preferred that the automatic oscillometric method be used for self-measured BP. Unfortunately, many of the marketed devices have not been appropriately validated and may not provide accurate readings. A list of independently validated devices can be found at www.dableducational.org. The preferred devices use arm cuffs. Finger cuffs are inaccurate and wrist cuffs often provide incorrect readings because of inappropriate technique. As a result, only arm devices are recommended by current guidelines [21, 22].

The reliability of reporting of home BP values by patients has been questioned in the past. This problem has been circumvented by the universal availability of a memory function in automated BP devices. Therefore, if the clinician has concerns about the values being reported, he can ask the patient to bring the machine and personally review the values recorded in the device memory.

Table 2.2 Indications for home BP and ABPM

Indication	HBP	ABPM	Comment
Identify white coat hypertension	++	+++	ABPM still the "gold-standard" when patients have HBP values that are "borderline" (125–135/80–85 mmHg)
Identify masked hypertension	++	+++	
Identify true resistant hypertension	++	+++	
Evaluate borderline office BP values without target organ damage	++	+++	
Evaluate nocturnal hypertension	–	+++	
Evaluate labile hypertension	++	++	HBP better for infrequent symptoms or paroxysms, ABPM better if frequent within a 24-h period
Evaluate hypotensive symptoms	+++	++	
Evaluate autonomic dysfunction	+	++	HBP useful to monitor orthostatic hypotension. ABPM useful to quantify supine hypertension and determine overall (average) BP levels
Clinical research (treatment, prognosis)	++	+++	

From Elliott W, Peixoto AJ and Bakris G. Primary and Secondary Hypertension. In: Skorecki K, Chetow G, Marsden P, Taal M, Yu A (Eds.), Brenner & Rector's The Kidney, 10th edition. Philadelphia: Elsevier 2016:1522–66, with permission

Table 2.3 Pros and cons of home BP and ABPM

Home BP		ABPM	
Pros	Cons	Pros	Cons
Multiplicity of measurements over a prolonged period of time	Requires patient training	Multiplicity of measurements	Inconvenient to patients, especially if multiple monitoring periods are necessary
Good reproducibility	Devices are possibly inaccurate	Excellent reproducibility	High cost
Elimination of the white coat effect	Patient reporting may be biased	Elimination of the white coat effect	Low reimbursement rates
Low cost	No reimbursement	BP measurement during sleep	
Increases patient engagement		Superior prognostic value	
Better prognostication than office BP			

For most patients, a BP log obtained over 7 days before each office visit provides reproducible information that allows good prognostication and treatment decisions [22]. We instruct our patients to obtain readings in duplicate (about 1 min apart), twice daily (in the morning before taking medications and in the evening before

Table 2.4 Accepted upper limits of normal for home and ambulatory blood pressure

24-hour ambulatory BP monitoring	
24-hour BP	131/79 mmHg
Awake BP	138/86 mmHg
Sleep BP	120/71 mmHg
Home BP monitoring	
Average BP[a]	133/82 mmHg

[a]Average of all values during the monitoring period, usually 7 days
Data based on equivalent of cardiovascular event rates observed at office BP of 140/90 mmHg. Based on data from Kikuya et al. [29] and Niiranen et al. [23]

dinner) for a 7-day period. In some clinical situations, more frequent or more prolonged monitoring may be needed. For example, patients with symptoms suggestive of intermittent hypotension may benefit from BP measurements during peak action of medications, such as in the mid-to-late morning or late evening, depending on the time when medications are taken. Patients with wide fluctuations in BP can be monitored more often to better quantify the overall BP variability, though we prefer to use 24-hour ABPM in such patients. Detailed guidelines on the use of home BP are available from the European Society of Hypertension [22] and the American Heart Association [21].

Normative values for home BP based on observed outcomes are now available [23]. These threshold levels were established using the observed cardiovascular event rates equivalent to those observed for office BP of 120/80 mmHg ("optimal") and 140/90 mmHg ("hypertension") in a large multinational cohort of patients [23]. Using this approach, the currently accepted level of "optimal" home BP is 121/78 mmHg, and the level defining "hypertension" is 133/82 mmHg (see Table 2.4).

Ambulatory Blood Pressure Monitoring

ABPM combines the ability to evaluate BP in the ambulatory setting with the unique feature of allowing the measurement of BP during sleep, which, as will be discussed below, provides additive prognostic information. ABPM is performed with a validated automated device (for a list, refer to www.dableducational.org) that is fitted on the patient using an appropriately sized cuff. ABP is usually performed over a 24-hour period, although most devices can run for longer periods of time as allowed by battery life and number of readings stored in the memory. In some clinical situations, 48-hour monitoring is quite useful, such as in patients undergoing hemodialysis, so that the entire interdialytic period can be evaluated. The device is programmed to inflate periodically; a typical measurement interval is every 20 min during the daytime (7 AM–11 PM) and every 30 min at night (11 PM–7 AM), though these schedules can be adjusted based on individual needs. The patient keeps a log of activities during the monitoring period including the time of going to bed and waking up and time of taking antihypertensive medications (if any). It is preferred that the periods designated as "night and day" reflect the actual periods of sleep and wakefulness obtained from the patient's diary. Most patients accept ABPM well, although sometimes sleep is affected (<10 % of cases) and rarely, patients have bruising or pain from the frequent cuff inflations. Up-to-date guidelines that include practical information on ABPM are available from the European Society of Hypertension [24, 25].

The generally accepted indications for ABPM are listed in Table 2.2. The most commonly used indication is to rule out white coat hypertension. In fact, it is this property that has made ABPM recommended for definitive initial diagnosis of hypertension by the British Hypertension Society [6] and the United States Preventive Services Task Force [8]. Another important clinical use is in the evaluation of patients with resistant hypertension. Mounting evidence indicates that almost 40 % of patients with "office resistance" have controlled BP levels on ABPM, i.e., "office resistance" [26]. Identification of patients with true resistance is important to identify those with increased risk of adverse cardiovascular and renal outcomes [27, 28].

Similar to home BP, outcomes-based normative values are available for ABPM (Table 2.4) [29]. When interpreting an ABPM recording, the clinician needs to take into account the total number of successful measurements; a generally accepted minimum of valid readings is 20 during wakefulness and 7 during sleep [25]. The key elements of the 24-hour BP profile are the awake, asleep, and overall 24-hour BP levels, as these are the prognostic determinants in hypertension.

The blood pressure decline during sleep ("dipping") is also calculated as the ratio between the asleep and awake BP. Normally, BP declines by ~15 % during sleep (i.e., a night/day ratio of 0.85). When evaluating the circadian BP profile based on the behavior of BP during sleep, four patterns are described:

1. Dipper: normal BP decline during sleep, arbitrarily defined as between 10 and 20 %.
2. Non-dipper: smaller than normal BP decline during sleep (between 0 and 10 %). This pattern is observed in 20–25 % of patients with essential hypertension, and with increasing frequency in patients with cardiovascular disease, kidney disease, and other causes of secondary hypertension.
3. Reverse dipper (also called "Riser"): BP increases during sleep. This pattern is often observed in patients with advanced kidney disease, sleep apnea, or autonomic dysfunction.
4. Extreme dipper: greater than normal BP fall during sleep (>20 %).

In large observational studies, extreme dippers have lower fatal and non-fatal cardiovascular event rates than those whose BP decreases by less <20 %. Reverse dippers, on the other hand, have significantly worse cardiovascular outcomes than all other patients [30].

Most software packages provide information on the 24-hour BP variability (defined as the standard deviation of systolic and diastolic BP for each of the monitoring periods) and the BP load (percentage of readings above a certain threshold). Although some data have linked high BP variability and high BP load to adverse outcomes, they do not appear to provide additional information beyond what is obtained from average BP values [31], so we give limited relevance to these values.

Integrating Home BP and ABPM into Clinical Decision Making

In deciding between home BP and ABPM, the clinician must take into account availability, costs, and patient preferences. For the initial evaluation of the patient, home BP is an adequate method, particularly in the primary care setting. In subspecialty practices, however, ABPM is more easily available and is particularly useful for patients with borderline home BP values. A systematic review of 20 studies compared the agreement between office, home and ABPM according to different BP thresholds [32]. Using a 24-hour BP average of 135/85 mmHg as the definition of HTN, an office BP of 140/90 mmHg has a sensitivity of 75 % (95 % CI, 61–85 %) and specificity of 75 % (95 % CI, 48–90 %) for the diagnosis of HTN. Likewise, a home BP average of 135/85 mmHg has a sensitivity of 86 % (95 % CI, 78–91 %) and a specificity of 62 % (95 % CI, 48–75 %) for the diagnosis. Therefore, neither office nor home BP has sufficient sensitivity or specificity for the diagnosis of HTN based on this analysis [32]. However, the use of different thresholds can produce adequate predictive values (positive and negative) that allow home BP to be integrated into the decision to obtain ABPM or not with greater precision [21]. A structured approach to this decision-making process is summarized below [21]:

- If office BP >140/90 mmHg, perform home BP monitoring.
- If home BP <125/76, continue to monitor (or continue same treatment).
- If home BP >135/85 mmHg, start treatment (or escalate therapy).
- If home BP between 125/76 and 135/85 mmHg, obtain ABPM.
- If 24-hour ABPM average <130/80 mmHg, continue same strategy. If higher, start or increase treatment.

Prognostic Relevance of Out-of-Office BP

Compared to isolated office BP measurements, home BP and ABPM generally demonstrate stronger associations with target organ damage (especially left ventricular hypertrophy and proteinuria) and cardiovascular and renal endpoints in hypertension [6, 33, 34]. There are several possible reasons for the better prognostic performance of home BP and ABPM. For example, home BP and ABPM include more readings, thus leading have lower variability and higher reproducibility of results, thus leading to a more precise determination of BP levels. Moreover, both techniques allow the detection of the white coat (high BP in the office, normal at home) and masked effects (normal BP in the office, high at home), which better reflect overall BP burden to the patient. White coat hypertension affects 20–30 % of patients with a diagnosis of office hypertension [35] and has generally been associated with similar cardiovascular outcomes as normotensive individuals [36], although recent data from the International Database of Home Blood Pressure in Relation to Cardiovascular Outcome (IDHOCO) indicated a 42 % increase in risk of CV events compared with those with normal BP in the office and at home, especially among untreated patients [37]. Interestingly, treated hypertensive patients who retained a "white coat effect" had the same overall risk as treated patients whose BP was controlled both at home and in the office. Masked hypertension, on the other hand, has a prevalence of 10–15 % in population studies and has been consistently associated with increased risk for adverse cardiovascular endpoints and mortality to a level that is identical to that of sustained hypertension [36]. Lastly, ABPM allows assessment of BP during sleep. Nighttime BP is a generally a slightly better marker of cardiovascular risk than daytime or 24-hour average BP [38–40].

In a meta-analysis of studies that took into account both office and ABPM in the assessment of cardiovascular events and mortality, only ABPM values, not office, were significant predictors of outcomes [39]. Along the same lines, a large cohort study that included simultaneous use of office and home BP to predict cardiovascular events and mortality, only home BP values were significant markers of risk [41]. The superiority of out-of-office methods over office BP has also been demonstrated in patients with resistant hypertension [28, 42], chronic kidney disease [27, 43–46], hemodialysis [47], and in the general population [48–50].

Clinical trials testing the use of office and out-of-office BP during hypertension treatment, however, have been unable to show any differences with respect to BP control or changes in left ventricular mass [51–53]. However, these studies were all relatively small and limited to 6–12 months in duration. A detailed analysis for the United States Agency for Healthcare Research and Quality demonstrated that very large sample sizes would be required for definitive clinical trials comparing office and home BP (between 6500 and 59,000 subjects followed for 10 years depending on the assumptions of baseline risk and differences between the two groups) [54], making it doubtful that such a randomized trial will be performed.

In summary, prospective cohort studies convincingly show the superiority of home BP and ABPM over office BP measurements for the diagnosis of hypertension and to predict hypertension-related outcomes. This evidence is already being incorporated into clinical practice guidelines for diagnosis of hypertension. Because it is unlikely that a definitive clinical trial will ever be performed in the treatment realm, decisions to use out-of-office BP for hypertension management are now made primarily on the basis of circumstantial evidence. We feel strongly that their use is warranted and our practice is to routinely use out-of-office BP as a guide to hypertension treatment. However, we acknowledge our practice is based on observational and not on clinical trial evidence.

Out-of-Office BP in Chronic Kidney Disease

Patients with CKD have a high prevalence of abnormal diurnal BP profiles, with decreased nocturnal BP dip [55]. Attention to this was raised by a landmark study in 1991 showing uniformly blunted circadian BP profiles in patients with CKD not on dialysis, patients on hemodialysis, and patients with a kidney transplant compared with controls matched for age, sex, office systolic BP and presence/absence

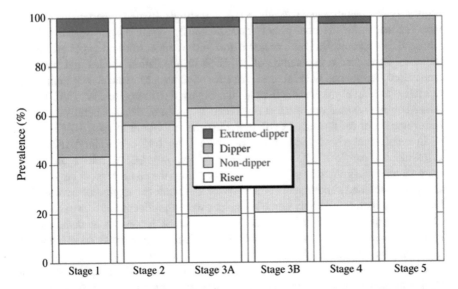

Fig. 2.1 Relative distribution of circadian BP profiles in patients with CKD. Prevalence of dipping classifications in terms of the sleep-time relative SBP decline—≥20 % (extreme-dipper), 10–20 % (dipper), 0–10 % (non-dipper), <0 % (riser)—of hypertensive patients with CKD in relation to stage (disease severity)—Stage 1: GFR ≥90 ml/min/1.73 m²; Stage 2: GFR 60–89 ml/min/1.73 m²; Stage 3A: GFR 45–59 ml/min/1.73 m²; Stage 3B: GFR 30–44 ml/min/1.73 m²; Stage 4: GFR 15–29 ml/min/1.73 m²; Stage 5: GFR <15 ml/min/1.73 m². Reproduced with permission from Hermida R et al., Nephrol Dial Transplant. 2014;29:1160–7

of antihypertensive drug therapy [56]. Average dipping during sleep (SBP%/DBP%) was 7 %/11 % in CKD patients (vs. 18 %/24 % in controls), 4 %/8 % in hemodialysis patients (vs. 14 %/24 % in controls), and 5 %/9 % in transplantation patients (vs. 13 %/18 % in controls) [56]. Since then, many studies have confirmed these observations. In an important analysis of the African American Study of Kidney Disease (AASK) in patients with hypertensive nephrosclerosis with an average GFR of 44 ml/min/1.73 m², there was an 80 % combined prevalence of non-dipping (41 %) or reverse dipping (39 %) [57]. Another large cohort study of CKD patients with less severe loss of renal function (average eGFR 59 ml/min/1.73 m²) showed a 61 % prevalence of non-dipping [58]. The prevalence of non-dipping, and more importantly, reverse dipping, which is associated with the highest cardiorenal risk, increases as eGFR falls [59] (see Fig. 2.1).

As in essential hypertension, home BP and ABPM have been tested in their predictive ability for adverse clinical outcomes in CKD. Several small studies suggested that the rate of loss of renal function and/or increase in proteinuria was greater in non-dipping than dipping patients with different causes of CKD [60], diabetic nephropathy [61], and IgA nephropathy [62]. However, more recent, larger studies have not confirmed the relevance of non-dipping to CKD progression after adjustments for average BP and other factors [43, 45].

The evaluation of risk of progression to dialysis or death was performed in a study of 217 male patients with CKD due to multiple etiologies, mostly diabetes and hypertension (baseline eGFR 45 ml/min/1.73 m²) [44]. After a median follow-up of 3.5 years, one standard deviation of home systolic BP (21 mmHg) was associated with 84% increased risk (95% CI = 1.46–2.32) of death or progression to ESRD after multiple relevant adjustments including office BP [44]. In a companion paper published shortly thereafter, the same authors presented ABPM data for the same cohort showing that one standard deviation increase in 24-hour systolic BP (17 mmHg) resulted in a 62% (95% CI − 1.21–2.18) increase in risk of dialysis or death after adjustment for clinic BP [43]. However, this prognostic advantage did not remain significant after adjustment for other clinical factors. Of the individual components of ABPM, only nighttime systolic BP was a significant predictor of death and dialysis risk on adjusted analyses (hazard ratio 1.79 for ESRD or death, 1.90 for death) [43].

In a multicenter study of 436 patients with CKD of varying etiologies, mostly hypertension, diabetes, and tubulointerstitial diseases (baseline eGFR 43 ml/min/1.73 m²), only ABPM, not office BP, was associated with cardiovascular events, progression to dialysis or death during 4.2 years of follow-up [46]. The same group of investigators recently published further data on outcomes based on the degree of BP control in the office, on ABPM, both or neither [63]. They considered office BP as being at goal if less than 140/90 mmHg, whereas ABPM was considered at goal if daytime BP was <135/85 mmHg and nighttime BP was <120/70 mmHg. Among the 489 study subjects, 17% were controlled both at home and office, 22% were controlled only on ABPM (i.e., a white coat effect), 15% only in the office (i.e., a masked effect), and 47% on neither ("uncontrolled"). The group with a "white coat effect" had similar risk of cardiovascular events, dialysis, and death as the referent group (controlled BP in both settings). Conversely, the "masked effect" and uncontrolled groups had 2.3 to 3.9-fold greater risk of negative outcomes than patients with controlled BP [63].

In a 5-year longitudinal analysis of 617 African-American patients with hypertensive nephrosclerosis found ABPM to be better than office BP for prediction of loss of renal function and cardiovascular events [45]. Both daytime and nighttime BPs were associated with increased risk of cardiovascular events despite adjustments for office BP and other variables. On the other hand, ABPM values were only associated with the composite renal endpoint (doubling of serum creatinine, dialysis, or death) in patients with controlled office BP (systolic BP <130 mmHg) [45].

In summary, similar to the general population, out-of-office BP measurements are better predictors of renal and cardiovascular outcomes in patients with CKD. However, the available data are not as strong as the studies are not as well powered as studies in other hypertensive populations, and several inconsistencies remain with respect to the prognostic role of individual ambulatory BP variables (i.e., daytime vs. nighttime vs. 24-hour average vs. dipping status).

Out-of-Office BP in Kidney Transplantation

Hypertension is present in the majority of kidney transplant recipients [64]. A recent study found only 16 % of recipients to be normotensive without the need for antihypertensive therapy [65]. This study also showed poor BP control in 44 %, while 10 % had white coat hypertension and 18 % had masked hypertension. Additionally, only 16 % of the recipients had a normal nocturnal dipping blood pressure pattern. This increased incidence of hypertension is in part a consequence of the immunosuppression regimen. In particular, corticosteroids and the calcineurin inhibitors (cyclosporine more so than tacrolimus) are associated with hypertension [66]. Furthermore, and consistent with native kidney disease, hypertension can be both a cause and a consequence of allograft renal insufficiency. A study addressing BP control by ABPM and office BP in 868 kidney transplant recipients found that only 34 % of participants had controlled ambulatory BP [64]. Circadian BP patterns showed a high proportion of reverse dippers (48 %) in addition to 34 % non-dippers, and only a small proportion (14 %) of normal dippers [64]. Another study compared office BP and ABPM in patients with CKD and patients with a kidney transplant [67]. The investigators hypothesized that the immunosuppressants would lead to a greater degree of hypertension compared to patients with CKD and similar levels of renal insufficiency. While the office-based BP levels were similar, ABPM identified a significant difference in both awake and asleep BP between the two groups (higher in transplant), and transplant recipients less often had a normal diurnal BP rhythm (21 % were dippers compared with 34 % of the CKD patients) [67]. In summary, nocturnal hypertension and non-dipping are common in transplant recipients, and likely occur to a greater extent than in patients with similar degrees of kidney dysfunction without a transplant.

Home BP monitoring has also been evaluated in kidney transplantation. Consistent with data from the general population, home BP in kidney transplant recipients better approximated ABPM than office BP readings (72 % concordance versus 54 %) [68]. Moreover, compared with ABPM reference data, HBPM was both more sensitive and specific at detecting hypertension than office-based BP measurements for the recipients studied.

Limited data are available to compare the prognostic relevance of out-of-office versus office BP in renal transplant recipients. ABPM correlates better with left ventricular mass than office BP in renal transplant patients [69, 70]. Small prospective studies have shown stronger associations between ABPM-derived BP values and serum creatinine levels [71, 72] and vascular injury in the allograft [72], although not all studies have corroborated this [73]. The only long-term study evaluating graft failure and cardiovascular events in renal transplant patients included 126 patients followed for 46 months [74]. In this study, the presence of a reverse dipper pattern on ABPM was associated with a 3.6-fold increase in risk of loss of allograft or cardiovascular event during follow-up ($P=0.02$). Neither office BP nor other measures derived from ABPM were associated with the outcomes in question [74]. In summary, the strength of the association between ABPM levels and clinical outcomes in renal transplantation is weak.

One relevant point related to renal transplantation is the increasing use of ABPM to evaluate potential kidney donors, as several studies indicate that donor candidates with hypertension are at risk for worsened BP control following kidney donation [75–77] and the prevalence of white coat hypertension may be as high as 62 % in this patient group [78, 79]. Therefore, the use of ABPM allows for better risk stratification prior to donation.

References

1. Peixoto AJ, Santos SF. Blood pressure management in hemodialysis: what have we learned? Curr Opin Nephrol Hypertens. 2010;19(6):561–6.
2. Weir MR, Burgess ED, Cooper JE, Fenves AZ, Goldsmith D, McKay D, et al. Assessment and management of hypertension in transplant patients. J Am Soc Nephrol. 2015;26:1248–60.
3. Smith RD, Levy P, Ferrario CM, Consideration of Noninvasive Hemodynamic Monitoring to Target Reduction of Blood Pressure Levels Study Group. Value of noninvasive hemodynamics to achieve blood pressure control in hypertensive subjects. Hypertension. 2006;47(4):771–7.
4. Taler SJ, Textor SC, Augustine JE. Resistant hypertension: comparing hemodynamic management to specialist care. Hypertension. 2002;39(5):982–8.
5. Covic A, Voroneanu L, Goldsmith D. Routine bioimpedance-derived volume assessment for all hypertensives: a new paradigm. Am J Nephrol. 2014;40(5):434–40.
6. National Institute for Health and Clinical Excellence. The clinical management of primary hypertension in adults: clinical guideline 127. NICE, 2011.
7. Mancia G, Fagard R, Narkiewicz K, Redon J, Zanchetti A, Bohm M, et al. 2013 ESH/ESC guidelines for the management of arterial hypertension: the Task Force for the management of arterial hypertension of the European Society of Hypertension (ESH) and of the European Society of Cardiology (ESC). J Hypertens. 2013;31(7):1281–357.
8. Piper MA, Evans CV, Burda BU, Margolis KL, O'Connor E, Whitlock EP. Diagnostic and predictive accuracy of blood pressure screening methods with consideration of rescreening intervals: a systematic review for the U.S. Preventive Services Task Force. Ann Intern Med. 2015;162(3):192–204.
9. United States Environmental Protection Agency. Eliminating mercury in hospitals. 2002 November 2002. Report No.
10. Pickering TG, Hall JE, Appel LJ, Falkner BE, Graves J, Hill MN, et al. Recommendations for blood pressure measurement in humans and experimental animals: Part 1: blood pressure measurement in humans: a statement for professionals from the Subcommittee of Professional and Public Education of the American Heart Association Council on High Blood Pressure Research. Hypertension. 2005;45(1):142–61.
11. Clark CE, Aboyans V. Interarm blood pressure difference: more than an epiphenomenon. Nephrol Dial Transplant. 2015;30(5):695–7.
12. Mehlsen J, Wiinberg N. Interarm difference in blood pressure: reproducibility and association with peripheral vascular disease. Int J Vas Med. 2014;2014:841542.
13. Judd E, Calhoun DA. Hypertension and orthostatic hypotension in older patients. J Hypertens. 2012;30(1):38–9.
14. Shibao C, Lipsitz LA, Biaggioni I, American Society of Hypertension Writing Group. Evaluation and treatment of orthostatic hypotension. J Am Soc Hypertens. 2013;7(4):317–24.
15. Wheeler DC, Becker GJ. Summary of KDIGO guideline. What do we really know about management of blood pressure in patients with chronic kidney disease? Kidney Int. 2013;83(3):377–83.
16. Freeman R, Wieling W, Axelrod FB, Benditt DG, Benarroch E, Biaggioni I, et al. Consensus statement on the definition of orthostatic hypotension, neurally mediated syncope and the postural tachycardia syndrome. Clin Auton Res. 2011;21(2):69–72.

17. Sharman JE, LaGerche A. Exercise blood pressure: clinical relevance and correct measurement. J Hum Hypertens. 2015;29(6):351–8.
18. Myers MG. Automated blood pressure measurement in routine clinical practice. Blood Press Monit. 2006;11(2):59–62.
19. Myers MG. The great myth of office blood pressure measurement. J Hypertens. 2012;30(10):1894–8.
20. Andreadis EA, Agaliotis GD, Angelopoulos ET, Tsakanikas AP, Chaveles IA, Mousoulis GP. Automated office blood pressure and 24-h ambulatory measurements are equally associated with left ventricular mass index. Am J Hypertens. 2011;24(6):661–6.
21. Pickering TG, Miller NH, Ogedegbe G, Krakoff LR, Artinian NT, Goff D, et al. Call to action on use and reimbursement for home blood pressure monitoring: executive summary: a joint scientific statement from the American Heart Association, American Society Of Hypertension, and Preventive Cardiovascular Nurses Association. Hypertension. 2008;52(1):1–9.
22. Parati G, Stergiou GS, Asmar R, Bilo G, de Leeuw P, Imai Y, et al. European Society of Hypertension practice guidelines for home blood pressure monitoring. J Hum Hypertens. 2010;24(12):779–85.
23. Niiranen TJ, Asayama K, Thijs L, Johansson JK, Ohkubo T, Kikuya M, et al. Outcome-driven thresholds for home blood pressure measurement: international database of home blood pressure in relation to cardiovascular outcome. Hypertension. 2013;61(1):27–34.
24. O'Brien E, Parati G, Stergiou G, Asmar R, Beilin L, Bilo G, et al. European Society of Hypertension position paper on ambulatory blood pressure monitoring. J Hypertens. 2013;31(9):1731–68.
25. Parati G, Stergiou G, O'Brien E, Asmar R, Beilin L, Bilo G, et al. European Society of Hypertension practice guidelines for ambulatory blood pressure monitoring. J Hypertens. 2014;32(7):1359–66.
26. de la Sierra A, Segura J, Banegas JR, Gorostidi M, de la Cruz JJ, Armario P, et al. Clinical features of 8295 patients with resistant hypertension classified on the basis of ambulatory blood pressure monitoring. Hypertension. 2011;57(5):898–902.
27. De Nicola L, Gabbai FB, Agarwal R, Chiodini P, Borrelli S, Bellizzi V, et al. Prevalence and prognostic role of resistant hypertension in chronic kidney disease patients. J Am Coll Cardiol. 2013;61(24):2461–7.
28. Salles GF, Cardoso CR, Muxfeldt ES. Prognostic influence of office and ambulatory blood pressures in resistant hypertension. Arch Intern Med. 2008;168(21):2340–6.
29. Kikuya M, Hansen TW, Thijs L, Bjorklund-Bodegard K, Kuznetsova T, Ohkubo T, et al. Diagnostic thresholds for ambulatory blood pressure monitoring based on 10-year cardiovascular risk. Circulation. 2007;115(16):2145–52.
30. Fagard RH, Thijs L, Staessen JA, Clement DL, De Buyzere ML, De Bacquer DA. Night-day blood pressure ratio and dipping pattern as predictors of death and cardiovascular events in hypertension. J Hum Hypertens. 2009;23(10):645–53.
31. Hansen TW, Thijs L, Li Y, Boggia J, Kikuya M, Bjorklund-Bodegard K, et al. Prognostic value of reading-to-reading blood pressure variability over 24 hours in 8938 subjects from 11 populations. Hypertension. 2010;55(4):1049–57.
32. Hodgkinson J, Mant J, Martin U, Guo B, Hobbs FD, Deeks JJ, et al. Relative effectiveness of clinic and home blood pressure monitoring compared with ambulatory blood pressure monitoring in diagnosis of hypertension: systematic review. BMJ. 2011;342:d3621.
33. Bliziotis IA, Destounis A, Stergiou GS. Home versus ambulatory and office blood pressure in predicting target organ damage in hypertension: a systematic review and meta-analysis. J Hypertens. 2012;30(7):1289–99.
34. Fuchs SC, Mello RG, Fuchs FC. Home blood pressure monitoring is better predictor of cardiovascular disease and target organ damage than office blood pressure: a systematic review and meta-analysis. Curr Cardiol Rep. 2013;15(11):413.
35. Kollias A, Ntineri A, Stergiou GS. Is white-coat hypertension a harbinger of increased risk? Hypertens Res. 2014;37(9):791–5.

36. Pierdomenico SD, Cuccurullo F. Prognostic value of white-coat and masked hypertension diagnosed by ambulatory monitoring in initially untreated subjects: an updated meta analysis. Am J Hypertens. 2011;24(1):52–8.
37. Stergiou GS, Asayama K, Thijs L, Kollias A, Niiranen TJ, Hozawa A, et al. Prognosis of white-coat and masked hypertension: International Database of HOme blood pressure in relation to Cardiovascular Outcome. Hypertension. 2014;63(4):675–82.
38. Fagard RH, Celis H, Thijs L, Staessen JA, Clement DL, De Buyzere ML, et al. Daytime and nighttime blood pressure as predictors of death and cause-specific cardiovascular events in hypertension. Hypertension. 2008;51(1):55–61.
39. Conen D, Bamberg F. Noninvasive 24-h ambulatory blood pressure and cardiovascular disease: a systematic review and meta-analysis. J Hypertens. 2008;26(7):1290–9.
40. Boggia J, Li Y, Thijs L, Hansen TW, Kikuya M, Bjorklund-Bodegard K, et al. Prognostic accuracy of day versus night ambulatory blood pressure: a cohort study. Lancet. 2007;370(9594):1219–29.
41. Niiranen TJ, Hanninen MR, Johansson J, Reunanen A, Jula AM. Home-measured blood pressure is a stronger predictor of cardiovascular risk than office blood pressure: the Finn-Home study. Hypertension. 2010;55(6):1346–51.
42. Redon J, Campos C, Narciso ML, Rodicio JL, Pascual JM, Ruilope LM. Prognostic value of ambulatory blood pressure monitoring in refractory hypertension: a prospective study. Hypertension. 1998;31(2):712–8.
43. Agarwal R, Andersen MJ. Prognostic importance of ambulatory blood pressure recordings in patients with chronic kidney disease. Kidney Int. 2006;69(7):1175–80.
44. Agarwal R, Andersen MJ. Prognostic importance of clinic and home blood pressure recordings in patients with chronic kidney disease. Kidney Int. 2006;69(2):406–11.
45. Gabbai FB, Rahman M, Hu B, Appel LJ, Charleston J, Contreras G, et al. Relationship between ambulatory BP and clinical outcomes in patients with hypertensive CKD. Clin J Am Soc Nephrol. 2012;7(11):1770–6.
46. Minutolo R, Agarwal R, Borrelli S, Chiodini P, Bellizzi V, Nappi F, et al. Prognostic role of ambulatory blood pressure measurement in patients with nondialysis chronic kidney disease. Arch Intern Med. 2011;171(12):1090–8.
47. Agarwal R, Peixoto AJ, Santos SF, Zoccali C. Out-of-office blood pressure monitoring in chronic kidney disease. Blood Press Monit. 2009;14(1):2–11.
48. Kikuya M, Ohkubo T, Asayama K, Metoki H, Obara T, Saito S, et al. Ambulatory blood pressure and 10-year risk of cardiovascular and noncardiovascular mortality: the Ohasama study. Hypertension. 2005;45(2):240–5.
49. Ohkubo T, Imai Y, Tsuji I, Nagai K, Kato J, Kikuchi N, et al. Home blood pressure measurement has a stronger predictive power for mortality than does screening blood pressure measurement: a population-based observation in Ohasama. Jpn J Hypertens. 1998;16(7):971–5.
50. Sega R, Facchetti R, Bombelli M, Cesana G, Corrao G, Grassi G, et al. Prognostic value of ambulatory and home blood pressures compared with office blood pressure in the general population: follow-up results from the Pressioni Arteriose Monitorate e Loro Associazioni (PAMELA) study. Circulation. 2005;111(14):1777–83.
51. Staessen JA, Byttebier G, Buntinx F, Celis H, O'Brien ET, Fagard R. Antihypertensive treatment based on conventional or ambulatory blood pressure measurement. A randomized controlled trial. Ambulatory Blood Pressure Monitoring and Treatment of Hypertension Investigators. JAMA. 1997;278(13):1065–72.
52. Staessen JA, Den Hond E, Celis H, Fagard R, Keary L, Vandenhoven G, et al. Antihypertensive treatment based on blood pressure measurement at home or in the physician's office: a randomized controlled trial. JAMA. 2004;291(8):955–64.
53. Verberk WJ, Kroon AA, Lenders JW, Kessels AG, van Montfrans GA, Smit AJ, et al. Self-measurement of blood pressure at home reduces the need for antihypertensive drugs: a randomized, controlled trial. Hypertension. 2007;50(6):1019–25.

54. Uhlig K, Patel K, Concannon TW, Balk EM, Ratichek SJ, Chang LKW, et al. Self-measured blood pressure: future research needs: identification of future research needs from comparative effectiveness review No 45. AHRQ Future Research Needs Papers. Rockville; 2012.

55. Peixoto AJ, White WB. Ambulatory blood pressure monitoring in chronic renal disease: technical aspects and clinical relevance. Curr Opin Nephrol Hypertens. 2002;11(5):507–16.

56. Baumgart P, Walger P, Gemen S, von Eiff M, Raidt H, Rahn KH. Blood pressure elevation during the night in chronic renal failure, hemodialysis and after renal transplantation. Nephron. 1991;57(3):293–8.

57. Pogue V, Rahman M, Lipkowitz M, Toto R, Miller E, Faulkner M, et al. Disparate estimates of hypertension control from ambulatory and clinic blood pressure measurements in hypertensive kidney disease. Hypertension. 2009;53(1):20–7.

58. Mojon A, Ayala DE, Pineiro L, Otero A, Crespo JJ, Moya A, et al. Comparison of ambulatory blood pressure parameters of hypertensive patients with and without chronic kidney disease. Chronobiol Int. 2013;30(1-2):145–58.

59. Hermida RC, Smolensky MH, Ayala DE, Fernandez JR, Moya A, Crespo JJ, et al. Abnormalities in chronic kidney disease of ambulatory blood pressure 24 h patterning and normalization by bedtime hypertension chronotherapy. Nephrol Dial Transplant. 2014;29(6):1160–7.

60. Timio M, Venanzi S, Lolli S, Lippi G, Verdura C, Monarca C, et al. "Non-dipper" hypertensive patients and progressive renal insufficiency: a 3-year longitudinal study. Clin Nephrol. 1995;43(6):382–7.

61. Farmer CK, Goldsmith DJ, Quin JD, Dallyn P, Cox J, Kingswood JC, et al. Progression of diabetic nephropathy--is diurnal blood pressure rhythm as important as absolute blood pressure level? Nephrol Dial Transplant. 1998;13(3):635–9.

62. Csiky B, Kovacs T, Wagner L, Vass T, Nagy J. Ambulatory blood pressure monitoring and progression in patients with IgA nephropathy. Nephrol Dial Transplant. 1999;14(1):86–90.

63. Minutolo R, Gabbai FB, Agarwal R, Chiodini P, Borrelli S, Bellizzi V, et al. Assessment of achieved clinic and ambulatory blood pressure recordings and outcomes during treatment in hypertensive patients with CKD: a multicenter prospective cohort study. Am J Kidney Dis. 2014;64(5):744–52.

64. Fernandez Fresnedo G, Franco Esteve A, Gómez Huertas E, Cabello Chaves V, Díz Gómez JM, Osorio Moratalla JM, et al. Ambulatory blood pressure monitoring in kidney transplant patients: RETENAL study. Transplant Proc. 2012;44(9):2601–2.

65. Czyżewski Ł, Wyzgał J, Kołek A. Evaluation of selected risk factors of cardiovascular diseases among patients after kidney transplantation, with particular focus on the role of 24-hour automatic blood pressure measurement in the diagnosis of hypertension: an introductory report. Ann Transplant. 2014;19:188–98.

66. Miller LW. Cardiovascular toxicities of immunosuppressive agents. Am J Transplant. 2002;2(9):807–18.

67. Azancot MA, Ramos N, Moreso FJ, Ibernon M, Espinel E, Torres IB, et al. Hypertension in chronic kidney disease: the influence of renal transplantation. Transplantation. 2014;98(5): 537–42.

68. Agena F, Prado Edos S, Souza PS, da Silva GV, Lemos FB, Mion D, et al. Home blood pressure (BP) monitoring in kidney transplant recipients is more adequate to monitor BP than office BP. Nephrol Dial Transplant. 2011;26(11):3745–9.

69. Covic A, Segall L, Goldsmith DJ. Ambulatory blood pressure monitoring in renal transplantation: should ABPM be routinely performed in renal transplant patients? Transplantation. 2003;76(11):1640–2.

70. Ferreira SR, Moises VA, Tavares A, Pacheco-Silva A. Cardiovascular effects of successful renal transplantation: a 1-year sequential study of left ventricular morphology and function, and 24-hour blood pressure profile. Transplantation. 2002;74(11):1580–7.

71. Jacobi J, Rockstroh J, John S, Schreiber M, Schlaich MP, Neumayer HH, et al. Prospective analysis of the value of 24-hour ambulatory blood pressure on renal function after kidney transplantation. Transplantation. 2000;70(5):819–27.

72. Wadei HM, Amer H, Taler SJ, Cosio FG, Griffin MD, Grande JP, et al. Diurnal blood pressure changes one year after kidney transplantation: relationship to allograft function, histology, and resistive index. J Am Soc Nephrol. 2007;18(5):1607–15.
73. Haydar AA, Covic A, Agharazili M, Jayawardene S, Taylor J, Goldsmith DJ. Systolic blood pressure diurnal variation is not a predictor of renal target organ damage in kidney transplant patients. Am J Transplant. 2003;4(2):244–7.
74. Ibernon M, Moreso F, Sarrias X, Sarrias M, Grinyo JM, Fernandez-Real JM, et al. Reverse dipper pattern of blood pressure at 3 months is associated with inflammation and outcome after renal transplantation. Nephrol Dial Transplant. 2012;27(5):2089–95.
75. Anderson CF, Velosa JA, Frohnert PP, Torres VE, Offord KP, Vogel JP, et al. The risks of unilateral nephrectomy: status of kidney donors 10 to 20 years postoperatively. Mayo Clin Proc. 1985;60(6):367–74.
76. Torres VE, Offord KP, Anderson CF, Velosa JA, Frohnert PP, Donadio JV, et al. Blood pressure determinants in living-related renal allograft donors and their recipients. Kidney Int. 1987;31(6):1383–90.
77. Talseth T, Fauchald P, Skrede S, Djøseland O, Berg KJ, Stenstrøm J, et al. Long-term blood pressure and renal function in kidney donors. Kidney Int. 1986;29(5):1072–6.
78. Ommen ES, Schröppel B, Kim JY, Gaspard G, Akalin E, de Boccardo G, et al. Routine use of ambulatory blood pressure monitoring in potential living kidney donors. Clin J Am Soc Nephrol. 2007;2(5):1030–6.
79. DeLoach SS, Meyers KE, Townsend RR. Living donor kidney donation: another form of white coat effect. Am J Nephrol. 2012;35(1):75–9.

Chapter 3
Pathophysiology of Hypertension in Chronic Kidney Disease and Dialysis

Karen A. Griffin, Aaron J. Polichnowski, and Anil K. Bidani

Introduction

The close association between hypertension and severe kidney disease has been recognized for over 100 years. Such an association is only to be expected given the central role played by the kidneys in chronic BP regulation [1–6]. BP is a product of cardiac output (CO) and total peripheral resistance (TPR), and although an exceedingly large number of perturbations can acutely increase BP by impacting one or both of these determinants, sustained hypertension can only result through the failure of the homeostatic mechanisms that restore normal BP. As emphasized by Guyton and his co-workers, while a variety of neurohormonal control systems including factors that influence vascular capacity and transcapillary fluid exchange can be effective over the short term (hours), the primary mechanism for the long-term BP homeostasis is through the regulation of body fluid volume by the kidneys because of its capacity for "infinite gain." The key component of this mechanism termed the renal body fluid feedback mechanism is the pressure natriuresis/diuresis phenomenon, i.e. the ability of the kidney to increase or decrease salt and water excretion in response to increases or decreases in renal perfusion pressure. Therefore, the development of all forms of sustained HTN almost by definition requires an impairment of pressure natriuresis. However, it bears emphasis that the normal kidneys are able to increase salt excretion by several-fold in response to increases in salt intake without an appreciable change in BP. Thus, the very frequency with which hypertension develops is indicative of the frequency with which the intrinsic renal and neurohormonal mechanisms fail to achieve the task of achieving sodium balance without a sustained increase in BP. This is perhaps not surprising given that the mammalian kidney has evolved to avidly conserve salt [7] and the very wide range of alterations

K.A. Griffin, MD (✉) • A.J. Polichnowski, PhD • A.K. Bidani, MD
Edward Hines Jr. VA Hospital and Loyola University Medical Center,
2160 South First Avenue, Bldg. 102, Room 3661, Maywood, IL 60153, USA
e-mail: kgriffi@lumc.edu

© Springer Science+Business Media New York 2016
A.K. Singh, R. Agarwal (eds.), *Core Concepts in Hypertension in Kidney Disease*, DOI 10.1007/978-1-4939-6436-9_3

that can blunt the ability/efficiency of sodium excretory mechanisms. In this context, it also needs to be acknowledged that despite extensive work, many aspects of the pressure natriuresis phenomenon remain to be fully explicated, particularly as they pertain to how the changes in BP are transmitted to and sensed by the kidneys so as to achieve the necessary adjustments in sodium excretion [8–11].

It is also of note that despite the intimate association of CKD and HTN, subtle neurohormonal, hemodynamic, and tubular Na reabsorption abnormalities can impair pressure natriuresis without a decrease in GFR and/or other detectable defects in renal function, as in fact is postulated to occur in individuals with essential HTN [4–6, 12, 13]. In general, renal vasoconstrictor mechanisms favor sodium reabsorption and increased BP while renal vasodilators favor sodium excretion and reduced BP even in the absence of GFR changes. The associated alterations in the pressure natriuresis relationships probably result from an altered BP sensing by the renal parenchyma as well as direct effects on tubular sodium reabsorption. But predictably, the presence of a reduced GFR and/or enhanced Na reabsorption in renal disease states likely magnifies the impact of such neurohormonal and hemodynamic determinants on the impairment of pressure natriuresis. Thus, it is not surprising that a strong correlation has been noted between the presence and severity of hypertension and the magnitude of the decline in renal function with the prevalence of HTN ranging between 60 and 100 % in patients with CKD [6, 14–17]. Nevertheless, significant variability is observed in the presence and severity of hypertension within and between renal disease etiologies, at any given reduction in GFR, likely reflecting differences in the other associated modulators of pressure natriuresis [4–6, 8–11]. In any event, the likely presence of multiple interacting mechanisms with the potential to impair pressure natriuresis and to reduce the efficiency of sodium excretion in CKD results in a hypertension that is more difficult to control and almost inevitably requires effective diuretic therapy in addition to other agents [4, 18–21].

Factors That Promote Hypertension in CKD By and large, these are the same factors that promote increased BP in individuals without CKD, but as noted earlier, their effects tend to be magnified in CKD. However, the two factors that play a particularly predominant role in the pathogenesis of HTN in CKD patients are salt and the activity of the renin–angiotensin–aldosterone system (RAAS). This is particularly true of ESRD patients on dialysis [22–26]. Therefore, these factors are discussed in somewhat greater detail.

Salt

Extensive studies in both humans and experimental animals have demonstrated a striking ability to adapt to very large increases in salt intake with only a mild and transient increase in BP, although some genetic and age-dependent individual variability is observed [4–6, 15]. This tolerance of large increases in salt intake without developing sustained HTN is a function of the ability to re-achieve sodium balance by increasing urinary sodium excretion with only modest and transient sodium retention [4–6, 15]. This is made possible through the suppression of the Na retention mechanism (RAAS) and activation of the natriuretic systems including ANP. By contrast, individuals with CKD exhibit progressive increases in BP salt sensitivity with increasing loss of renal function [6, 14, 15]. The most extreme illustration of this phenomenon is provided by individuals with ESRD, particularly those without kidneys, in whom BP becomes extremely sensitive to changes in sodium intake and blood volume [22–26]. However, it bears emphasis that salt sensitivity is a continuous rather than a categorical phenotype [4, 6, 27] and there is considerable variability in the BP response to salt supplementation even in individuals with CKD, depending upon the pathophysiology associated with the underlying renal disease and its severity.

The different patterns of steady-state pressure natriuresis relationships that have been observed when HTN is due to renal mechanisms are schematically depicted in Fig. 3.1a [3–5]. As illustrated in the schematic, most forms of renal dysfunction other than those due to a generalized increase in preglomerular resistance are associated with increased BP salt sensitivity. However, the precise pattern and degree of salt sensitivity differs between the different mechanisms of renal HTN. This variability is believed to result from the differences in the degree to which the two common postulated pathways to salt sensitivity are being impacted: (1) loss of functional nephrons and (2) RAAS responsiveness [3–5]. In this context, it may be important to separate the effects of RAAS activation on BP per se from that on salt sensitivity of BP. While RAAS activation per se increases BP, it is the ability of salt to further modulate RAAS that determines salt sensitivity. As illustrated in Fig. 3.1b, increased BP salt sensitivity is observed somewhat counterintuitively, both with RAAS blockade and with continuous angiotensin II infusions. Accordingly in states of generalized preglomerular vasoconstriction (e.g., scleroderma and advanced hypertensive nephrosclerosis), it is the ability of RAAS to be suppressed by further increases in salt intake that renders the HTN in such states to be salt-insensitive. However, if the increases in preglomerular resistances are patchy or focal as in early hypertensive nephrosclerosis, renin release and RAAS suppressability are also non-homogenous and therefore BP tends to exhibit variable salt sensitivity [3–5, 12]. Similarly, in states of reduced glomerular capillary filtration coefficient (K_f) (e.g., glomerulonephritis), HTN develops due to the initial reductions in GFR, salt retention, and RAAS activation. But once HTN is established, the volume expansion suppresses RAAS and renders it less responsive to further changes in salt intake and thereby makes the BP more salt sensitive. Similarly, the increased sodium retention due to primary increases in tubular sodium reabsorption lead to volume expansion and RAAS suppression, resulting in salt-sensitive HTN. The clearest illustration of such a mechanism, although not directly relevant to CKD states, is provided by the monogenic forms of HTN. All of these involve mutations that result in an initial increase in distal renal tubular Na absorption, blunted pressure natriuresis, and salt-sensitive HTN [4–6, 28]. By contrast, in CKD states, the increased tubular Na reabsorption is more likely to be secondary to increased RAAS activation. Although

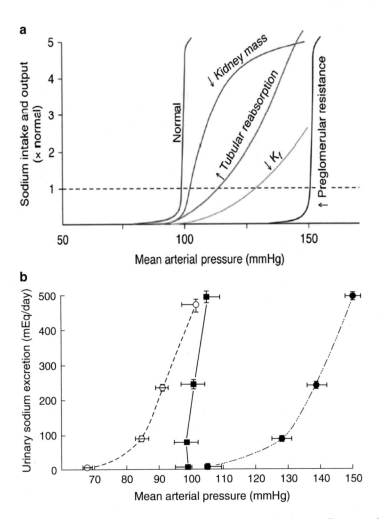

Fig. 3.1 (a) Steady-state relationships between arterial pressure and urinary sodium excretion and sodium intake for subjects with normal kidneys and four general types of renal dysfunction that cause hypertension: decreased kidney mass, increased reabsorption in distal and collecting tubules, reductions in glomerular capillary filtration coefficient (K_f), and increased preglomerular resistance. Note that increased preglomerular resistance causes *salt-insensitive* hypertension, whereas the other renal abnormalities cause *salt-sensitive* hypertension [4]. From Hall JE, Granger JP, do Carmo JM, da Silva AA, Dubinion J, George E, Hamza S, Speed J, Hall ME. Hypertension: Physiology and pathophysiology. Compr Physiol. 2012;2:2393–2442. Copyright Wiley 2012, used with permission. (b) Relationship between mean arterial pressure and sodium excretion (as an index of sodium intake) after steady state was achieved at four levels of sodium intake in dogs. Sodium intakes ranging from approximately 5–500 mEq/day were provided under normal conditions with a functional renin–angiotensin system, after blockade of Ang II formation with chronic angiotensin-converting enzyme (ACE) inhibitor, and after infusing Ang II continuously at 5 ng/kg/min to prevent plasma Ang II levels from being suppressed on the high-salt diet. Note the sensitivity of blood pressure to sodium intake when Ang II levels are prevented from changing [5]. From Brands MW. Chronic blood pressure control. Compr Physiol. 2012;2:2481–2494. Copyright Wiley 2012, used with permission

the loss of functional nephrons in CKD also promotes BP salt sensitivity, the degree of actual BP salt sensitivity observed is likely to depend on the etiopathogenesis of the underlying renal disease, the extent of RAAS activation and its suppressability. This is most clearly illustrated in experimental models of renal mass reduction (RMR). Strikingly different chronic BP responses are observed despite equivalent 70–80 % reductions in renal mass and GFR produced by infarction vs surgical excision of renal tissue [4, 29, 30]. In the surgical excision models of RMR, both in the rat and the dog, HTN does not develop on a normal salt diet perhaps because compensatory increases in SNGFR and tubular reabsorption are relatively balanced and the RAAS is suppressed due to the increased NaCl delivery to the macula densa. However, BP becomes very sensitive to increased salt intake as RAAS cannot be further suppressed. By contrast, when comparable RMR is achieved by infarction as in the conventional 5/6 renal ablation model, there is increased non-suppressible focal renin release from the peri-infarct areas and the animals rapidly develop HTN that is relatively salt-insensitive [4, 31, 32]. These considerations emphasize that in most renal diseases, a combination of interacting mechanisms are likely to be operative that influence the severity of HTN and its salt sensitivity. Furthermore, such patterns may not be fixed and may change over time with the evolution/progression of the renal disease. However, as noted earlier, with the development of ESRD, HTN largely becomes salt and volume dependent and the influence of the other HTN promoting mechanisms, including RAAS and increased sympathetic activity becomes quantitatively reduced [6, 22–26]. Nevertheless, these determinants often modify the relationships between volume expansion, cardiac output, and peripheral resistance resulting in significant individual variability in BP and its response to dialytic fluid removal.

Although the preceding discussion has emphasized the central role played by renal mechanisms of salt homeostasis in the pathogenesis of sustained hypertension, it also needs to be emphasized that not all states of impaired salt homeostasis and salt retention result in hypertension even in individuals with CKD. In general, salt retention tends to cause hypertension only when it results in an increase in effective circulatory volume as distinct from an increase in total extracellular fluid volume or even absolute blood volume. Accordingly, salt retention does not lead to hypertension in states of increased vascular capacity and/or altered Starling forces at the peripheral capillaries which favor increased leakage of fluids into the interstitial compartment and/or into the peritoneal space [4, 6]. Recently, it has been suggested that salt sensitivity even in the monogenic syndromes due to increased distal tubular sodium absorption is dependent not only on the sodium retention but also on a concomitant failure to reduce peripheral resistance (increase in vascular capacity) [33]. Evidence has also been obtained recently to indicate a significant macrophage regulated and VEGF-C dependent subcutaneous storage capacity for sodium which may additionally buffer and modulate sodium retention and BP increases in sodium excess states, including those with ESRD [34–36].

In any event, although controversy persists as to the advisability of more rigorous salt restriction measures in the general population [37], there is clear evidence of their usefulness and importance in the CKD population with HTN [38, 39].

Renin–Angiotensin–Aldosterone System

As is evident from the preceding discussion, RAAS plays a central and critical role in BP and volume homeostasis [3–6, 40, 41]. This hormonal cascade is initiated by the release of renin, a rate-limiting enzyme that catalyzes hydrolysis of angiotensin (Ang) I from the N-terminus of angiotensinogen. Renin is released from the juxtaglomerular cells (JG) of the renal afferent arteriole in response to a number of stimuli including, but not limited to, decreased renal perfusion pressure, reduced chloride concentration at the macula densa cells, sympathetic nerve stimulation via β-1 adrenergic receptors, and negative feedback by Ang II on the JG cells. As depicted in Fig. 3.2, Ang I is hydrolyzed by the angiotensin-converting enzyme (ACE) to form the potent vasoconstrictor, Ang II. Although a number of other biologically active enzymatic products and components of this hormonal cascade have been described [42, 43], Ang II is the primary effector of both short term and long-term BP regulation by this system [3–5]. These effects are mediated both through its direct vasoconstrictive pressor effects and through its stimulatory effects on renal tubular sodium reabsorption. Both effects are primarily mediated through the AT_1 receptor, although there is evidence that under certain conditions effects mediated

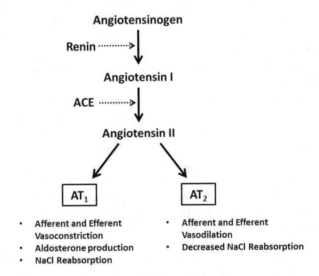

Fig. 3.2 Renin–angiotensin system (RAS) signaling cascade [42–46, 49–51]. Angiotensinogen is converted to Angiotensin I by the rate-limiting enzyme, renin. Angiotensin I is then converted to Angiotensin II by angiotensin-converting enzyme (ACE). It is now well recognized that most organs have all the components necessary to produce Angiotensin II locally. In the kidney, Angiotensin II acts on two major receptors, AT_1 and AT_2, which can be found on most major cell types. The primary effects of AT_1 stimulation are afferent and efferent vasoconstriction and NaCl reabsorption. Angiotensin II also promotes the release of aldosterone from the adrenal cortex, which further increases sodium reabsorption via its actions on principal cells in the distal tubule and collecting ducts. In contrast, AT_2 stimulation promotes afferent and efferent vasodilation and natriuresis

by AT_2 receptors may be natriuretic and BP lowering [44–46]. In any event, by virtue of its potent vasoconstrictor effects on the systemic and renal vasculature via the AT_1 receptor, Ang II contributes to the maintenance of BP during states of circulatory depression (hypotension) and/or volume depletion. The renal vasoconstrictive effects additionally potentiate the stimulatory effects of Ang II on Na reabsorption by most nephron segments leading to Na and volume conservation. The sodium conservation is further enhanced through the stimulation of aldosterone biosynthesis by Ang II (vide infra).

In this context, it is worth noting that the kidney is unique in that its tissue concentrations of Ang II exceed what would be delivered by arterial blood flow and there is substantial evidence that renal Ang II may be largely generated locally from angiotensinogen delivered from the circulation as well as that produced by the proximal tubule cells. All components required to generate intrarenal Ang II are present along the nephron [47–49]. There is also evidence that activation of intrarenal RAAS may be particularly relevant to tubular sodium reabsorption in the pathogenesis of salt-sensitive hypertension [50, 51]. In normal individuals when RAAS is fully functional and appropriately responsive to volume/Na and BP signals, the chronic renal pressure natriuresis relationship is quite steep and large changes in sodium intake can be achieved with minimal BP change. By contrast, when RAAS is inappropriately activated and/or is poorly suppressible by further increases in salt intake or perfusion pressure, pressure natriuresis is impaired and salt-sensitive hypertension develops, as is the case in most individuals with CKD.

Of note, despite the very frequent participation of RAAS in the pathogenesis of hypertension in CKD, the aspect that has received the greatest emphasis is its postulated role in mediating BP-independent renal damage and CKD progression [19, 45, 52, 53]. Two sets of mechanisms are postulated for these adverse effects of Ang II on renal injury. It is widely believed that Ang II predominantly causes efferent arteriolar constriction, resulting in disproportionate P_{GC} elevations and progressive glomerulosclerosis (GS) [19, 54]. However, such selective efferent constriction has typically been observed in states of low perfusion pressure and reduced macula densa flow (e.g., renal artery stenosis, hypovolemia), which stimulate not only renin release but also concurrent cyclooxygenase-2-mediated prostaglandin (PG) E_2 release from the macula densa [55]. PGE2 attenuates afferent but not efferent responses to angiotensin II [56] (see Fig. 3.3). This results in selective efferent constriction and a context-appropriate preferential preservation of glomerular filtration rate and glomerular capillary pressure P_{GC} in renal hypoperfusion states [45, 57]. Hence the sensitivity to nonsteroidal anti-inflammatory drug (NSAID) induced acute renal failure in such states. It is unlikely that a selective angiotensin II-mediated efferent constriction is a feature of ambient glomerular hemodynamics in the volume-replete normotensive or the volume-expanded hypertensive CKD states. Moreover, substantial evidence indicates that pathogenic glomerular hypertension in CKD models is primarily a consequence of an impairment of the autoregulatory responses of the dilated afferent arterioles that normally protect the glomerular capillaries from transmission of systemic BP elevations, episodic or sustained [57–59]. Moreover, when exogenous Ang II is administered, clear evidence of both afferent

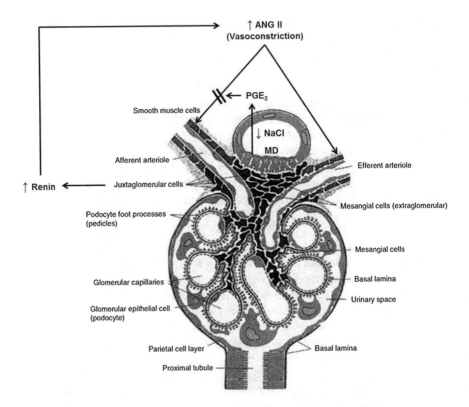

Fig. 3.3 Schematic illustration of the interactions between Angiotensin II (ANG II) and prostaglandin E2 (PGE$_2$) in regulating afferent arteriolar vasoconstriction at the juxtaglomerular apparatus (JGA) in states of renal hyperperfusion with reduced tubular flow and NaCl delivery at the macula densa (MD). The reduced NaCl delivery stimulates the release of both renin [4–6, 40] and PGE$_2$ [55]. PGE$_2$ attenuates the afferent arteriole myogenic responses to ANG II [56]. As shown in the diagram, the JGA consists of juxtaglomerular cells which secrete renin, the MD, and the extraglomerular mesangial cells. Adapted from Hunley TE, et al. in Avner ED, ed. Pediatric Nephrology, Sixth Edition, Vol 1, Springer-Verlag New York 2010

and efferent constriction as well as reduction in glomerular BP transmission is seen [60]. The second set of mechanisms believed to mediate the deleterious effects of Ang II in CKD involve several BP-independent tissue injury and fibrosis pathways [52, 53]. While such pathways have indeed been demonstrated in-vitro, it has been difficult to demonstrate the BP independence of such effects in-vivo when BP measurements have been performed adequately. By contrast, there is fairly unambiguous evidence of BP-dependent renoprotection by RAAS blockade [58, 59].

As noted earlier, Ang II, via the AT$_1$ receptor, also stimulates the production of aldosterone by the zona glomerulosa of the adrenal cortex, the powerful Na retaining hormone that contributes to the development of hypertension via the actions of the mineralocorticoid receptor on ENaC channels promoting the reabsorption of sodium and water along the distal tubules and collecting ducts [4, 5]. Its impact on the pressure natriuresis pattern is very similar to that of Ang II [3–5, 10]. In addition to these slower genomic effects mediated through the MR receptor, more rapid non-genomic renal effects have also been described but their role in long-term BP homeostasis is unclear [5, 61]. More recently, pathways for salt-sensitive HTN that are mediated through the MR receptor independent of aldosterone have also been postulated [62–64]. Of note, although Ang II and plasma aldosterone tend to parallel each other except in primary mineralcorticoid excess states, this may not hold true in CKD states. Angiotensin II and extracellular potassium levels, the two major regulators of aldosterone secretion may frequently change in different directions in CKD and utilize signaling pathways to differentially impact NaCl cotransporter activity [65].

Sympathetic Nervous System

While the aforementioned volume expansion and RAAS activity are the predominant mediators of hypertension in CKD/ESRD patients, activation of the sympathetic nervous system (SNS) is also recognized to play a significant role in this patient population [66–68]. Elevations in BP by the SNS can be achieved by exerting both inotropic and chronotropic effects on cardiac output and through vasoconstrictive effects on the vasculature, in addition to the effects mediated by the activation of renal nerves (via infra) [4–6, 66–70].

Central Sympathetic Nervous System

Sustained overactivity of the sympathetic nervous system has been observed in several types of human hypertension including, but not limited to, obesity, obstructive sleep apnea, early type 2 diabetes, heart failure, and chronic kidney disease/ESRD [67]. This may be the result of deactivation of inhibitory neural inputs (e.g., baroreceptors), activation of excitatory neural inputs (e.g., carotid body chemoreceptors, renal afferents), or stimulation by circulating angiotensin II, that activates excitatory brainstem neurons that are devoid of a blood–brain barrier [67, 71]. Both excitatory and inhibitory synaptic inputs received by the nucleus tractus solitarious (NTS) project to the rostral ventrolateral medulla, and from there preganglionic sympathetic fibers synapse in the adrenal medulla or the paravertebral sympathetic chain ganglia. Postganglionic fibers releasing norepinephrine innervate the heart, blood vessels, and kidney.

Renal Sympathetic Nervous System

The renal sympathetic nerves contribute to hypertension through multiple pathways that include renal vasoconstriction via α_{1A} adrenergic receptors on renal arterial resistance vessels, stimulation of renin release via β_1 adrenergic receptors on juxtaglomerular granular cells, and increased renal sodium and water reabsorption via

α_{1B} adrenergic receptors on renal tubular epithelial cells [4–6, 70, 71]. Increasing activity of SNS is seen with declining renal function. This is due to the fact that the kidney is richly innervated with sensory afferents projecting centrally to the nucleus tractus solitaries (NTS) evoking reflex sympathetic excitation. These afferents can be activated by ischemic (adenosine) or uremic (urea) metabolites and have been implicated in the pathogenesis of hypertension observed with renovascular disease or CKD, respectively [6, 72–74]. The renal SNS also contributes to salt-dependent hypertension by shifting the pressure natriuresis curve to the right. Of note, the renal responses to sympathetic nerve stimulation are frequency dependent and can therefore be additively activated with the lowest frequency stimulating only sodium reabsorption, with the addition of renin release at the next highest frequency, and at the highest frequencies sodium reabsorption and renin release are accompanied by reductions in RBF and GFR [70, 71].

Endothelial Dysfunction, Nitric Oxide, and Oxidative Stress

Among its numerous biological functions, the vascular endothelium is also the site of synthesis of several vasoactive molecules including nitric oxide (NO) and reactive oxygen species (ROS) which are intimately involved in the regulation of vascular tone and BP. Although the term endothelial dysfunction has been used to refer to alterations of vascular function in several pathological states [75–77], the present discussion is primarily limited to the role of NO loss and oxidant stress in the pathogenesis and pathophysiology of hypertension in CKD/ESRD states [78–82]. Loss of NO, particularly in the medullary circulation, has been shown to increase renal vascular resistance, enhance the sensitivity to other vasoconstrictions, augment renal salt reabsorption, and impair pressure natriuresis. Such NO deficiency can occur through multiple mechanisms including decreased endothelial arginine transport, altered NO synthase (NOS) expression, decreased NO bioavailability due to increased scavenging by ROS and/or NOS inhibition by endogeneous inhibitors including the NOS inhibitor, asymmetric dimethyl arginine (ADMA), the levels which are increased in CKD states [4, 78–82]. ROS also promote salt-sensitive hypertension, partly through limiting NO availability and partly through direct effects on the renal microvasculature and renal tubules that increase vasoconstriction, particularly in the medulla, enhance sodium reabsorption, and impair pressure natriuresis relationships. As GFR declines with CKD, the effects of NO loss and increased ROS become further potentiated, setting up a vicious cycle.

Endothelin

One of the more potent systemic and renal vasoconstrictors produced by the endothelium is endothelin (ET-1). Receptors for ET-1 are located throughout the body with the greatest concentration being located in the lungs and kidney. ET-1 acts on both endothelin A (ET_A) and endothelin B (ET_B) receptors. ET_A effects are vasoconstrictive and prohypertensive, while ET_B activation results in medullary vasodilation and natriuresis [4, 6, 83]. Thus depending on the location and type of receptor activated, ET-1 can elicit a chronic hypertensive state or have an antihypertensive effect [4, 6, 84]. Sodium increases ET-1 expression in the kidney and the absence of ET-1 action on ET_B receptors results in salt-dependent hypertension [85–87]. In patients with renal disease and ESRD, plasma ET-1 levels are increased and correlate with BP [6, 88]. Supporting a role for ET-1 in CKD hypertension are the antihypertensive effects of selective ET_A receptor blockade which has therefore emerged as a potential target for the treatment of hypertension in patients with CKD/ESRD [6, 89, 90]. Interestingly, treatment of anemia in patients with renal disease using human recombinant erythropoietin also has been shown to have adverse effects on endothelial function by increasing ET-1 production and increasing BP.

Dopamine and Renalase

Renal dopamine is natriuretic and is estimated to potentially impact approximately 50 % of excreted sodium. Additionally, renal dopamine counteracts the effect of angiotensin II, thus making dopamine an important contributor to sodium homeostasis and BP regulation [91–94]. A high-salt diet stimulates renal dopamine synthesis and excretion while a low salt diet has the opposite effect. Dopamine exerts its natriuretic effect through the activation of D1-like dopamine receptors in the proximal tubule which in turn reduces the activity of the Na/H exchanger (NHE3) by increasing its internalization. There is also evidence to suggest that the renal vascular natriuretic response to D1-like receptor stimulation may differ between hypertensive and normotensive individuals. However, the contribution of the system to CKD hypertension is probably mediated through changes in the activity of renalase. Renalase is a secreted amine oxidase that metabolizes circulating catecholamines, including dopamine [94, 95]. Renalase is highly expressed in the proximal tubule and is not only secreted in the blood but is also secreted in the urine. The activity of renalase is much higher in the urine than in the plasma. Recent data indicate that renalase deficiency is associated with increased BP and elevated circulating catecholamines. This may occur through the action of urinary renalase on urinary catecholamines thereby regulating dopamine concentration in luminal fluid and modulating proximal tubular sodium transport. Prior to the discovery of renalase it was thought that luminal dopamine levels could only be regulated prior to secretion into the tubular lumen as the two enzymes that play an important role in the catabolism of dopamine, monoamine oxidase (MAO), and carboxy-O-methyl-transferase (COMT) are intracellular. However, inhibition of MAO and COMT does not have a significant impact on dopamine-dependent natriuresis in experimental models suggesting a role for renalase in the metabolizing and regulation of dopamine levels in the tubular lumen [96]. Studies in the renalase knockout mouse model which exhibit an elevated BP have also provided support for these concepts [95]. Increased dietary sodium has also been shown to inhibit renalase protein expression in experimental models of CKD and salt-sensitive hypertension while administration of recombinant renalase has been shown to decrease BP in these models [96, 97]. Moreover, blood levels of renalase are significantly reduced in end-stage renal disease patients [97, 98].

Other Pressor Factors

A discussion of the multiple other factors that have the potential to cause hypertension in CKD/ESRD patients is beyond the scope of this chapter. However, some of the factors that may be of particular relevance in CKD patients are briefly discussed.

Parathyroid Hormone

Although the hypertension in most patients with CKD is primarily due to other factors, it has been suggested that the secondary hyperparathyroidism usually present in these patients may be contributory [99, 100]. Patients with primary hyperparathyroidism (PHPT) also often have hypertension, but the mechanisms have not been fully elucidated. It has been suggested that in addition to the activation of the sympathetic RAAS, elevated serum and intracellular calcium levels may lead to an increase in vascular smooth muscle tone [101]. However, the relationship of these mechanisms in PHPT to the hypertension in the majority of CKD patients who tend to be normo- or hypocalcemic remains to be established.

Vitamin D

Patients with CKD often have reduced synthesis of calcitriol, the active form of vitamin D. Studies in animal models have suggested that vitamin D may play a role in the hypertension, left ventricular hypertrophy and diastolic dysfunction, and albuminuria observed in CKD states [102–105]. Some of the evidence comes from studies in vitamin D receptor knockout mice which develop elevated BP and left ventricular hypertrophy thought to be due to the loss of normal suppression of RAAS by vitamin D [103–105]. A relationship between vitamin D and BP has also been suggested on epidemiologic grounds based on the observation that the incidence of hypertension increases at higher latitudes where low UV irradiation levels exist [106]. Similarly, studies by Harburg et al. have also shown that dark skin pigmentation affects UV light penetration and reduces the cutaneous synthesis of vitamin D which is also associated with a higher BP in these populations [107]. However, more recent work by Liu et al. showing that the skin is capable of modulating systemic NO bioavailability by its release from cutaneous stores with UV exposure has provided an alternative explanation for these associations. This effect may account for the latitudinal and seasonal variations of BP that are independent of vitamin D and may confound interpretations of previous work examining the relationship between vitamin D and BP [108]. Similarly, although several epidemiological studies have supported an association between Vitamin D deficiency and hypertension [102, 109], clinical trials of Vitamin D supplementation have yielded negative results [110].

Calcium

Over the years there has been considerable debate as to the role of dietary and non-dietary calcium supplementation and its effects on hypertension. In addition to the direct vasoconstrictive effects of hypercalcemia [111], calcium has been shown to modulate the enzymatic activities that integrate the balance of synthesis and degradation of the dominant second messenger for renin secretion, cAMP [112]. Acting primarily through adenylyl cyclase V activity, calcium does not directly control renin secretion but rather modulates the degree of response to the classic renin-stimulating pathways of the renal baroreceptor, macula densa, and renal nerves. Unlike most secretory cells, with the exception of the chief cells of the parathyroid gland, intracellular and extracellular calcium concentration exhibits an inverse relationship with cAMP-stimulated renin secretion, a response known as the "calcium paradox." Taken together, these data suggest that calcium indirectly affects renin secretion by decreasing adenylyl cyclase activity in the JG cells and thereby reducing the synthesis of cAMP and the release of renin [112–115]. A Cochrane Review of 13 randomized, controlled trials of 485 hypertensive subjects found calcium supplementation to be associated with a statistically significant decrease of systolic BP of −2.5 mmHg. However, the authors concluded that evidence for a causal association between calcium supplementation and reduction of BP was weak and may be compromised by potential bias. Larger and longer duration, double-blind placebo-controlled trials are therefore needed [116], particularly since adverse cardiovascular effects of calcium supplementation have also been reported [117].

Hypokalemia

Dietary potassium seems to affect BP independent of sodium intake. Our modern diet is relatively high in salt (NaCl) and low in potassium compared to the diets consumed by our evolutionary ancestors. The results of the recent Prospective Urban Rural Epidemiology (PURE) trial in 102,216 adults from 18 countries conducted to examine the association between sodium intake and BP have shown a low potassium diet to be strongly associated with elevated BP and potassium excretion to be inversely associated with systolic BP [118]. A high potassium diet and intravenous potassium infusions have both been shown to suppress thiazide sensitive sodium chloride cotransporter (NCC) activity result in kaliuresis and natriuresis. A low K diet has the opposite effects [119–122]. Recent experimental data have shown that dietary potassium deficiency and hypokalemia lead to hyperpolarization of the distal convoluted tubule membrane and activation of NCC via WNK. This response represents an attempt to limit potassium losses even at the expense of raising the BP [123].

Uric Acid

Although uric acid (UA) has not been conventionally considered as a pressor factor, the association between increased UA levels and hypertension has been long known. Recent experimental and clinical studies have suggested that uric acid may play a primary role in the pathogenesis of hypertension [124–127]. However, there has been considerable controversy regarding the role of hyperuricemia in the pathogenesis of hypertension and not all guidelines have included uric acid as a risk factor of concern [128, 129]. Nevertheless, considerable inferential evidence is accumulating particularly with respect to its role in the pathogenesis in the metabolic syndrome [124–127]. However, UA levels are commonly elevated in CKD but their specific contribution to hypertension in CKD patients remains unclear. The uncertainty has persisted as there has been no double-blinded, placebo-controlled trial of urate lowering medications in CKD, due to the potentially life-threatening side effects of allopurinol.

Translating Mechanisms to Patients

Obesity

The growing epidemic of obesity [130] is widely recognized to not only contribute to hypertension, diabetes, and CKD but also to be an independent risk factor for the pathogenesis and progression of CKD [131–137]. Hypertension related to obesity is on an upward trend with approximately two thirds of Americans being classified as overweight (body mass index [BMI] >25) or obese (BMI >30). The pathogenesis of hypertension associated with obesity is multifactorial and in large part attributed to activation of the sympathetic nervous system (SNS), increased RAAS activity, release of cytokines from adipose tissues, and enhanced salt and water reabsorption [131, 133–136]. Several mechanisms contribute to SNS activation including increased leptin levels, insulin resistance, obstructive sleep apnea (OSA) (vide-infra), and endothelial dysfunction [131, 134, 135, 137–139]. The prohypertensive contributions of these mechanisms are further reinforced and exaggerated by the presence of CKD.

Obstructive Sleep Apnea

The pathogenesis of the OSA associated hypertension is believed to depend on periodic asphyxia as a result of repeated episodes of upper airway collapse, which stimulates muscle sympathetic nerve activity and BP [140–142]. It is thought that these sympathetic responses to acute episodes of hypoxia are altered over time, and lead to an enhanced chemoreflex activity and alteration in arterial baroreflex control that play a role in the pathogenesis of the chronic sympatho-excitation observed with

OSA. With time, the intermittent nocturnal sympathetic nerve activation gives rise to daytime activation of SNS even though arterial oxygenation and carbon dioxide levels are normal during this time [143]. The resulting effect is both daytime and nighttime hypertension. Of interest, animal studies have also shown that renal and adrenal denervation prevents the rise in BP from OSA by preventing the increase in sympathetic nerve activity (SNA) [144, 145]. Recommended treatment is the use of continuous positive airway pressure (CPAP) as it blunts nocturnal muscle SNA and its attendant elevations in nocturnal blood pressure. In addition to normalizing BP, the use of CPAP reduces daytime sleepiness and when used long-term, decreases muscle SNA [146, 147].

Metabolic Syndrome

The metabolic syndrome is defined by the International Diabetes Federation as having a waist circumference ≥94 cm for men and ≥80 cm for women, plus any two of the following four factors: triglyceride level ≥150 mg/dL (1.7 mmol/L), HDL cholesterol <40 mg/dL (1.03 mmol/L) in males and <50 mg/dL (1.29 mmol/L) in females, BP ≥130/85 mmHg, or fasting plasma glucose ≥100 mg/dL (5.6 mmol/L) [148]. Given the definition, the prevalence rate of hypertension in metabolic syndrome of up to 75 % is not surprising [149]. Its multifactorial pathogenesis is also not unexpected given the number of hypertensinogenic conditions frequently associated with the metabolic syndrome that include but are not limited to central obesity and insulin resistance [134, 139, 149, 150]. Consistent with this is the observation that individuals with the metabolic syndrome have a ~5.5-fold risk of diabetes and twofold risk of new hypertension as compared to individuals without the metabolic syndrome [151].

Diabetes Mellitus

The prevalence of hypertension in individuals with diabetes is approximately twice that of nondiabetics and increases with age [152]. Although the majority of diabetics have essential hypertension and obesity as the etiology of their elevated BP, the development of diabetic nephropathy and CKD per se can lead to elevations in BP [152]. The mechanisms as in most forms of CKD likely depend on volume expansion due to sodium and water retention associated with reduced renal function. While there is frequently evidence of suppression of peripheral RAS, it is believed that the degree of suppression is either not proportional to the volume expansion or that there is an activation of the intrarenal RAS, which contributes to the development of hypertension [153–155]. However, as noted earlier, it is the BP-independent deleterious effects of RAS activation in accelerating the progression of diabetic nephropathy that have received greater emphasis [156–159]. Nevertheless, the evidence of BP independence of the benefits is less definitive than has been implied [19, 58, 160]. Either the BP has been significantly lower in the RAS blockade group or calcium channel blockers have been used in the comparator group which can independently adversely impact CKD progression through its deleterious effects on renal autoregulation [19, 59, 160, 161]. Of note, evidence for therapeutic superiority of RAS blockade was not seen in the diabetic individuals enrolled in the renal ALLHAT trial [162]. Moreover, trials of dual RAS blockade not only do not confer additional benefits but in fact increase the risk of adverse events [163–165]. Therefore, dual RAS blockade is no longer recommended. However, the use of single RAS blockade when combined with appropriate diuretic therapy is very effective as antihypertensive therapy supporting the role of volume/RAS dependent mechanisms in the pathogenesis of diabetic nephropathy associated hypertension.

An additional mechanism that has been postulated to contribute specifically to hypertension in the diabetic CKD patients is that of insulin resistance [149, 150, 166, 167]. However, a number of experimental studies by Hall and co-workers have failed to demonstrate a hypertensive effect of chronic insulin infusion under several conditions including preexisting impairment of renal function [168, 169]. Consistent with these observations, patients with insulinomas and insulin resistance also do not exhibit hypertension [170, 171]. Diabetic individuals, however, are more prone to developing isolated systolic hypertension due to their hyperlipidemia and athero-sclerotic vascular disease [166]. In addition, the progressive accumulation of atherosclerotic plaques can result in narrowing of the renal arteries and the development of renovasular hypertension [172]. Diabetics, especially those with more advanced disease may exhibit supine hypertension with orthostatic hypotension. These individuals often have autonomic dysfunction that impairs their ability to adequately increase peripheral vascular resistance and heart rate when changing position from a supine to more upright posture [173].

Hyperaldosteronism

The contribution of secondary aldosteronism to increased sodium reabsorption, volume expansion, impaired pressure natriuresis, and hypertension was discussed earlier. Therefore, this discussion is confined to primary aldosteronism which was first described by Conn in 1955 and had a prevalence rate of <1 % in the general hypertensive population [174]. The prevalence of hyperaldosteronism seems to have increased since the 1990s and has been estimated to range from ~5 to 15 % in the general and selective hypertensive populations [175]. It has been reported to be ~20 % in patients presenting with resistant hypertension, defined as BP that remains elevated despite the use of three antihypertensive medications with one being a diuretic. Although not fully understood, this increase in prevalence is in part due to the recognition that not all patients with hyperaldosteronism present with hypokalemia and the inclusion of hypertensive individuals with normokalemia when screening for hyperaldosteronism has in part contributed to the increased prevalence rate.

Another contributing factor is the association of obesity with elevated aldosterone levels due to release of factors from adipocytes that function as aldosterone secretagogues [176]. Aldosterone primarily acts on the mineralocorticoid receptor stimulating serum and glucocorticoid-inducible kinase expression resulting in phosphorylation of the ubiquitin ligase, NEDD4 [177]. This leads to reduced ubiquitylation of ENaC resulting in its accumulation at the plasma membrane and enhanced sodium reabsorption across principal cells. Although there is evidence that increased ENaC activation and Na reabsorption may be present in certain proteinuric individuals [178, 179], there is limited evidence of an increase in the incidence of primary aldosteronism in CKD population.

Renovascular Disease

Only a brief discussion primarily focused on the pathophysiology of hypertension in renovascular disease is provided here as the overall subject is addressed more comprehensively in a separate chapter. Seminal work using experimental models of unilateral and bilateral renal artery stenosis dating back to the original studies of Goldblatt have established the essentials of the pathogenesis of hypertension in renovascular disease [4, 180–186]. These studies have demonstrated the critical role of the interactions between RAS and volume status in the pathogenesis of renovascular hypertension and its sensitivity to RAS blockade. With unilateral renovascular disease and a normal contralateral kidney, hypertension develops initially because of the increased renin release from the stenosed kidney due to decreased renal perfusion pressure and ischemia. While there is increased salt and water retention by the ipsilateral stenosed kidney, there is increased salt and water excretion by the normal contralateral kidney in response to the increased perfusion pressure. Thus, volume expansion is prevented but the pressure natriuresis relationship to the normal contralateral kidney is nevertheless impaired due to an exposure to the increased systemic levels of angiotensin II. There is also evidence of recruitment of other pressor mechanisms such as activation of the SNS and increased oxidative stress, etc. [187, 188]. Because hypertension is primarily dependent on the increased renin release from the stenosed kidney, it is at least initially very responsive to RAS blockade. By contrast with bilateral renal vascular disease, the lack of escape from the salt retention by both kidneys results in volume expansion and the conversion of a renin-dependent to a volume-dependent hypertensive state, which is poorly responsive to RAS blockade. The same pathophysiology is observed with renal artery stenosis of a solitary kidney. However, in both instances, induction of volume depletion by salt restriction or diuretics restores the renin dependency of hypertension and its responsiveness to RAS blockade. However, it is of note that over time, even the unilateral renal artery stenosis hypertension becomes poorly responsive to RAS blockade. Such a change is believed to be due to the development of either gradually increasing volume expansion or the development of hypertensive renal damage in the previously normal unprotected contralateral kidney, thus resulting in a pathophysiology very similar to that in bilateral renal artery stenosis models. Studies in human renovascular disease have in general confirmed these pathophysiological insights [185, 188, 189]. Such studies have also indicated that hemodynamically significant renal artery stenosis resulting in increased renin release is only observed with a translesional pressure gradient of 10–20 % and a decrease in luminal cross sectional area of 70–80 % [190, 191]. However, the pathogenesis of hypertension in most human renovascular disease seems somewhat more complex because it is generally due to atherosclerotic disease, occurs in older individuals and often in the presence of essential hypertension as well as other comorbidities. Moreover, the very presence of CKD (elevated serum creatinine) indicates bilateral renal disease, either renovascular or due to other etiologies. Such complexity is also indicated by the relatively poor response in clinical trials to renovascular angioplasty and stenting [192–194]. And, if anything, the results have been even more disappointing with respect to recovery of renal function after such interventions even though there are often documented improvements in renal blood flow and perfusion. This has suggested that the pathogenesis of ischemic nephropathy is similarly complex in the setting of atherosclerotic renal vascular disease, which is the subject of ongoing investigations [192–194].

References

1. Guyton AC. The surprising kidney fluid mechanism for pressure control—its infinite gain! Hypertension. 1990;16:725–30.
2. Guyton AC. Blood pressure control—special role of the kidneys and body fluids. Science. 1991;252:1813–6.
3. Cowley Jr AW. Long-term control of arterial blood pressure. Physiol Rev. 1992;72:231–300.
4. Hall JE, Granger JP, do Carmo JM, da Silva AA, Dubinion J, George E, Hamza S, Speed J, Hall ME. Hypertension: physiology and pathophysiology. Compr Physiol. 2012;2:2393–442.
5. Brands MW. Chronic blood pressure control. Compr Physiol. 2012;2:2481–94.
6. Wadel HM, Textor SC. The role of the kidney in regulating arterial blood pressure. Nat Rev Nephrol. 2012;8:602–9.
7. Smith HW. From fish to philosopher. 1st ed. Boston: Little Brown; 1953. p. 264.
8. Romero JC, Knox FG. Mechanisms underlying pressure-related natriuresis: the role of the renin-angiotensin and prostaglandin systems. State of the art lecture. Hypertension. 1988;11:724–38.
9. Firth JD, Raine AEG, Ledingham JGG. The mechanism of pressure natriuresis. J Hypertens. 1990;8:97–103.
10. Hall JE, Mizelle HL, Hildebrandt DA, Brands MW. Abnormal pressure natriuresis. A cause or a consequence of hypertension? Hypertension. 1990;15:547–59.
11. Evans RG, Majid DSA, Eppel GA. Mechanisms mediating pressure natriuresis: what we know and what we need to find out. Clin Exp Pharm Physiol. 2005;32:400–9.
12. Laragh JH. Nephron heterogeneity: clue to the pathogenesis of essential hypertension and effectiveness of angiotensin-converting enzyme inhibitor treatment. Am J Med. 1989;87 Suppl 68:2S–14.
13. Johnson RJ, Rodriguez-Iturbe B, Nakagawa T, Kang D-H, Feig DI, Herrera-Acosta J. Subtle renal injury is likely a common mechanism for salt-sensitive essential hypertension. Hypertension. 2005;45:326–30.

14. Koomans HA, Roos JC, Boer P, Geyskes GG, Mess EJD. Salt sensitivity of blood pressure in chronic renal failure: evidence for renal control of body fluid distribution in man. Hypertension. 1982;4:190–7.
15. Koomans HA, Roos JC, Dorhout Mees EJ, Delawi IM. Sodium balance in renal failure. A comparison of patients with normal subjects under extremes of sodium intake. Hypertension. 1985;7:714–21.
16. Buckalew Jr VM, Berg RL, Wang SR, Porush JG, Rauch S, Schulman G. Prevalence of hypertension in 1,795 subjects with chronic renal disease: the modification of diet in renal disease study baseline cohort. Modification of diet in renal disease study group. Am J Kidney Dis. 1996;28:811–21.
17. National Kidney Foundation. K/DOQI clinical practice guidelines for chronic kidney disease: evaluation, classification, and stratification. Am J Kidney Dis. 2002;39:S1–S266.
18. Vasavada N, Agarwal R. Role of excess volume in the pathophysiology of hypertension in chronic kidney disease. Kidney Int. 2003;64:1772–9.
19. Bidani AK, Griffin KA. Pathophysiology of hypertensive renal damage: implications for therapy. Hypertension. 2004;44:595–601.
20. Platinga LC, Miller 3rd ER, Stevens LA, Saran R, Messer K, Flowers N, Geiss L, Powe NR, Center for Disease Control and Prevention Chronic Kidney Disease Surveillance Team. Blood pressure control among persons without and with chronic kidney disease: US trends and risk factors 1999–2006. Hypertension. 2009;54:47–56.
21. Sarafidis PA, Li S, Chen SC, Collins AJ, Brown WW, Klag MJ, Bakris GL. Hypertension awareness, treatment, and control in chronic kidney disease. Am J Med. 2008;121:332–40.
22. Coleman TG, Bower JD, Langford HG, Guyton AC. Regulation of arterial pressure in the anephric state. Circulation. 1970;42:509–14.
23. Agarwal R. Systolic hypertension in hemodialysis patients. Semin Dial. 2003;16:334.
24. Horl MP, Horl WH. Hemodialysis-associated hypertension: pathophysiology and therapy. Am J Kidney Dis. 2002;39:227–44.
25. Wilson J, Shah T, Nissenson AR. Role of sodium and volume in the pathogenesis of hypertension in hemodialysis. Semin Dial. 2004;27:260–4.
26. Blankestijn PJ, Lightenberg G. Volume-independent mechanisms of hypertension in hemodialysis patients: clinical implications. Semin Dial. 2004;17:265–9.
27. Weinberger MH. Salt sensitivity of blood pressure in humans. Hypertension. 1996;27(3 Pt. 2):481–490.
28. Lifton RP, Gharavi AG, Geller DS. Molecular mechanisms of human hypertension. Cell. 2001;104:545–56.
29. Langston JB, Guyton AC, Douglas BH, Dorsett PE. Effect of changes in salt intake on arterial pressure and renal function in partially nephrectomized dogs. Circ Res. 1963;12:508–12.
30. Griffin KA, Picken M, Bidani AK. Method of renal mass reduction is a critical modulator of subsequent hypertension and glomerular injury. J Am Soc Nephrol. 1994;4:2023–31.
31. Correa-Rotter R, Hostette TH, Manivel JC, Rosenberg ME. Renin expression in renal ablation. Hypertension. 1992;20:483–90.
32. Griffin KA, Picken MM, Churchill M, Churchill P, Bidani AK. Functional and structural correlates of glomerulosclerosis after renal mass reduction in the rat. J Am Soc Nephrol. 2000;11:497–506.
33. Kurtz TW, Dominiczak AF, DiCarlo SE, Pravenec M, Morris Jr RC. Molecular-based mechanisms of Mendelian forms of salt-dependent hypertension. Questioning the prevailing theory. Hypertension. 2015;65:932–41.
34. Machnik A, Neuhofer W, Jantsch J, Dahlmann A, Tammela T, Machura K, Park J-K, Beck F-X, Muller DN, Derer W, Goss J, Ziomber A, Dietsch P, Wagner H, van Rooijen N, Kurtz A, Hilgers KF, Alitalo K, Eckardt K-U, Luft FC, Kerjaschki D, Titze J. Macrophages regulate salt-dependent volume and blood pressure by a vascular endothelial growth factor-C-dependent buffering mechanism. Nat Med. 2009;15:545–52.
35. Titze J. A different view on sodium balance. Curr Opin Nephrol Hypertens. 2015;24:14–20.

36. Dahlmann A, Dorfelt K, Eicher F, Linz P, Kopp C, Mossinger I, Horn S, Buschges-Seraphin B, Wabel P, Hammon M, Cavallaro A, Echardt KU, Kotanko P, Levin NW, Johannes B, Uder M, Luft FC, Muller DN, Titze JM. Magnetic resonance-determined sodium removal from tissue stores in hemodialysis patients. Kidney Int. 2015;87:434–41.

37. Aaron KJ, Sanders PW. Role of dietary salt and potassium intake in cardiovascular health and disease: a review of the evidence. Mayo Clin Proc. 2013;88:987–95.

38. He FJ, MacGregor GA. Salt, blood pressure and cardiovascular disease. Curr Opin Cardiol. 2007;22:298–305.

39. Heerspink HJL, Navis G, Ritz E. Salt intake in kidney disease—a missed therapeutic opportunity? Nephrol Dial Transplant. 2012;27:3435–42.

40. Navar LG, Inscho EW, Majid DSA, Imig JD, Harrison-Bernard LM, Mitchell KD. Paracrine regulation of the renal microcirculation. Physiol Rev. 1996;76:425–536.

41. Semoes E, Silva AC, Flynn JT. The renin angiotensin aldosterone system in 2011: role in hypertension and chronic kidney disease. Pediatr Nephrol. doi:10.1007/s00467-0211-2002-y.

42. Reudelhuber TL. The renin-angiotensin system: peptides and enzymes beyond angiotensin II. Curr Opin Nephrol Hypertens. 2005;14:155–9.

43. Ferrario CM. Role of angiotensin II in cardiovascular disease therapeutic implications of more than a century of research. J Renin Angiotensin Aldosterone Syst. 2006;7(1):3–14.

44. Carey RM, Siragy HM. Newly recognized components of the renin-angiotensin system: potential roles in cardiovascular and renal regulation. Endocr Rev. 2003;24(3):261–71.

45. Griffin KA, Bidani AK. Angiotensin II type 2 receptor in chronic kidney disease: the good side of angiotensin II? Kidney Int. 2009;75(10):1006–8.

46. Benndorf RA, Krebs C, Hirsch-Hoffman B, Schwedhelm E, Cieslar G, Schmidt-Haupt R, Steinmetz OM, Meyer-Schwesinger C, Thaiss F, Haddad M, Fehr S, Hellmann A, Helmchen U, Hein L, Ehmke H, Stahl RA, Boger RH, Wenzel UO. Angiotensin II type 2 receptor deficiency aggravates renal injury and reduces survival in chronic kidney disease in mice. Kidney Int. 2009;75(10):1039–49.

47. Casarini DE, Boim MA, Stella RC, Krieger-Azzolini MH, Krieger JE, Schor N. Angiotensin I-converting enzyme activity in tubular fluid along the rat nephron. Am J Physiol. 1997;272(3 Pt 2):F405–9.

48. Kobori H, Nangaku M, Navar LG, Nishiyama A. The intrarenal renin-angiotensin system: from physiology to the pathobiology of hypertension and kidney disease. Pharmacol Rev. 2007;59(3):251–87.

49. Navar LG, Prieto MC, Satou R, Kobori H. Intrarenal angiotensin II and its contribution to the genesis of chronic hypertension. Curr Opin Pharmacol. 2011;11:180–6.

50. Crowley SD, Gurley SB, Herrera MJ, Ruiz P, Griffiths R, Kumar AP, Kim HS, Smithies O, Le TH, Coffman TM. Angiotensin II causes hypertension and cardiac hypertrophy through its receptors in the kidney. Proc Natl Acad Sci. 2006;103:17985–90.

51. Giani JF, Shah KH, Khan Z, Bernstein EA, Shen XA, McDonough AA, Gonzalez-Villalobos RA, Bernstein KE. The intrarenal generation of angiotensin II is required for experimental hypertension. Curr Opin Pharm. 2015;21:73–81.

52. Harris RC, Neilson EG. Toward a unified theory of renal progression. Annu Rev Med. 2006;57:365–80.

53. Ruster C, Wolf G. Renin-angiotensin-aldosterone system and progression of renal disease. J Am Soc Nephrol. 2006;17:2985–91.

54. Brenner BM. Nephron adaptation to renal injury or ablation. Am J Physiol. 1985;249:F324–37.

55. Peti-Peterdi J, Komlosi P, Fuson AL, Guan Y, Schneider A, Qi Z, Redha R, Rosivall L, Breyer MD, Bell PD. Luminal NaC1 delivery regulates basolateral PGE2 release from macula densa cells. J Clin Invest. 2003;112:76–82.

56. Tang L, Loutzenhiser K, Loutzenhiser R. Biphasic actions of prostaglandin E(2) on the renal afferent arteriole: role of EP(3) and EP(4) receptors. Circ Res. 2000;86:663–70.

57. Loutzenhiser R, Griffin K, Williamson G, Bidani A. Renal autoregulation: new perspectives regarding the protective and regulatory roles of the underlying mechanisms. Am J Physiol. 2006;290:R1153–67.

58. Griffin KA, Bidani AK. Progression of renal disease: the renoprotective specificity of renin angiotensin system blockade. Clin J Am Soc Nephrol. 2006;1:1054–65.
59. Bidani AK, Polichnowski AJ, Loutzenhiser R, Griffin KA. Renal microvascular dysfunction, hypertension and CKD progression. Curr Opin Nephrol Hypertens. 2013;22:1–9.
60. Polichnowski AJ, Griffin KA, Picken MM, Licea-Vargas H, Long J, Williamson GA, Bidani AK. Hemodynamic basis for the limited renal injury in rats with angiotensin II-induced hypertension. Am J Physiol. 2015;308:F252–60.
61. Funder JW. Minireview: aldosterone and the cardiovascular system: genomic and nongenomic effects. Endocrinology. 2006;147:5564–7.
62. Funder JW. Reconsidering the roles of the mineralcorticoid receptor. Mol Cell Endocrinol. 2009;301:2–6.
63. Shibata S, Mu SY, Kawarazaki H, Muraoka K, Ishizawa K, Yoshida S, Kawarazaki W, Takeuchi M, Ayuzawa N, Miyoshi J, Takai Y, Ishikawa A, Shimiosawa T, Ando K, Nagase M, Fujita T. Rac1 GTPase in rodent kidneys is essential for salt-sensitive hypertension via a mineralcorticoid receptor-dependent pathway. J Clin Invest. 2011;121:3233–43.
64. Shibata S, Nagase M, Yoshida S, Kawarazaki W, Kurihara H, Tanaka H, Miyoshi J, Takai Y, Fujita T. Modification of mineralcorticoid receptor function by Rac1 GTPase: implication in proteinuric kidney disease. Nat Med. 2008;14:1370–6.
65. Pessoa SB, van der Lubbe N, Verdonk K, Roks AJ, Hoom EJ, Danser AH. Key developments in renin-angiotensin-aldosterone system inhibition. Nat Rev Nephrol. 2013;9:26–36.
66. Converse Jr RL, Jacobsen TN, Toto RD, Jost CM, Cosentino F, Fouad-Tarazi F, Victor RG. Sympathetic overactivity in patients with chronic renal failure. N Engl J Med. 1992;327:1912–28.
67. Victor RG, Shafiq MM. Sympathetic neural mechanisms in human hypertension. Curr Hypertens Rep. 2008;10:241–7.
68. Esler M, Lambert E, Schlaich M. Chronic activation of the sympathetic nervous system is the dominant contributor to systemic hypertension. J Appl Physiol. 2010;109:1996–8.
69. Schlaich MP, Lambert E, Kaye DM, Krozowski Z, Campbell DJ, Lambert G, Hastings J, Aggarwal A, Esler MD. Sympathetic augmentation in hypertension: role of nerve firing, norepinephrine reuptake, and angiotensin neuromodulation. Hypertension. 2004;43:169–75.
70. DiBona GF. Physiology in perspective: the wisdom of the body. Neural control of the kidney. Am J Physiol. 2005;289:R633–41.
71. Johns EJ, Kopp UC, DiBona GF. Neural control of renal function. Compr Physiol. 2011;1:731–67.
72. Ye S, Ozgur B, Campese VM. Renal afferent impulses, the posterior hypothalamus, and hypertension in rats with chronic renal failure. Kidney Int. 1997;51:722–7.
73. Klein IH, Ligtenberg G, Oey PL, Koomans HA, Blankestijn PJ. Sympathetic activity is increased in polycystic kidney disease and is associated with hypertension. J Am Soc Nephrol. 2001;12:2427–33.
74. Neumann J, Ligtenberg G, Klein II, Koomans HA, Blankestijn PJ. Sympathetic hyperactivity in chronic kidney disease: pathogenesis, clinical relevance, and treatment. Kidney Int. 2004;65:1568–76.
75. Gimbrone Jr MA. Vascular endothelium: an integrator of pathophysiologic stimuli in atherosclerosis. Am J Cardiol. 1995;75:67B–70.
76. Cai H, Harrison DG. Endothelial dysfunction in cardiovascular diseases: the role of oxidant stress. Circ Res. 2000;87:840–4.
77. Modlinger PS, Wilcox CS, Aslam S. Nitric oxide, oxidative stress, and progression of chronic renal failure. Semin Nephrol. 2004;24:354–65.
78. Rodriguez-Iturbe B, Vaziri ND, Herrera-Acosta J, Johnson RJ. Oxidative stress, renal infiltration of immune cells, and salt-sensitive hypertension: all for one and one for all. Am J Physiol. 2004;286:F606–16.
79. Baylis C. Nitric oxide deficiency in chronic kidney disease. Am J Physiol. 2008;294:F1–9.
80. Wilcox CS. Asymmetric dimethylarginine and reactive oxygen species. Unwelcome twin visitors to the cardiovascular and kidney disease tables. Hypertension. 2012;59(Pt. 2):375–81.

81. Cowley Jr AW, Mori T, Mattson D, Zou A-P. Role of renal NO production in the regulation of medullary blood flow. Am J Physiol. 2003;284:R1355–69.
82. Cowley Jr AW, Abe M, Mori T, O'Connor PM, Ohsaki Y. Reactive oxygen species as important determinants of medullary flow, sodium excretion, and hypertension. Am J Physiol. 2015;308:F179–97.
83. Clavell AL, Stingo AJ, Margulies KB, Brandt RR, Burnett Jr JC. Role of endothelin receptor subtypes in the in vivo regulation of renal function. Am J Physiol. 1995;268:F455–60.
84. Rautureau Y, Schiffrin EL. Endothelin in hypertension: an update. Curr Opin Nephrol Hypertens. 2012;21:128–36.
85. Kohan DE. The renal medullary endothelin system in control of sodium and water excretion and systemic blood pressure. Curr Opin Nephrol Hypertens. 2006;15:34–40.
86. Gariepy CE, Ohuchi T, Williams SC, Richardson JA, Yanagisawa M. Salt-sensitive hypertension in endothelin-B receptor-deficient rats. J Clin Invest. 2000;105:925–33.
87. Ahn D, Ge Y, Stricklett PK, Gill P, Taylor D, Hughes AK, Yanagisawa M, Miller L, Nelson RD, Kohan DE. Collecting duct-specific knockout of endothelin-1 causes hypertension and sodium retention. J Clin Invest. 2004;114:504–11.
88. Koyama H, Tabata T, Nishzawa Y, Inoue T, Morii H, Yamaji T. Plasma endothelin levels in patients with uraemia. Lancet. 1989;1:991–2.
89. Goddard J, Johnston NR, Hand MF, Cumming AD, Rabelink TJ, Rankin AJ, Webb DJ. Endothelin-A receptor antagonism reduces blood pressure and increases renal blood flow in hypertensive patients with chronic renal failure: a comparison of selective and combined endothelin receptor blockade. Circulation. 2004;109:1186–93.
90. Lariviere R, Level M. Endothelin-1 in chronic renal failure and hypertension. Can J Physiol Pharmacol. 2003;81:607–21.
91. Aperia A. Dopamine action and metabolism in the kidney. Curr Opin Nephrol Hypertens. 1994;3:39–45.
92. O'Connell DP, Ragsdale NV, Boyd DG, Felder RA, Carey RM. Differential human renal tubular responses to dopamine type 1 receptor stimulation are determined by blood pressure status. Hypertension. 1997;29(1 Pt 1):115–22.
93. Bobulescu IA, Quinones H, Gisler SM, Di Sole F, Hu MC, Shi M, Zhang J, Fuster DG, Wright N, Mumby M, Moe OW. Acute regulation of renal Na+/H+ exchanger NHE3 by dopamine: role of protein phosphatase 2A. Am J Physiol. 2010;298:1205–13.
94. Wang X, Villar VA, Armando I, Eisner GM, Felder RA, Jose PA. Dopamine, kidney, and hypertension: studies in dopamine receptor knockout mice. Pediatr Nephrol. 2008;23:2131–46.
95. Xu J, Li G, Wang P, Velazquez H, Yao X, Li Y, Wu Y, Peixoto A, Crowley S, Desir GV. Renalase is a novel, soluble monoamine oxidase that regulates cardiac function and blood pressure. J Clin Invest. 2005;115:1275–80.
96. Pestana M, Sampaio-Maia B, Moreira-Rodrigues M, et al. Expression of relanase in ¾ nephrectomy rat model. NDT Plus. 2009;2(Suppl 2):ii55.
97. Desir GV. Role of renalase in the regulation of blood pressure and the renal dopamine system. Curr Opin Nephrol Hypertens. 2011;20:31–6.
98. Desir GV, Wang L, Peixoto AJ. Human renalase: a review of its biology, function, and implications for hypertension. J Am Soc Hypertension 2012;6:417–26.
99. Slatopolsky E, Brown A, Dusso A. Pathogenesis of secondary hyperparathyroidism. Kidney Int. 1999;73:S14–9.
100. Cunningham J, Locatelli F, Rodriguez M. Secondary hyperparathyroidism: pathogenesis, disease progression, and therapeutic options. Clin J Am Soc Nephrol. 2011;6:913–21.
101. Gennari C, Nami R, Gonnelli S. Hypertension and primary hyperparathyroidism: the role of adrenergic and renin-angiotensin-aldosterone systems. Miner Electrolyte Metab. 1995;21:77–81.
102. Melamed ML, Thadhani RI. Vitamin D therapy in chronic kidney disease and end stage renal disease. Clin J Am Soc Nephrol. 2012;7:358–65.
103. Li YC, Kong J, Wei M, Chen ZF, Liu SQ, Cao LP. 1,25-Dihydroxyvitamin D(3) is a negative endocrine regulator of the renin-angiotensin system. J Clin Invest. 2002;110:229–38.

104. Xiang W, Kong J, Chen S, Cao LP, Qiao G, Zheng W, Liu W, Li X, Gardner DG, Li YC. Cardiac hypertrophy in vitamin D receptor knockout mice: role of the systemic and cardiac renin-angiotensin systems. Am J Physiol. 2005;288:E125–32.
105. Li YC. Vitamin D, in chronic kidney disease. Contrib Nephrol. 2013;1080:98–109.
106. Rostand SG. Ultraviolet light may contribute to geographic and racial blood pressure differences. Hypertension. 1997;30(2 Pt 1):150–6.
107. Harburg E, Gleibermann L, Roeper P, Schork MA, Schull WJ. Skin color, ethnicity, and blood pressure I: Detroit blacks. Am J Public Health. 1978;68(12):1177–83.
108. Liu D, Fernandez BO, Hamilton A, Lang NN, Gallagher JM, Newby DE, Feelisch M, Weller RB. UVA irradiation of human skin vasodilates arterial vasculature and lowers blood pressure independently of nitric oxide synthase. J Invest Dermatol. 2014;134(7):1839–46.
109. Forman JP, Giovannucci E, Holmes MD, Bischoff-Ferrari HA, Tworoger SS, Willett WC, Curhan GC. Plasma 25-hydroxyvitamin D levels and risk of incident hypertension. Hypertension. 2007;49(5):1063–9.
110. Veberidge LA, Struthers AD, Khan F, Jorde R, Scragg R, Macdonald HM, Alvarez JA, Boxer RS, Dalbeni A, Gepner AD, Isbel NM, Larsen T, Nagpal J, Petchey WG, Stricker H, Strobel F, Tangpricha V, Toxqui L, Vaquero MP, Wamberg L, Zittermann A, Witham MD, D-PRESSURE Collaboration. Effect of Vitamin D supplementation on blood pressure: a systematic review and meta-analysis incorporating individual patient data. JAMA Intern Med. 2015;175:745–54.
111. Pargger H, Kaufmann MA, Drop LJ. Renal vascular hyperresponsiveness to elevated ionized calcium in spontaneously hypertensive rat kidneys. Intensive Care Med. 1998;24:61–70.
112. Churchill PC. Second messengers in renin secretion. Am J Physiol. 1985;249:F175–84.
113. Ortiz-Capisano MC, Ortiz PA, Harding P, Garvin JL, Beierwaltes WH. Decreased intracellular calcium stimulates renin release via calcium-inhibitable adenylyl cyclase. Hypertension. 2007;49:162–9.
114. Beierwaltes WH. The role of calcium in the regulation of renin secretion. Am J Physiol. 2010;298:F1–11.
115. Kurtz A. Renin release: sites, mechanisms, and control. Annu Rev Physiol. 2011;73:377–99.
116. Dickinson HO, Nicolson DJ, Cook JV, Campbell F, Beyer FR, Ford GA, Mason J. Calcium supplementation for the management of primary hypertension in adults. Cochrane Database Syst Rev. 2006;2, CD004639.
117. Bolland MJ, Barber PA, Doughty RN, Mason B, Horne A, Ames R, Gamble GD, Grey A, Reid IR. Vascular events in healthy older women receiving calcium supplementation: randomised controlled trial. Br Med J. 2008;336:262–6.
118. Mente A, O'Donnell MJ, Rangarajan S, McQueen MJ, Poirier P, Wielgosz A, Morrison H, Li W, Wang X, Di C, Mony P, Devanath A, Rosengren A, Oguz A, Zatonska K, Yusufali AH, Lopez-Jaramillo P, Avezum A, Ismail N, Lanas F, Puoane T, Diaz R, Kellshadi R, Iqbal R, Yusuf R, Chifamba J, Khatib R, Teo K, Yusuf S. PURE investigators. Association of urinary sodium and potassium excretion with blood pressure. N Engl J Med. 2014;371:601–11.
119. Frindt G, Palmer LG. Effects of dietary K on cell-surface expression of renal ion channels and transporters. Am J Physiol. 2010;299(4):F890–7.
120. Rengarajan S, Lee DH, Oh YT, Delpire E, Youn JH, McDonough AA. Increasing plasma [K+] by intravenous potassium infusion reduces NCC phosphorylation and drives kaliuresis and natriuresis. Am J Physiol. 2014;306(9):F1059–68.
121. Castaneda-Bueno M, Cervantes-Perez LG, Rojas-Vega L, Arroyo-Garza I, Vazquez N, Moreno F, Gamba G. Modulation of NCC activity by low and high K(+) intake: insights into the signaling pathways involved. Am J Physiol. 2014;306(12):F1507–19.
122. Vitzthum H, Seniuk A, Schulte LH, Muller ML, Hetz H, Ehmke H. Functional coupling of renal K+ and Na+ handling causes high blood pressure in Na+ replete mice. J Physiol. 2014;592(Pt 5):1139–57.
123. Terker AS, Zhang C, McCormick JA, Lazelle RA, Zhang C, Meermeier NP, Siler DA, Park HJ, Fu Y, Cohen DM, Weinstein AM, Wang WH, Yang CL, Ellison DH. Potassium modulates

electrolyte balance and blood pressure through effects on distal cell voltage and chloride. Cell. 2015;21(1):39–50.

124. Mazzali M, Kanbay M, Segal MS, Shflu M, Jalal D, Feig FI, Johnson RJ. Uric acid and hypertension: cause or effect? Curr Rheumatol Rep. 2010;12(2):108–17.

125. Parsa A, Brown E, Weir MR, Flink JC, Shuldiner AR, Mitchell BD, McArdle PF. Genotype-based changes in serum uric acid affect blood pressure. Kidney Int. 2012;81(5):502–7.

126. Johnson RJ, Titte S, Cade JR, Rideout BA, Oliver WJ. Uric acid, evolution and primitive cultures. Semin Nephrol. 2005;25(1):3–8.

127. Nakagawa T, Hu H, Zharikov S, Tuttle K, Short RA, Glushakova O, Ouyang X, Feig DI, Block ER, Herrera-Acosta J, Patel JM, Johnson RJ. A causal role for uric acid in fructose-induced metabolic syndrome. Am J Physiol. 2006;290(3):F625–31.

128. Pearson TA, Blair SN, Daniels SR, Eckel RH, Fair JM, Fortmann SP, Franklin BA, Godlstein LB, Greenland P, Grundy SM, Hong Y, Miller NH, Lauer RM, Ockene IS, Sacco RL, Sallis Jr JF, Smith Jr SC, Stone NJ, Taubert KA. AHA guidelines for primary prevention of cardio-vascular disease and stroke: 2002 update: consensus panel guide to comprehensive risk reduction for adult patients without coronary or other atherosclerotic vascular diseases. American Heart Association Science Advisory and Coordinating Committee. Circulation 2002;106(3):388–91.

129. Chobanian AV, Bakris GL, Black HR, Cushman WC, Green LA, Isso Jr JL, Jones DW, Materson BJ, Oparil S, Wright Jr JT, Roccella EJ, National Heart, Lung and Blood Institute Joint National Committee on Prevention, Detection, Evaluation and Treatment of High Blood Pressure, National High Blood Pressure Education Program Coordinating Committee. National Heart, Lung, and Blood Institute Joint National Committee on Prevention, Detection, Evaluation, and Treatment of High Blood Pressure; National High Blood Pressure Education Program Coordinating Committee. The Seventh Report of the Joint National Committee on Prevention, Detection, Evaluation and Treatment of High Blood Pressure: the JNC 7 report. JAMA. 2003;289(19):2560–72.

130. Flegal KM, Carroll MD, Ogden CL, Curtin LR. Prevalence and trends in obesity among US adults, 1999–2008. JAMA. 2010;303(3):235–41.

131. Hall JE, Kuo JJ, da Silva AA, de Paula RB, Liu J, Tallam L. Obesity-associated hypertension and kidney disease. Curr Opin Nephrol Hypertens. 2003;12:195–200.

132. Bagby SP. Obesity-initiated metabolic syndrome and the kidney: a recipe for chronic kidney disease. J Am Soc Nephrol. 2004;15:2775–91.

133. Wahba IM, Mak RH. Obesity and obesity-initiated metabolic syndrome: mechanistic links to chronic kidney disease. Clin J Am Soc Nephrol. 2007;2:550–62.

134. Griffin KA, Kramer H, Bidani AK. Adverse renal consequences of obesity. Am J Physiol. 2008;94:F685–96.

135. Landsberg L, Aronne LJ, Bellin LJ, Burke V, Igel LI, Lloyd-Jones D, Sowers J. Obesity-related hypertension: pathogenesis, cardiovascular risk, and treatment. J Clin Hypertens. 2013;15:14–33.

136. Wickman C, Kramer H. Obesity and kidney disease: potential mechanisms. Semin Nephrol. 2013;33:14–22.

137. Hall ME, do Carmo JM, da Silva AA, Juncos LA, Wang Z, Hall JE. Obesity, hypertension and chronic kidney disease. Int J Nephrol Renovasc Dis. 2014;7:75–88.

138. Goodfriend TL. Obesity, sleep apnea, aldosterone, and hypertension. Curr Hypertens Rep. 2008;10(3):222–6.

139. Sarzani R, Salvi F, Dessi-Fulgheri P, Rappelli A. Renin-angiotensin system, natriuretic pep-tides, obesity, metabolic syndrome, and hypertension: an integrated view in humans. J Hypertens. 2008;26(5):831–43.

140. Somers VK, Dyken ME, Clary MP, Abboud FM. Sympathetic neural mechanisms in obstruc-tive sleep apnea. J Clin Invest. 1995;96(4):1897–904.

141. Narkiewicz K, Pesek CA, Kato M, Phillips BG, Davison DE, Somers VK. Baroreflex control of sympathetic nerve activity and heart rate in obstructive sleep apnea. Hypertension. 1998;32(6):1039–43.

142. Malpas SC. Sympathetic nervous system overactivity and its role in the development of cardiovascular disease. Physiol Rev. 2010;90(2):513–67.
143. Carlson JT, Hedner J, Elam M, Ejnell H, Sellgren J, Wallin BG. Augmented resting sympathetic activity in awake patients with obstructive sleep apnea. Chest. 1993;103(6):1763–8.
144. Bao G, Metreveli N, Li R, Taylor A, Fletcher EC. Blood pressure response to chronic episodic hypoxia: role of the sympathetic nervous system. J Appl Physiol. 1997;83(1):95–101.
145. Fletcher EC, Bao G, Li R. Renin activity and blood pressure in response to chronic episodic hypoxia. Hypertension. 1999;34(2):309–14.
146. Donadio V, Liguori R, Vetrugno R, Conti M, Elam M, Wallin BG, Karlsson T, Buglardini E, Baruzzi A, Montagna P. Daytime sympathetic hyperactivity in OSAS is related to excessive daytime sleepiness. J Sleep Res. 2007;16(3):327–32.
147. Narkiewicz K, Kato M, Phillips BG, Pesek CA, Davison DE, Somers VK. Nocturnal continuous positive airway pressure decreases daytime sympathetic traffic in obstructive sleep apnea. Circulation. 1999;100(23):2332–5.
148. Alberti KG, Zimmet P, Shaw J, IDF Epidemiology Task Force Consensus Group. The metabolic syndrome—a new worldwide definition. Lancet. 2005;366(9491):1059–62.
149. Reaven GM. Relationships among insulin resistance, type 2 diabetes, essential hypertension, and cardiovascular disease: similarities and differences. J Clin Hypertens. 2011; 13:238–43.
150. Reaven GM. Insulin resistance and its consequences. In: LeRoith D, Taylor SI, Olefasky JM, editors. Diabetes mellitus: a fundamental and clinical text. 3rd ed. Philadelphia: Lippincott, Williams and Wilkins; 2004. p. 899–915.
151. Franklin SS. Hypertension in the metabolic syndrome. Vol. IV: Metabolic syndrome and related disorders. Irvine: Mary Ann Liebert, Inc.; 2005. pp. 287–98.
152. Epstein M, Sowers JR. Diabetes mellitus and hypertension. Hypertension. 1992;19(5): 403–18.
153. Anderson S, Jung FF, Ingelfinger JR. Renal renin-angiotensin system in diabetes: functional, immunohistochemical, and molecular biological correlations. Am J Physiol. 1993;34:F477–86.
154. Ye M, Wysocki J, William J, Soler MJ, Cokie I, Batlle D. Glomerular localization and expression of angiotensin-converting enzyme 2 and angiotensin-converting enzymes: implications for albuminuria in diabetes. J Am Soc Nephrol. 2006;17:3067–75.
155. Duryasula RV, Shankland SJ. Activation of a local renin-angiotensin system in podocytes by glucose. Am J Physiol. 2008;294:F830–9.
156. Lewis EJ, Hunsicker LG, Bain RP, Rohde RD. The effect of angiotensin-converting-enzyme inhibition on diabetic nephropathy. N Engl J Med. 1993;329(20):1456–62.
157. Brenner BM, Cooper ME, de Zeeuw D, Keane WF, Mitch WE, Parving HH, Remuzzi G, Snapinn SM, Zhang Z, Shahinfar S. RENAAL Study Investigators. Effects of losartan on renal and cardiovascular outcomes in patients with type 2 diabetes and nephropathy. N Engl J Med. 2001;345(12):861–9.
158. Lewis EJ, Hunsicker LG, Clarke WR, Berl T, Pohl MA, Lewis JB, Ritz E, Atkins RC, Rohde R, Raz I, Collaborative Study Group. Renoprotective effect of the angiotensin-receptor antagonist irbesartan in patients with nephropathy due to type 2 diabetes. N Engl J Med. 2001;345(12):851–60.
159. Kunz R, Friedrich C, Wobers M, Mann JFE. Meta-analysis: effect of monotherapy and combination therapy with inhibitors of the renin-angiotensin system on proteinuria in renal disease. Ann Intern Med. 2008;148:30–48.
160. Bidani AK, Griffin KA. The benefits of renin-angiotensin blockade in hypertension are dependent on blood-pressure lowering. Nat Clin Pract Nephrol. 2006;2(10):542–3.
161. Griffin KA, Bidani AK. Potential risks of calcium channel blockers in chronic kidney disease. Curr Cardiol Rep. 2008;10(6):448–55.
162. ALLHAT Officers and Coordinators for the ALLHAT Collaborative Research Group, The Antihypertensive and Lipid-Lowering Treatment to Prevent Heart Attack Trial. Major outcomes in high-risk hypertensive patients randomized to angiotensin-converting enzyme

inhibitor or calcium channel blocker vs. diuretic: the antihypertensive and lipid-lowering treatment to prevent heart attack trial (ALLHAT). JAMA. 2002;288:2981–97.

163. ONTARGET Investigators, Yusuf S, Teo KK, Pogue J, Dyal L, Copland I, Schumacher H, Dagenais G, Sleight P, Anderson C. Telmisartan, ramipril, or both in patients at high risk for vascular events. N Engl J Med. 2008;358(15):1547–59.

164. Fried LF, Emanuele N, Zhang JH, Brophy M, Conner TA, Duickworth W, Leehey DJ, McCullough PA, O'Connor t, Palevsky PM, Reilly RF, Seliger SL, Warren SR, Watnick S, Peduzzi P, Guarino P, VA NEPHRON-D Investigators. Combined angiotensin inhibition for the treatment of diabetic nephropathy. N Engl J Med. 2013;369(20):1892–903

165. Parving HH, Brenner BM, McMurray JJV, de Zeeuw D, Haffner SM, Solomon SD, Chaturvedi N, Persson F, Desai AS, Nicolaides M, Richard Z, Xiang Z, Brunel P, Pfeffer MA, ALTITUDE Investigators. Cardiorenal end points in a trial of aliskiren for type 2 diabetes. New Engl J Med. 2012;367(23):2204–13.

166. DeFronzo RA, Ferrannini E. Insulin resistance. A multifaceted syndrome responsible for NIDDM, obesity, hypertension, dyslipidemia, and atherosclerotic cardiovascular disease. Diabetes Care. 1991;14(3):173–94.

167. Wang CC, Goalstone ML, Draznin B. Molecular mechanisms of insulin resistance that impact cardiovascular biology. Diabetes. 2004;53:2735–40.

168. Hall JE, Brands MW, Mizelle HL, Gaillard CA, Hildebrandt DA. Chronic intrarenal hyperinsulinemia does not cause hypertension. Am J Physiol. 1991;260:F663–9.

169. Hall JE, Brands MW, Zappe DH, Galicia MA. Insulin resistance, hyperinsulinemia, and hypertension: cause, consequences, or merely correlation? Proc Soc Exp Biol Med. 1995;208:317–29.

170. Pontiroli AE, Alberetto M, Pozza G. Patients with insulinoma show insulin resistance in the absence of arterial hypertension. Diabetologia. 1992;35:294–5.

171. Sawicki PT, Baba T, Berger M, Starke A. Normal blood pressure in patients with insulinoma despite hyperinsulinemia and insulin resistance. J Am Soc Nephrol. 1992;3:S64–8.

172. Sawicki PT, Kaiser S, Heinemann L, et al. Prevalence of renal artery stenosis in diabetes mellitus: an autopsy study. J Intern Med. 1991;229:489–92.

173. Onrot J, Goldberg MR, Hollister AS, et al. Management of chronic orthostatic hypotension. Am J Med. 1986;80:454–64.

174. Conn JW. Primary aldosteronism, a new clinical syndrome. J Lab Clin Med. 1955;45:3–17.

175. Calhoun D. Aldosteronism and hypertension. Clin J Am Soc Nephrol. 2006;1:1039–45.

176. Ehrhart-Bornstein M, Lamounier-Zepter V, Schraven A, Langenbach J, Willenberg HS, Barthel A, Hauner H, McCann SM, Scherbaum WA, Bornstein SR. Human adipocytes secrete mineralocorticoid-releasing factors. Proc Natl Acad Sci U S A. 2003;100:14211–6.

177. Staub O, Rotin D. Role of Ubiquitylation in cellular membrane transport. Physiol Rev. 2006;86:669–707.

178. Svenningsen P, Bistrup C, Friis UG, Bertog M, Haerteis S, Krueger B, Stubbe J, Jensen ON, Thiesson HC, Uhrenholt TR, Jespersen B, Jensen BL, Korbmacher C, Skott O. Plasmin in nephrotic urine activates the epithelial sodium channel. J Am Soc Nephrol. 2009;20:299–310.

179. Svenningsen P, Uhrenholt TR, Palarasah Y, Skodt K, Jensen BL, Skott O. Prostasin-dependent activation of epithelial Na+ channels by low plasmin concentrations. Am J Physiol. 2009;297:R1733–41.

180. Goldblatt H, Lynch J, Hanzal RF, Summerville WW. Studies on experimental hypertension: I. The production of persistent elevation of systolic blood pressure by means of renal ischemia. J Exp Med. 1934;59:347–79.

181. Brunner HR, Kirschman JD, Sealey JE, Larah JH. Hypertension of renal origin: evidence for two different mechanisms. Science. 1971;174:1344–6.

182. Miller Jr ED, Samuels AI, Haber E, Barger AC. Inhibition of angiotensin conversion in experimental renovascular hypertension. Science. 1972;177:1108–9.

183. Gavras H, Brunner HR, Vaughan Jr ED, Laragh JH. Angiotensin-sodium interaction in blood pressure maintenance of renal hypertensive and normotensive rats. Science. 1973;180:1369–71.

184. Gavras H, Brunner HR, Thurston H, Laragh JH. Reciprocation of renin dependency with sodium volume dependency in renal hypertension. Science. 1975;188:1316–7.
185. Brown JJ, Davies DL, Morton JJ, Robertson JI, Cuesta V, Lever AF, Padfield PL, Trust P. Mechanism of renal hypertension. Lancet. 1976;1:1219–21.
186. Textor SC, Smith-Powell L. Post-stenotic arterial pressures, renal haemodynamics and sodium excretion during graded pressure reduction in conscious rats with one- and two-kidney coarctation hypertension. J Hypertens. 1988;6:311–9.
187. DiBona GF, Kopp UC. Neural control of renal function. Physiol Rev. 1997;77(1):75–197.
188. Garovic VD, Textor SC. Renovascular hypertension and ischemic nephropathy. Circulation. 2005;112:1362–74.
189. Textor SC, Novick A, Mujais SK, Ross R, Bravo EL, Fouad FM, Tarazi RC. Responses of the stenosed and contralateral kidneys to [Sar1, Thr8] all in human renovascular hypertension. Hypertension. 1983;5:796–804.
190. De Bruyne B, Manoharan G, Pijls NH, et al. Assessment of renal artery stenosis severity by pressure gradient measurements. J Am Coll Cardiol. 2006;48:1851–5.
191. Baumgartner I, Lerman LO. Renovascular hypertension: screening and modern management. Eur Heart J. 2011;32(13):1590–8.
192. Textor SC, Misra S, Oderich GS. Percutaneous revascularization for ischemic nephropathy. The past, present, and future. Kidney Int. 2013;83:28–40.
193. Kwon SH, Lerman LO. Atherosclerotic renal artery stenosis: current status. Adv Chronic Kidney Dis. 2015;22:224–31.
194. Textor SC, Lerman LO. Paradigm shifts in atherosclerotic renovascular disease: where are we now? J Am Soc Nephrol. 2015;26:2074–80.

Chapter 4
Syndromes of Renovascular Hypertension

Sandra M. Herrmann and Stephen C. Textor

Introduction

The central role of the kidney in the regulation of blood pressure was first established by the seminal studies of Loesch and Goldblatt in 1933 and 1934, respectively. They described the rise in arterial pressure that followed clamping of renal arteries in dogs [1, 2]. The mechanisms underlying this form of hypertension were elucidated following the pivotal discovery of the renal pressor system by Page and Braun-Menendez [3–5]. These findings led to the first surgical nephrectomy to cure hypertension in the late 1930s [6]. The concept of surgical treatment for renovascular hypertension (RVH) was appealing, since antihypertensive medications were not available until later. However, not all patients remained normotensive 1 year post surgery [7]. Therefore, there was great interest in defining this disease process, as well as those patients who would benefit from either nephrectomy or, eventually, renal revascularization. Over the last few decades, marked by the aging of the population and advances in imaging technology and therapy, there has been a paradigm shift in occlusive renovascular disease (RVD). Despite compelling evidence in recent clinical trials favoring medical therapy, experienced clinicians still recognize the need for renal artery revascularization in high-risk patients, such as those presenting with flash pulmonary edema, accelerated hypertension, and a rapid decline in renal function [8–11]. Therefore, it is important to understand the mechanisms and implications of renal artery stenosis, as well as the risks and benefits of renal artery revascularization in addition to medical therapy.

S.M. Herrmann, MD • S.C. Textor, MD (✉)
Nephrology and Hypertension Division, Mayo Clinic,
200, First Street SW, Rochester, MN, USA
e-mail: stextor@mayo.edu

© Springer Science+Business Media New York 2016
A.K. Singh, R. Agarwal (eds.), *Core Concepts in Hypertension in Kidney Disease*, DOI 10.1007/978-1-4939-6436-9_4

Epidemiology and Causes of Renovascular Disease

Renovascular disease is a major cause of secondary hypertension. It accounts for 1–5 % of hypertension cases in the general population, and reaches a prevalence of 20–40 % in highly selected referral populations [12, 13]. The vast majority of renal artery lesions (90 %) are caused by atherosclerosis, followed by variants of fibromuscular disease (FMD). Far less common causes include vasculitis, dissection, radiation, and extrinsic compression by tumors [14, 15] (see Fig. 4.1).

Atherosclerotic renovascular disease (ARVD) is typically seen in patients older than 65 years of age, often in conjunction with a number of comorbidities and progressive loss of renal function. Fibromuscular dysplasia, on the other hand, is commonly seen in women 15–50 years of age, not related to atherosclerosis and/or inflammation and involving only a few additional vascular territories, mainly the carotid arteries [16, 17]. Multiple subtypes of FMD have been described, depending upon the portion of the vessel wall that is primarily involved. Medial fibroplasia, which is characterized by its classic "string of beads" appearance, represents the most common dysplastic lesion. This is followed by perimedial fibroplasia, characterized by a homogeneous collar of elastic tissue at the junction of the media and the adventitia. This subtype may also produce a "beaded" renal artery appearance, but luminal dimensions are typically much smaller than normally seen. Intimal and adventitial hyperplasia account for less than 10 % and 1 % of the other cases of FMD, respectively [17]. The natural history of FMD tends to be more predictable than that of ARVD. Usually, FMD responds well to angioplasty and does not culminate in renal failure unless complicated by dissection or occasionally thrombosis [14]. The other miscellaneous causes of renal artery stenosis are fairly less common and include acute occlusion by an embolus or dissection of the aorta or renal artery, as illustrated in Table 4.1.

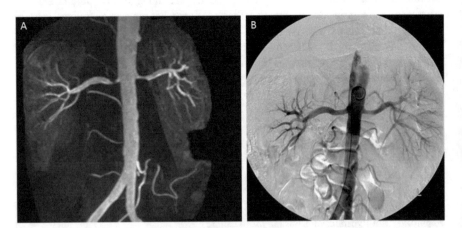

Fig. 4.1 High-grade renal artery stenosis after radiation therapy with accelerated hypertension (**a**) resolved after revascularization (**b**). The magnetic resonance angiogram (MRA) and post-stent pictures are from a patient with accelerated hypertension presenting more than 20 years after radiation for testicular cancer that resolved after revascularization

Table 4.1 Causes of renovascular disease

Unilateral renal artery disease
Unilateral atherosclerotic renal artery stenosis
Unilateral fibromuscular dysplasias
Renal artery aneurism
Arterial embolus
Arteriovenous fistula (e.g., congenital, traumatic)
Segmental arterial occlusion (e.g., posttraumatic, radiation, thrombi)
Extrinsic compression of renal artery (e.g., tumor)
Bilateral renal artery disease or solitary functional kidney
Renal artery stenosis to a solitary kidney
Bilateral renal artery stenosis
Aortic coarctation
Systemic vasculitis (e.g., polyarteritis nodosa, Takayasu's arteritis)
Vascular occlusion due to endovascular stent graft
Atheroembolic disease

Physiopathology of Renovascular Hypertension

Evidence from experimental renovascular models demonstrate that the renin–angiotensin–aldosterone system (RAAS) and sodium retention play a major role in RVH. The precise role of each depends in part on whether a contralateral, nonstenotic kidney is present. Seminal studies in animals performed by Mueller et al. [18] have shown that partial ligation of one renal artery reduces perfusion and glomerular filtration rate (GFR); this culminates in reduced excretion of salt and water. If the normal nonstenotic contralateral kidney is now removed, the stenotic kidney still promptly excretes the same amount of salt and water as both kidneys combined. Furthermore, there is little increase in GFR. Howard and colleagues [19] found similar results in patients, showing that reduced renal blood flow and consequently reduced perfusion pressure to the stenotic kidney was associated with a reduced water and sodium excretion as compared to the nonstenotic contralateral kidney. These studies underscored both the effect of the stenotic kidney in excretory function and the importance of the contralateral kidney in restoring homeostasis. As the renal perfusion pressure decreases and the fraction of salt and water absorbed in the proximal tubule increases, therefore, the kidney supplied by a narrowed artery excretes a lesser quantity of urine and sodium [20].

Unilateral Renovascular Disease

Unilateral renovascular hypertension in humans corresponds to the animal model of two-kidney one-clip (2K1C) Goldblatt hypertension, in which a normal, contralateral kidney is present (see Fig. 4.2a). The clipped kidney secretes renin, an enzyme localized in the juxtaglomerular cells of the kidney, which acts on its substrate angiotensinogen and leads to increased angiotensin I production. Angiotensin-converting enzyme located in the pulmonary capillary bed acts on angiotensin I to cleave off two amino acids to generate the eight amino-acid peptide angiotensin II. Angiotensin II acts as a potent vasoconstrictor, which leads to elevation in blood pressure [21]. Angiotensin II also acts indirectly through the central nervous system [22] and stimulates secretion of aldosterone by the adrenal cortex [23]. The rise in blood pressure stimulates pressure natriuresis by the intact contralateral kidney, which restores volume. Accordingly, the presence of the intact kidney prevents significant sodium retention. Thus, hypertension in unilateral disease is not primarily volume dependent, but is "angiotensin-dependent," and tests of both renin release and function demonstrate the effects of reduced perfusion to the stenotic kidney. Lateralization of renal vein renin secretion to the hypoperfused kidney as compared to the contralateral kidney (renin ratio levels >1.5) and asymmetric radionucleotide renography showing delayed uptake magnified in the presence of captopril have been utilized to predict the response to revascularization. This model is most closely related to the early phase (see below) of rapidly developing renovascular hypertension, such as that associated with renal artery dissection.

Based on pathophysiology and reversibility of hypertension, hypertension in the 2K1C model can be better understood by considering three phases: acute, intermediate, and chronic. Phase I, also called the acute phase, occurs between 2 and 4 weeks after clipping and is characterized by elevated plasma renin activity and angiotensin II. Phase II, the intermediate phase occurs between 5 and 9 weeks after clipping, wherein renin levels start to decline, but blood pressure remains elevated; removal of the clip or angiotensin II blockade still produces decline in blood pressure. Phase III, or chronic phase, eventually develops beyond 9 weeks after clipping of renal artery. This phase is associated with reduced renin activity and angiotensin levels, but sustained hypertension. Removal of the clip in this phase no longer lowers the blood pressure [21]. It may be surprising that removal of the instigating lesion is no longer capable of restoring normotension in the chronic phase. Mechanisms that have been proposed for maintenance of hypertension include increased oxidative stress, inflammation, and structural vascular changes [24, 25].

RVD rarely affects both kidneys to an equal degree. Hence, the kidney with more significant stenosis can lose viable function, as the contralateral unaffected kidney is capable of adaptive changes, developing hypertrophy, and undergoing a compensatory rise in single-kidney GFR, albeit to varying degrees. As a result, overall GFR may not change [26]. Unilateral ARVD is often accompanied by a progressive increase in oxidative stress and inflammation, especially in an atherosclerotic milieu. These effects are reflected by increased circulating and renal venous inflammatory biomarkers, evident not only from the stenotic kidney, but also from

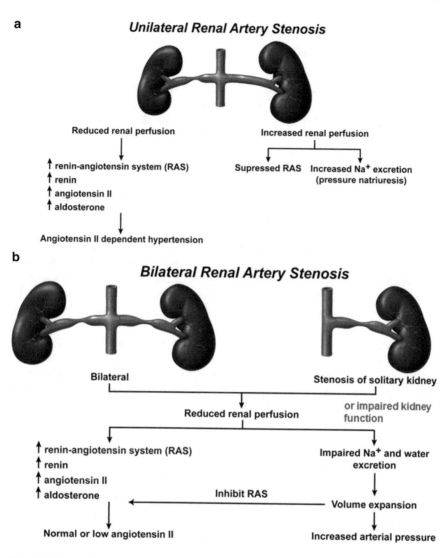

Fig. 4.2 Schematic view of two-kidney one-clip (**a**) and one-kidney one-clip (**b**) renovascular hypertension. The presence of a contralateral kidney exposed to elevated perfusion pressures in two-kidney one-clip hypertension tend to allow pressure natriuresis to ensue while ongoing stimulation of renin release from the stenotic kidney. The one-kidney model (or bilateral renal vascular disease) eventually produces sodium retention and a fall in renin level with minimal evidence of angiotensin dependence, unless sodium depletion occurs

the contralateral kidney [24, 27]. The long-term pro-inflammatory effects of elevated blood pressure and resultant renal damage—affecting both the stenotic and the contralateral kidney—likely are the result of complex interactions, including changes in renal hemodynamics, hormonal and sympathetic nervous activity in conjunction with increased oxidative stress, and inflammation leading to structural changes and fibrosis [28].

Bilateral Renovascular Disease or Stenosis to a Solitary Functioning Kidney

The one-kidney one-clip (1K1C) model corresponds to bilateral renovascular disease or stenosis to a solitary functioning kidney in humans (see Fig. 4.2b). Circumstantial evidence suggests that both renin and volume factors are involved. In this model, the contralateral kidney is removed. Decreased renal perfusion triggers initial RAAS activation and sodium retention. Without a contralateral kidney, pressure natriuresis can no longer occur, and sodium retention becomes the primary mechanism supporting hypertension. The volume expansion associated with sodium retention inhibits renin secretion such that renin activity level is normal or low in this model [29]. Following clipping of the renal artery, glomerular filtration pressure is maintained distal to the stenosis by angiotensin II-mediated vasoconstriction preferentially on the efferent glomerular arterioles, which helps to maintain GFR despite reduced perfusion [30]. Therefore, administration of antihypertensive medications such as angiotensin-converting enzyme (ACE) inhibitors and angiotensin receptor blockers (ARBs) in patients with bilateral stenosis or solitary stenotic kidney potentially causes worsening of renal function due to disruption of this mechanism.

Undoubtedly, the RAAS is a primary driver for the development of renovascular hypertension in both models. Animal models that lack angiotensin receptors (AT1 receptor knockout animals), for example, fail to develop hypertension despite renal artery clipping [31]. However, other mechanisms play a substantial role in at least some of these patients (see Fig. 4.3).

Renovascular Syndromes

Reduced renal perfusion provokes chronic stimulation of the RAAS and renal adrenergic nerves, and downstream adverse effects besides hypertension [32]. For example, angiotensin II has been implicated, in animal studies, in the development of renal damage by enhancing the effects of inflammatory chemokines and factors promoting fibrosis [33]. Combined with severely decreased perfusion and evolving hypoxia, ischemic nephropathy develops, ultimately with irreversible kidney damage [32]. Furthermore, chronic RAAS activity is implicated in the development of abnormal left ventricular remodeling, which leads to cardiac dysfunction [34]. Cardiac output is frequently elevated in patients with RVD, and demonstrates exaggerated responses to hypertension and to drugs that suppress sympathetic adrenergic function [20]. Heart failure and flash pulmonary edema are two of the clinical syndromes associated with RVD (see Table 4.2).

The clinical manifestations of RVD are protean. New onset of hypertension in a young female patient should raise suspicion for secondary causes of hypertension, including renovascular hypertension. As such, sudden development of accelerated

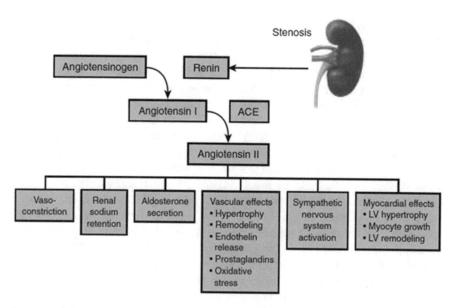

Fig. 4.3 Schematic view of activation of the renin–angiotensin system in occlusive vascular disease. Decreased renal perfusion to the kidney provokes renin release by juxtaglomerular cells in the kidney, which leads to increased circulating and local angiotensin II; a downstream effect follows, which includes arteriolar vasoconstriction, sodium retention, and elevated systemic vascular resistance. Studies implicate angiotensin II in many other pathways of vascular and cardiac smooth muscle remodeling, activation of inflammatory and fibrogenic cytokines, and induction of other vasoactive systems. *ACE* indicates angiotensin-converting enzyme, *LV* left ventricular. Adapted from: Garovic VD, Textor SC. Circulation. 2005;112:1362–1374

Table 4.2 Clinical syndromes associated with renovascular disease

Onset of hypertension before age 30 or after age 50
Accelerated, resistant, malignant hypertension
Deterioration of renal function in response to renin–angiotensin blockade   Flash pulmonary edema   Progressive renal failure   Refractory congestive heart failure

hypertension (sometimes associated with hyponatremic-hypertensive syndrome in a patient not known to be hypertensive, or with previously well-controlled hypertension) can be seen in RVD, especially in patients with acute unilateral renal artery occlusion [35, 36].

By far, the most common presentation of RVD is progressive worsening of pre-existent hypertension. This may be accompanied by a small increase in serum creatinine concentration. RVD is especially common in patients with resistant hypertension. A review of patients older than 50 years of age referred to a hypertension center were found to have secondary causes in 12.5 %, the most common of which was RVD (35 %) [37]. Another usual clinical feature of RVD is worsening kidney function after initiation of renin–angiotensin blockade therapy, which decreases systemic blood pressure and magnifies the already reduced renal perfusion provoked by the critical artery lesion. This usually is functional and reversible after discontinuation of the of renin–angiotensin blockade therapy [38]. Intolerance of these agents due to renal dysfunction can be particularly significant in bilateral or solitary kidney RVD and renal artery revascularization should be considered in order to facilitate their re-introduction [39]. Bilateral RVD should also be considered in patients with a history of "flash" or episodic pulmonary edema, especially in patients with heart failure with a preserved ejection fraction (HFpEF) [40]. In one study, congestive heart failure was present in one-third of patients with ARVD and renal dysfunction. Referral of these patients for renal artery revascularization resulted in improvement of congestive heart failure (CHF) control and reduced number of hospitalizations [41]. Progressive renal dysfunction presenting with advanced renal failure is also another clinical presentation of RVD. Hypertension is usually present in these cases. Using data from the United States Renal Data System (USRDS), Guo et al. [42] discovered the presence of ARVD in 11.2 % of patients aged 67 years or older at dialysis inception between 1996 and 2001. However, renal failure was attributed to ARVD in less than half of these patients. Anecdotal cases and observational series indicate that some patients may have some stabilization or improvement of kidney function after revascularization, although this is uncommon [43, 44]. Prospective randomized trials have failed to show compelling benefits of revascularization compared with current medical therapy. The only caveat with these studies is that a subgroup of high-risk patients, including those with episodes of flash pulmonary edema and rapidly deteriorating GFR and accelerated hypertension, were not included in prospective trials and may have experienced reduced mortality rates with effective renal revascularization [11].

Diagnostic Approach in Renovascular Hypertension

Many patients are diagnosed with hypertension and treated with first-line therapy for hypertension without screening for RVD. Indeed, such screening is not indicated unless the patient presents with clinical symptoms suggestive of RVD, as illustrated in Table 4.2. The tools for screening allow for greater diagnostic sensitivity and accuracy than ever before, due to advances in noninvasive imaging techniques. In the past, most lesions were detected with the goal of identifying lesions suitable for revascularization. Results of recent randomized clinical trials have modified this practice, favoring medical therapy as the initial mode of therapy [8–10].

It is worth emphasizing that the presence of a renovascular lesion does not translate necessarily into functional importance. Studies in humans using progressive balloon occlusion show that renin release does not occur until the pressure distal to the lesion falls at least 10–20 % below the pressure proximal to the lesion [45]. Some degree of renal artery stenosis is incidentally identified in patients who are undergoing vascular imaging for different reasons [46, 47]. The great majority of these stenotic lesions is minor, and does not produce a degree of obstruction hemo-dynamically significant enough to cause RVH. Actually, many patients have moder-ate ARVD that remains clinically silent for several years. However, occlusive vascular disease progresses in a subset of patients with ARVD, which can cause progressive tissue injury and accelerating hypertension, in which case a benefit from revascularization can be noted. Identification of patients who would benefit from further evaluation, however, remains challenging. Selecting patients for fur-ther studies depends on the commitment to act upon the results of those tests. Clinicians need to ascertain when medical therapy alone is insufficient and further tests are to be pursued with the intention of restoring renal blood flow to a kidney that remains viable [48]. Several clinical features should be considered in this con-text, particularly for the subset of patients with high-risk presentations [11, 49].

Imaging procedures are important for diagnosis, the choice of diagnostic imag-ing technique for RVD depends on patient characteristics, local availability, and expertise and is discussed further below.

Imaging

Duplex Doppler Ultrasonography

Ultrasonography is widely accepted as the first-line diagnostic imaging test because of its availability and cost. Duplex Doppler renal ultrasonography combines grey-scale imaging from traditional ultrasound with a Doppler technique to assess renal blood flow velocities, evaluating renal morphology and the presence of significant stenosis. With experienced operators, it is an excellent initial imaging study, with up to 95% sensitivity and 90% specificity in dedicated laboratories, providing both structural and functional assessment of the kidneys [50, 51]. In a patient with normal cardiac function, peak systolic velocities (PSV) in the main renal artery range between 60 and 100 cm/s. In a region of focal vascular disease, the reduced cross-sectional area of the stenotic segment causes increased blood velocity to maintain flow. Although relationships between PSV and the degree of vessel occlusion are approxi-mate, PSV levels above 180–200 cm/s translate into more than 60% lumen occlusion and are considered "hemodynamically significant." [52] (See Fig. 4.4a.) The Cardiovascular Outcomes in Renal Atherosclerotic Lesions (CORAL) trial required PSV values above 300 cm/s for entry by ultrasound criteria [10]. A more accurate method may be to calculate the ratio of the renal artery to aorta velocities (RA:aorta). A threshold of >3.5:1 ratio suggests relatively high-grade RVD. However, overlying bowel gas and complex anatomy may make assessment of the entire renal arterial tree technically difficult. Alternatively, evaluating the renal segmental arteriolar bed distal to the stenotic lesion, where the peak velocity is decreased, allows identification of the loss of the normal sharp upstroke of velocity in systole causing parvus tardus waveform indicative of upstream vascular obstruction [53] (see Fig. 4.4b).

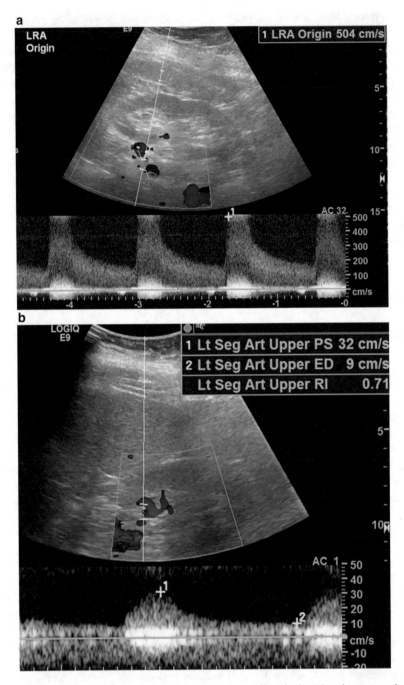

Fig. 4.4 Duplex ultrasound showing renal artery peak systolic velocity (**a**) and parvus tardus in left segmental artery (**b**): **a** shows elevated peak systolic velocity of more than 500 cm/s of the left renal artery (LRA). PSV levels above 180–200 cm/s translate into more than 60 % lumen occlusion and are considered "hemodynamically significant." **b** demonstrates parvus tardus (*arrow*), note the slope of the systolic upstroke and absence of early systolic peak associated with diminished amplitude of the waveform

Another parameter obtained with Doppler ultrasound is the evaluation of resistive index (RI). The RI is defined as height of the PSV minus height of the end-diastolic velocity (EDV) divided by the PSV [RI = (PSV − EDV)/PSV] and reflects the status of the flow characteristics in the renal microcirculation beyond the main renal arteries. RI < 0.8, in conjunction with clinical findings, has been promoted as a useful parameter to predict benefit after revascularization [54, 55]. However, similar outcomes have been reported independent of renal parenchymal values for RI greater than or less than 0.8 [56]. In our experience, lower RI likely is associated with better preserved renal flow characteristics and likely better kidney functional outcomes, but this alone is rarely decisive as to whether or not to proceed with renal artery revascularization. Situations that one may consider revascularization despite RI > 0.8 include patients with RVD without atrophic kidney presenting with recurrent flash pulmonary edema, rapidly declining kidney function, and/or refractory hypertension.

Computed Tomography and Magnetic Resonance Angiography

Although catheter angiography remains the gold standard for imaging of the renal vascular system, it is costly, invasive, and adds the risks that come with intra-arterial instrumentation. It is commonly reserved for endovascular procedures, such as balloon angioplasty and stenting. Advances in computed tomography angiography (CTA) and magnetic resonance angiography (MRA) have allowed for more precise evaluation of RVD and may be undertaken to define vascular anatomy, functional characteristics, and abnormalities within the kidneys.

CTA is noninvasive and provides excellent spatial and temporal resolution for imaging of the renal arteries and surrounding tissues, making it sensitive for diagnosis of other secondary causes of hypertension, such as adrenal disease and other atherosclerotic disease [57]. Recent studies indicate that the risk of contrast-induced changes in renal function from intravenous dosing is extremely low using standard volume expansion, possibly no different from a non-contrast CT, even among those with impaired kidney function [58–60]. Although gadolinium contrast-enhanced MRA provides excellent functional and structural vascular imagingmagnetic resonance angiography (MRA) of the kidney, the use of gadolinium for patients with any reduction in estimated glomerular filtration rate (eGFR) has virtually disappeared out of concern for the potential toxicity related to nephrogenic systemic fibrosis (an eGFR of 40 mL/min/m² was defined by the American College of Radiology on MR safety as the cutoff below which no gadolinium should be given). CTA and MRA are of comparable accuracy, reaching sensitivity and specificity >90 % in a number of single-center studies compared with catheter angiography [61, 62].

Intra-Arterial Angiography

Intra-arterial angiography is considered the gold standard for the diagnosis of renal artery stenosis, but it is invasive and likely not indicated as the primary and initial diagnostic methodology. It should be reserved to confirm the occlusive vascular lesion and to perform renal artery revascularization. Besides the concern of interobserver variability in estimating stenosis severity, angiography per se does not provide reliable functional or hemodynamic information. However, measuring the pressure gradient during angiography overcomes these limitations and allows for functional evaluation of the hemodynamic significance prior to revascularization [63]. Gradients above 22 mmHg are usually in agreement of estimating stenosis of 50 %, and there is a curvilinear relationship between the systolic resting gradient and systolic blood pressure [64]. The level of translesional pressure gradient helps to determine the hemodynamic significance of an apparent occlusive lesion. Due to the invasive nature of intra-arterial angiography and its associated possible risks, such as vascular injury and bleeding, it should not be used as a screening method [65].

Radionucleotide Renography

After the injection of radioisotopes, the kidney can be visualized and the contribution of each kidney to the glomerular filtration can be estimated. The two most common radiolabelled pharmaceutical agents used are Tc99m-MAG3 (mercaptoacetyltriglycine) and Tc99m-DTPA (diethylenetriamine pentaacetic acid), with the former being more reliable in renal insufficiency (MAG3 is secreted effectively by the proximal tubule, whereas DTPA is excreted by glomerular filtration). Any prescribed ACE inhibitor or ARB therapy must be discontinued 2–5 days previously. The criteria for RVD include (a) a decrease in the percentage of uptake of the isotope by the affected kidney to <40 % of the total; (b) delayed time to peak uptake of the isotope to >10–11 min, well above the normal value of 6 min; and (c) delayed excretion of the isotope with retention at 25 min or >20 % [48]. The addition of captopril and comparison with a baseline (non-captopril) renogram allows estimation of the functional role of angiotensin in maintaining glomerular filtration and exaggerates hemodynamic differences between a kidney with stenosis and one without [66]. This test provides no information about the cause of the stenosis, nor does it reliably distinguish unilateral from bilateral RVD, since asymmetry can be presented if one side is more affected than the other [67, 68]. The sensitivity of renal renography ranges from 58 to 95 % and its specificity ranges from 17 to 100 %, even when studies were performed in selected patients who had an intervention based on positive results on angiography [62]. Moreover, renogram sensitivity decreases with the decline of renal function, especially when creatinine reaches levels >2 mg/dL or CKD stage 4 or 5 [69]. The role of renography in the current era is best used to determine split renal function prior to proceeding with therapeutic nephrectomy for RVD, however, captopril renogram is not recommended by current American College of Cardiology-American Heart Association guidelines for the management of patients suspected of having RVD [49].

Selection of Therapy

Medical Therapy for Renovascular Disease

Our understanding of therapy for ARVD has changed substantially over the last 15–20 years, and its management for specific patients is more controversial than ever before. In the past, the lack of effective antihypertensive drug therapy led to more widespread efforts to identify and reverse RVH by means of either surgical or endovascular renal revascularization. Several prospective, randomized controlled trials in the last decade, however, indicate that many patients with ARVD can achieve satisfactory blood pressure control for years with current medical therapy alone [8–10]. Management of systemic atherosclerotic disease should be achieved with widespread administration of statins, aspirin, and smoking cessation. The development of specific clinical features over time, including progressive vascular occlusion, worsening of kidney function while taking ACE/ARB therapy, accelerated hypertension, and recurrent pulmonary edema, warrant consideration for revascularization and suggest that the atherosclerotic process has advanced [11, 70].

It is important to reiterate that ARVD is part of the continuum of atherosclerotic cardiovascular disease (ASCVD). Patients with significant ARVD, as outlined in the CORAL trial, are far more likely to die from cardiovascular causes than to develop renal failure. The main goal of therapy is the prevention of events such as stroke and acute myocardial infarction, which can have a direct impact on survival [10]. Glucose control is also important. Hypertensive patients with ARVD of any extent, compared with hypertensive patients without ARVD, carry a substantially increased risk for future cardiovascular events, which indicates that systemic hypertension is both a manifestation of ARVD and a risk factor for the progression and downstream consequences of ARVD. Therefore, even in patients with low-grade ARVD, aggressive pharmacological treatment strategies should be adopted as a preventive measure [71].

With the current availability of broad-spectrum antihypertensives, the ability to control blood pressure in patients with ARVD has been greatly improved. Failure to achieve goal blood pressure in early trials was associated with treatment crossover rates to the interventional arm up to 40%, whereas the crossovers in recent trials (ASTRAL and CORAL) were below 10% [72, 73]. Angiotensin-converting enzyme inhibitors and angiotensin II receptor blockers are considered as first-line drugs. If goal blood pressure is not reached, one may add a thiazide diuretic, calcium channel blocker, β[beta] blocker, or aldosterone antagonist [49, 72]. The use of a protocol-driven approach produced excellent overall blood pressure control in the CORAL trial [10]. A caveat to recognize is the possible decline in renal function with ACE/ARB therapy, especially with bilateral ARVD or solitary kidney.

On the other hand, reduction in renal perfusion pressure distal to the stenosis, especially if encountered on a chronic basis, can lead to cortical hypoxia, microvascular rarefaction, and development of interstitial inflammation, tubular atrophy, and irreversible fibrosis [74–76]. Decline in GFR by 20 % or doubling of serum creatinine, also known as a "renal event" in clinic trials, can be noted in 1 in 5 patients over 2–4 years [8, 9]. Progression is more likely in patients with bilateral renal artery stenosis or stenosis of a solitary functioning kidney [77]. Also, the rate of progression of ARVD is much greater in these patients (60 %) than the usual rate of 35 % at 3 years, and more than 50 % at 5 years [78, 79] (see Fig. 4.5).

The rate of occlusion is 2 % at 1 year, 5 % at 2 years, and may be as high as 15 % at 5 years [80]. Thus, without physical intervention, patients with ARVD are at risk of progression of stenosis to the point of complete occlusion, ischemic nephropathy to the point of end-stage renal disease, and acute kidney failure with antihypertensive therapy, especially with renin–angiotensin inhibition. The only question remaining to the clinicians is: Which patients should be referred for revascularization and at which time?

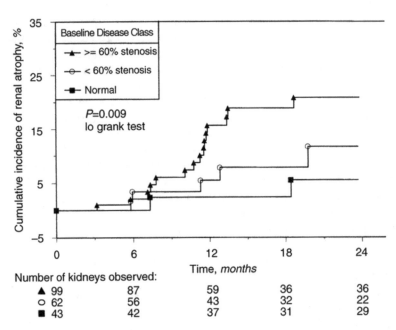

Fig. 4.5 Cumulative incidence of renal atrophy in atherosclerotic renovascular disease, as measured by renal artery Doppler ultrasonography. Standard error is 10 % through 24 months for all plots. (*Filled triangle*) indicates ≥60 % stenosis; (*open circle*), <60 % stenosis; (*filled square*), no stenosis. $P=0.009$, log rank test. Reprinted with permission from Caps MT, Zierler E, Polissar NL, et al. Risk of atrophy in kidneys with atherosclerotic renal artery stenosis. Kidney Int. 1998;53(3):735–42

Revascularization Therapies for Renovascular Disease

Various surgical interventions to control RVH have been pursued in the past, but largely were replaced by the introduction of catheter-based intervention, also known as percutaneous transluminal renal angioplasty (PTRA), by Andreas Gruentzig in 1978 [81]. Although not widely accepted initially, PTRA with stenting has now become the main mode of revascularization for patients with ARVD. Stenting yields higher procedural success and long-term patency rates, especially for ostial lesions, and is more effective in terms of improving blood pressure and stabilizing or improving renal function over time [65, 82–87]. In general, the maximum antihypertensive response is observed within 2 days, and the final durable outcome within 2–4 weeks. The blood pressure-reducing effects in more recent trials ranged between 8 and 16 mmHg, but not necessarily reduction of the number of antihypertensive medications [8, 9].

The ideal candidate for PTRA is the patient who has ARVD with either drug intolerance or has refractory hypertension, recurrent flash pulmonary edema, refractory heart failure, or rapid decline of renal function [11].

Similarly, patients with renal artery FMD undergoing PTRA have beneficial long-term effects, however the longer the duration of the hypertension or higher the patients' age the less the benefit of PTRA and more adverse the prognosis of renovascular hypertension in this population [88].

The main risks of the procedure include bleeding at the access site, retroperitoneal hematoma, and renal artery dissection. Other, more serious complications of the procedure include renal artery perforation, requiring surgery, and renal artery thrombosis contributing to acute kidney injury, otherwise seen with atheroembolization or as a contrast reaction. Depending on the extent of structural damage, acute kidney injury in this setting can be reversible or irreversible.

With the introduction of drug-eluting stents, acute restenosis rates have declined from 9–76 % to 0–4 %, and late restenosis from 25–45 % to 3–39 % compared to angioplasty alone [86]. In-stent restenosis, nevertheless, should be suspected clinically with a rise in blood pressure and the need for intensive antihypertensive therapy. These patients should undergo duplex ultrasonography, and decisions on repeat intervention should follow the general considerations, also taking into account that restenosis rates may be higher with bare-metal stents [89, 90].

Retreatment with angioplasty with or without repeat stenting (preferably drug-eluting stents) can be attempted, but the restenosis rate after repeat intervention is higher.

In the current era, surgical renal revascularization surgery is preferred only for selected patients with complex anatomic lesions [91, 92], including multiple small renal arteries, early primary branching of the main renal artery, requirement for aortic reconstruction near the renal arteries for other indications (such as aneurysm repair or severe aortoiliac occlusive disease), or to avoid manipulation of a highly diseased aorta or failed endovascular stents, including repeated in-stent restenosis [49, 93]. For unilateral ARVD nephrectomy can be performed in cases with nearly complete renal artery occlusion and a small atrophic kidney, or otherwise single bypass grafting (either aorto-renal or, in case of a diseased aorta, hepato-renal or spleno-renal bypass) or unilateral repair with contralateral nephrectomy of a non-functioning, atrophic kidney [94]. Surgical intervention leads to improvement in hypertension in up to 95 % of patients [95]. It can even grant a "cure" in those without concomitant essential (primary) hypertension or intrarenal vascular disease (nephrosclerosis) of the contralateral kidney due to chronic (usually >5 years) exposure to hypertension [96]. Compared with PTRA, surgery used to have a higher primary success rate (approaching 100 %) and a fivefold lower restenosis rate (4 %) at 2 years. However, with improvement in techniques and the possibilities of repeat intervention, the outcomes have become quite similar.

In distinction from PTRA, surgery has a tangible mortality risk that varies from less than 2.5–10 % depending on age, comorbidities (especially the severity of the extrarenal ASCVD), and surgical extent and experience [16, 73, 94, 95, 97, 98]. Independent risk factors for in-hospital mortality are age, history of chronic kidney disease, heart failure, or chronic lung disease, each increasing the risk twofold. As such, the ideal candidate is the younger individual (<65 years) without symptomatic coronary or cerebrovascular disease and who requires renal artery surgery only.

In more recent randomized controlled trials, it has been shown that patients with ARVD will escape early detection as a result of diminished enthusiasm for vascular intervention. This will certainly be appropriated for most of the patients with patients with ARVD, as suggested by CORAL and the other cohorts [8–10]. However, progressive occlusive vascular disease associated with clinical manifestations, including progression of chronic renal disease and recurrent pulmonary edema out of proportion to the degree of cardiac disease, will continue to develop. The role of nephrologists is to recognize this subgroup of patients at risk of developing ischemic nephropathy and other high-risk manifestations of ARVD at a time when they still may benefit from revascularization with or without adjunctive maneuvers.

Summary

Renal vascular disease is a common cause of hypertension, particularly ARVD, in the elderly population. It can manifest from asymptomatic disease, be found incidentally by imaging studies, or be identified clinically by presenting with renovascular syndromes such as accelerated hypertension, flash pulmonary edema, and/or progressive renal dysfunction. It is of paramount importance that the clinician evaluate the significance of the RVD in the individual bases and weight the risk and benefits of renal artery revascularization versus medical therapy alone. Management of ASCVD and hypertension is the main goal of medical therapy. However, patients with a high risk of progression, such as patients with significant renal artery stenosis with bilateral disease or solitary kidney are likely to benefit from revascularization of the kidney by decreasing the risk of developing circulatory congestion and/or

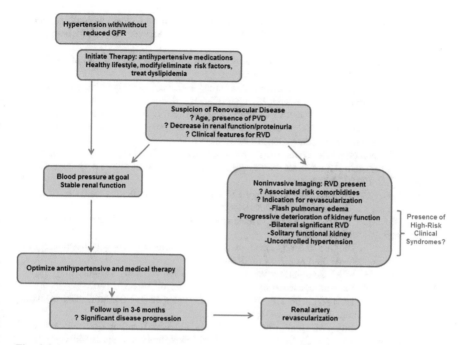

Fig. 4.6 Management of renovascular hypertension and ischemic nephropathy. Algorithm summarizing the management scheme for patients with renovascular hypertension and/or ischemic nephropathy. *GFR* indicates glomerular filtration rate, *PVD* peripheral vascular disease, *RVD* renovascular disease

progression of renal dysfunction. Follow-up is necessary, even after revascularization, due to potential restenosis or disease recurrence. An algorithm for the management of ARVD is provided for guidance (see Fig. 4.6).

References

1. Loesch J. Ein Beitrag zur experimentellen Nephritis und zum arteriellen Hochdruck I. Die Veränderungen im Blutdruck. II. Die Veränderungen in der Blutchemie. Zentralblatt für Innere Medizin. 1933;7:144–69.
2. Goldblatt H, Lynch J, Hanzal RF, Summerville WW. Studies on experimental hypertension: I. The production of persistent elevation of systolic blood pressure by means of renal ischemia. J Exp Med. 1934;59:347–79.
3. Braun-Menéndez E, Fasciolo JC, Leloir LF, Muñoz JM. La sustancia hipertensora de la sangre del riñón isquemiado. Rev Soc Argent Biol. 1939;15:420–5.
4. Page IH, Helmer OM. A crystalline pressor substance (angiotonin) resulting from the reaction between renin and renin-activator. J Exp Med. 1940;71:29–42.
5. Braun-Menendez E, Page IH. Suggested revision of nomenclature--angiotensin. Science. 1958;127:242.
6. Butler AM. Chronic pyelonephritis and arterial hypertension. J Clin Invest. 1937;16:889–97.
7. Smith HW. Unilateral nephrectomy in hypertensive disease. J Urol. 1956;76:685–701.

8. Bax L, Woittiez AJ, Kouwenberg HJ, et al. Stent placement in patients with atherosclerotic renal artery stenosis and impaired renal function: a randomized trial. Ann Intern Med. 2009;150:840–8. W150-1.
9. Wheatley K, Ives N, Gray R, et al. Revascularization versus medical therapy for renal-artery stenosis. N Engl J Med. 2009;361:1953–62.
10. Cooper CJ, Murphy TP, Cutlip DE, et al. Stenting and medical therapy for atherosclerotic renal-artery stenosis. N Engl J Med. 2014;370:13–22.
11. Ritchie J, Green D, Chrysochou C, Chalmers N, Foley RN, Kalra PA. High-risk clinical presentations in atherosclerotic renovascular disease: prognosis and response to renal artery revascularization. Am J Kidney Dis. 2014;63:186–97.
12. Olin JW, Piedmonte MR, Young JR, DeAnna S, Grubb M, Childs MB. The utility of duplex ultrasound scanning of the renal arteries for diagnosing significant renal artery stenosis. Ann Intern Med. 1995;122:833–8.
13. Chrysochou C, Kalra PA. Epidemiology and natural history of atherosclerotic renovascular disease. Prog Cardiovasc Dis. 2009;52:184–95.
14. Dubel GJ, Murphy TP. The role of percutaneous revascularization for renal artery stenosis. Vasc Med. 2008;13:141–56.
15. Lao D, Parasher PS, Cho KC, Yeghiazarians Y. Atherosclerotic renal artery stenosis--diagnosis and treatment. Mayo Clin Proc. 2011;86:649–57.
16. Safian RD, Textor SC. Renal-artery stenosis. N Engl J Med. 2001;344:431–42.
17. Slovut DP, Olin JW. Fibromuscular dysplasia. N Engl J Med. 2004;350:1862–71.
18. Mueller CB, Surtshin A, Carlin MR, White HL. Glomerular and tubular influences on sodium and water excretion. Am J Phys. 1951;165:411–22.
19. Howard JE, Berthrong M, Gould DM, Yendt ER. Hypertension resulting from unilateral renal vascular disease and its relief by nephrectomy. Bull Johns Hopkins Hosp. 1954;94:51–85.
20. Dustan HP. Physiologic consequences of renal arterial stenosis. N Engl J Med. 1969;281:1348–54.
21. Treadway KK, Slater EE. Renovascular hypertension. Annu Rev Med. 1984;35:665–92.
22. Reid IA. Interactions between ANG II, sympathetic nervous system, and baroreceptor reflexes in regulation of blood pressure. Am J Phys. 1992;262:E763–78.
23. Black HR, Glickman MG, Schiff Jr M, Pingoud EG. Renovascular hypertension: pathophysiology, diagnosis, and treatment. Yale J Biol Med. 1978;51:635–54.
24. Lerman LO, Nath KA, Rodriguez-Porcel M, et al. Increased oxidative stress in experimental renovascular hypertension. Hypertension. 2001;37:541–6.
25. Lupu AN, Maxwell MH, Kaufman JJ, White FN. Experimental unilateral renal artery constriction in the dog. Circ Res. 1972;30:567–74.
26. Textor SC. Atherosclerotic renal artery stenosis: flaws in estimated glomerular filtration rate and the problem of progressive kidney injury. Circ Cardiovasc Interv. 2011;4:213–5.
27. Eirin A, Gloviczki ML, Tang H, et al. Chronic renovascular hypertension is associated with elevated levels of neutrophil gelatinase-associated lipocalin. Nephrol Dial Transplant. 2012;27:4153–61.
28. Juncos LA, Chandrashekar KB, Lopez-Ruiz AF, Juncos LI, editors. Interaction between stenotic and contralateral kidneys: unique features of each in unilateral disease. 1st ed. London: Springer; 2014.
29. Gavras H, Brunner HR, Thurston H, Laragh JH. Reciprocation of renin dependency with sodium volume dependency in renal hypertension. Science. 1975;188:1316–7.
30. Pickering TG. Renovascular hypertension: etiology and pathophysiology. Semin Nucl Med. 1989;19:79–88.
31. Cervenka L, Horacek V, Vaneckova I, et al. Essential role of AT1A receptor in the development of 2K1C hypertension. Hypertension. 2002;40:735–41.
32. Textor SC, Lerman LO. Paradigm shifts in atherosclerotic renovascular disease: where are we now? J Am Soc Nephrol. 2015;26:2074–80.
33. Chade AR, Rodriguez-Porcel M, Grande JP, et al. Mechanisms of renal structural alterations in combined hypercholesterolemia and renal artery stenosis. Arterioscler Thromb Vasc Biol. 2003;23:1295–301.

34. Wright JR, Shurrab AE, Cooper A, Kalra PR, Foley RN, Kalra PA. Left ventricular morphology and function in patients with atherosclerotic renovascular disease. J Am Soc Nephrol. 2005;16:2746–53.
35. Agarwal M, Lynn KL, Richards AM, Nicholls MG. Hyponatremic-hypertensive syndrome with renal ischemia: an underrecognized disorder. Hypertension. 1999;33:1020–4.
36. Atkinson AB, Davies DL, Leckie B, et al. Hyponatraemic hypertensive syndrome with renal-artery occlusion corrected by captopril. Lancet. 1979;2:606–9.
37. Calhoun DA, Jones D, Textor S, et al. Resistant hypertension: diagnosis, evaluation, and treatment: a scientific statement from the American Heart Association Professional Education Committee of the Council for High Blood Pressure Research. Circulation. 2008;117:e510–26.
38. Hackam DG, Spence JD, Garg AX, Textor SC. Role of renin-angiotensin system blockade in atherosclerotic renal artery stenosis and renovascular hypertension. Hypertension. 2007;50:998–1003.
39. Chrysochou C, Foley RN, Young JF, Khavandi K, Cheung CM, Kalra PA. Dispelling the myth: the use of renin-angiotensin blockade in atheromatous renovascular disease. Nephrol Dial Transplant. 2012;27:1403–9.
40. Messerli FH, Bangalore S, Makani H, et al. Flash pulmonary oedema and bilateral renal artery stenosis: the Pickering syndrome. Eur Heart J. 2011;32:2231–5.
41. Kane GC, Xu N, Mistrik E, Roubicek T, Stanson AW, Garovic VD. Renal artery revascularization improves heart failure control in patients with atherosclerotic renal artery stenosis. Nephrol Dial Transplant. 2010;25:813–20.
42. Guo H, Kalra PA, Gilbertson DT, et al. Atherosclerotic renovascular disease in older US patients starting dialysis, 1996 to 2001. Circulation. 2007;115:50–8.
43. Textor SC. Attending rounds: a patient with accelerated hypertension and an atrophic kidney. Clin J Am Soc Nephrol. 2014;9:1117–23.
44. Dorros G, Jaff M, Mathiak L, He T. Multicenter Palmaz stent renal artery stenosis revascularization registry report: four-year follow-up of 1,058 successful patients. Catheter Cardiovasc Interv. 2002;55:182–8.
45. De Bruyne B, Manoharan G, Pijls NH, et al. Assessment of renal artery stenosis severity by pressure gradient measurements. J Am Coll Cardiol. 2006;48:1851–5.
46. Rihal CS, Textor SC, Breen JF, et al. Incidental renal artery stenosis among a prospective cohort of hypertensive patients undergoing coronary angiography. Mayo Clin Proc. 2002;77:309–16.
47. Olin JW, Melia M, Young JR, Graor RA, Risius B. Prevalence of atherosclerotic renal artery stenosis in patients with atherosclerosis elsewhere. Am J Med. 1990;88:46N–51.
48. Herrmann SM, Textor SC. Diagnostic criteria for renovascular disease: where are we now? Nephrol Dial Transplant. 2012;27:2657–63.
49. Hirsch AT, Haskal ZJ, Hertzer NR, et al. ACC/AHA 2005 Practice Guidelines for the management of patients with peripheral arterial disease (lower extremity, renal, mesenteric, and abdominal aortic): a collaborative report from the American Association for Vascular Surgery/ Society for Vascular Surgery, Society for Cardiovascular Angiography and Interventions, Society for Vascular Medicine and Biology, Society of Interventional Radiology, and the ACC/ AHA Task Force on Practice Guidelines (Writing Committee to Develop Guidelines for the Management of Patients With Peripheral Arterial Disease): endorsed by the American Association of Cardiovascular and Pulmonary Rehabilitation; National Heart, Lung, and Blood Institute; Society for Vascular Nursing; TransAtlantic Inter-Society Consensus; and Vascular Disease Foundation. Circulation 2006;113:e463–654.
50. Rabbia C, Valpreda S. Duplex scan sonography of renal artery stenosis. Int Angiol. 2003;22:101–15.
51. Spyridopoulos TN, Kaziani K, Balanika AP, et al. Ultrasound as a first line screening tool for the detection of renal artery stenosis: a comprehensive review. Med Ultrason. 2010;12:228–32.
52. Weinberg I, Jaff MR. Renal artery duplex ultrasonography. In: Lerman LO, Textor SC, editors. Renal vascular disease. London: Springer; 2014. p. 211–29.

53. Sarkodieh JE, Walden SH, Low D. Imaging and management of atherosclerotic renal artery stenosis. Clin Radiol. 2013;68:627–35.
54. Radermacher J, Chavan A, Bleck J, et al. Use of Doppler ultrasonography to predict the outcome of therapy for renal-artery stenosis. N Engl J Med. 2001;344:410–7.
55. Santos S, Leite LR, Tse TS, Beck R, Lee RA, Shepherd RF. Renal resistance index predicting outcome of renal revascularization for renovascular hypertension. Arq Bras Cardiol. 2010;94:452–6.
56. Garcia-Criado A, Gilabert R, Nicolau C, et al. Value of Doppler sonography for predicting clinical outcome after renal artery revascularization in atherosclerotic renal artery stenosis. J Ultrasound Med. 2005;24:1641–7.
57. Liu PS, Platt JF. CT angiography of the renal circulation. Radiol Clin N Am. 2010;48:347–65. viii-ix.
58. Lufft V, Hoogestraat-Lufft L, Fels LM, et al. Contrast media nephropathy: intravenous CT angiography versus intraarterial digital subtraction angiography in renal artery stenosis: a prospective randomized trial. Am J Kidney Dis. 2002;40:236–42.
59. McDonald RJ, McDonald JS, Carter RE, et al. Intravenous contrast material exposure is not an independent risk factor for dialysis or mortality. Radiology. 2014;273:714–25.
60. McDonald JS, McDonald RJ, Comin J, et al. Frequency of acute kidney injury following intravenous contrast medium administration: a systematic review and meta-analysis. Radiology. 2013;267:119–28.
61. Rountas C, Vlychou M, Vassiou K, et al. Imaging modalities for renal artery stenosis in suspected renovascular hypertension: prospective intraindividual comparison of color Doppler US, CT angiography, GD-enhanced MR angiography, and digital substraction angiography. Ren Fail. 2007;29:295–302.
62. Vasbinder GB, Nelemans PJ, Kessels AG, Kroon AA, de Leeuw PW, van Engelshoven JM. Diagnostic tests for renal artery stenosis in patients suspected of having renovascular hypertension: a meta-analysis. Ann Intern Med. 2001;135:401–11.
63. Mangiacapra F, Trana C, Sarno G, et al. Translesional pressure gradients to predict blood pressure response after renal artery stenting in patients with renovascular hypertension. Circ Cardiovasc Interv. 2010;3:537–42.
64. Gross CM, Kramer J, Weingartner O, et al. Determination of renal arterial stenosis severity: comparison of pressure gradient and vessel diameter. Radiology. 2001;220:751–6.
65. Zeller T, Frank U, Muller C, et al. Predictors of improved renal function after percutaneous stent-supported angioplasty of severe atherosclerotic ostial renal artery stenosis. Circulation. 2003;108:2244–9.
66. Kumar R, Padhy AK, Machineni S, Pandey AK, Malhotra A. Individual kidney glomerular filtration rate in the interpretation of non-diagnostic curves on captopril renography. Nucl Med Commun. 2000;21:637–43.
67. Mann SJ, Pickering TG, Sos TA, et al. Captopril renography in the diagnosis of renal artery stenosis: accuracy and limitations. Am J Med. 1991;90:30–40.
68. Roccatello D, Picciotto G, Rabbia C, Pozzato M, De Filippi PG, Piccoli G. Prospective study on captopril renography in hypertensive patients. Am J Nephrol. 1992;12:406–11.
69. Prigent A, Chaumet-Riffaud P. Clinical problems in renovascular disease and the role of nuclear medicine. Semin Nucl Med. 2014;44:110–22.
70. de Leeuw PW, Postma CT, Kroon AA. Treatment of atherosclerotic renal artery stenosis: time for a new approach. JAMA. 2013;309:663–4.
71. Dechering DG, Kruis HM, Adiyaman A, Thien T, Postma CT. Clinical significance of low-grade renal artery stenosis. J Intern Med. 2010;267:305–15.
72. Tullis MJ, Caps MT, Zierler RE, et al. Blood pressure, antihypertensive medication, and atherosclerotic renal artery stenosis. Am J Kidney Dis. 1999;33:675–81.
73. Dworkin LD, Cooper CJ. Clinical practice. Renal-artery stenosis. N Engl J Med. 2009;361:1972–8.
74. Veniant M, Heudes D, Clozel JP, Bruneval P, Menard J. Calcium blockade versus ACE inhibition in clipped and unclipped kidneys of 2K-1C rats. Kidney Int. 1994;46:421–9.

75. Keddis MT, Garovic VD, Bailey KR, Wood CM, Raissian Y, Grande JP. Ischaemic nephropathy secondary to atherosclerotic renal artery stenosis: clinical and histopathological correlates. Nephrol Dial Transplant. 2010;25:3615–22.
76. Gloviczki ML, Glockner JF, Crane JA, et al. Blood oxygen level-dependent magnetic resonance imaging identifies cortical hypoxia in severe renovascular disease. Hypertension. 2011;58:1066–72.
77. Chabova V, Schirger A, Stanson AW, McKusick MA, Textor SC. Outcomes of atherosclerotic renal artery stenosis managed without revascularization. Mayo Clin Proc. 2000;75:437–44.
78. Pohl MA, Novick AC. Natural history of atherosclerotic and fibrous renal artery disease: clinical implications. Am J Kidney Dis. 1985;5:A120–30.
79. Caps MT, Zierler RE, Polissar NL, et al. Risk of atrophy in kidneys with atherosclerotic renal artery stenosis. Kidney Int. 1998;53:735–42.
80. Strandness Jr DE. Natural history of renal artery stenosis. Am J Kidney Dis. 1994;24:630–5.
81. Jerie P. Thirty years of the balloon catheter—A. Gruntzig and percutaneous balloon angioplasty. Cas Lek Cesk. 2004;143:866–71.
82. Tuttle KR, Chouinard RF, Webber JT, et al. Treatment of atherosclerotic ostial renal artery stenosis with the intravascular stent. Am J Kidney Dis. 1998;32:611–22.
83. Blum U, Krumme B, Flugel P, et al. Treatment of ostial renal-artery stenoses with vascular endoprostheses after unsuccessful balloon angioplasty. N Engl J Med. 1997;336:459–65.
84. Rocha-Singh K, Jaff MR, Rosenfield K. Evaluation of the safety and effectiveness of renal artery stenting after unsuccessful balloon angioplasty: the ASPIRE-2 study. J Am Coll Cardiol. 2005;46:776–83.
85. van de Ven PJ, Beutler JJ, Kaatee R, et al. Transluminal vascular stent for ostial atherosclerotic renal artery stenosis. Lancet. 1995;346:672–4.
86. van de Ven PJ, Kaatee R, Beutler JJ, et al. Arterial stenting and balloon angioplasty in ostial atherosclerotic renovascular disease: a randomised trial. Lancet. 1999;353:282–6.
87. Rees CR, Palmaz JC, Becker GJ, et al. Palmaz stent in atherosclerotic stenoses involving the ostia of the renal arteries: preliminary report of a multicenter study. Radiology. 1991;181:507–14.
88. Alhadad A, Mattiasson I, Ivancev K, Gottsater A, Lindblad B. Revascularisation of renal artery stenosis caused by fibromuscular dysplasia: effects on blood pressure during 7-year follow-up are influenced by duration of hypertension and branch artery stenosis. J Hum Hypertens. 2005;19:761–7.
89. Rocha-Singh K, Jaff MR, Kelley EL. Renal artery stenting with noninvasive duplex ultrasound follow-up: 3-year results from the RENAISSANCE renal stent trial. Catheter Cardiovasc Interv. 2008;72:853–62.
90. Chi YW, White CJ, Thornton S, Milani RV. Ultrasound velocity criteria for renal in-stent restenosis. J Vasc Surg. 2009;50:119–23.
91. Stanley JC, David M. Hume memorial lecture. Surgical treatment of renovascular hypertension. Am J Surg. 1997;174:102–10.
92. Novick AC. Long-term results of surgical revascularization for renal artery disease. Urol Clin N Am. 2001;28:827–31. x.
93. Stout CL, Glickman MH. Renal artery stent infection and pseudoaneurysm management. Ann Vasc Surg. 2010;24:114 e13–7.
94. Aurell M, Jensen G. Treatment of renovascular hypertension. Nephron. 1997;75:373–83.
95. Lawrie GM, Morris Jr GC, Glaeser DH, DeBakey ME. Renovascular reconstruction: factors affecting long-term prognosis in 919 patients followed up to 31 years. Am J Cardiol. 1989;63:1085–92.
96. Hughes JS, Dove HG, Gifford Jr RW, Feinstein AR. Duration of blood pressure elevation in accurately predicting surgical cure of renovascular hypertension. Am Heart J. 1981;101:408–13.
97. Hansen KJ, Starr SM, Sands RE, Burkart JM, Plonk Jr GW, Dean RH. Contemporary surgical management of renovascular disease. J Vasc Surg. 1992;16:319–30. discussion 330-1.
98. Novick AC. Current concepts in the management of renovascular hypertension and ischemic renal failure. Am J Kidney Dis. 1989;13:33–7.

Chapter 5
Resistant Hypertension in Chronic Kidney Disease

Panagiotis I. Georgianos and Pantelis A. Sarafidis

Introduction

Resistant hypertension was first formally defined in the seventh report of the US Joint National Committee on Prevention, Detection, Evaluation of High Blood Pressure (JNC-7) as failure to achieve goal blood pressure (BP) <140/90 mmHg [or <130/80 mmHg for patients with chronic kidney disease (CKD) and diabetes] in patients who are adherent to maximal tolerated doses of ≥3 antihypertensive medications, including a diuretic [1]. Following this definition, those who are able to reach goal BP on treatment with ≥4 antihypertensive drugs are commonly classified as having controlled resistant hypertension [1]. In addition, the term "refractory hypertension" was introduced for patients who meet the definition of resistant hypertension, but their BP remains uncontrolled despite the use of ≥4 antihypertensive medications at maximally tolerated doses [2–4].

Prior to these definitions, the prevalence of resistant hypertension in the general population was poorly defined, since relevant data on the epidemiology of resistant hypertension were obtained from indirect sources, such as cross-sectional studies on hypertension control, large retrospective studies from tertiary referral centers, and hypertension outcome trials [5]. In recent years, large-scaled population studies including detailed records of the prescribed antihypertensive medication, although suffering from inherent limitations related to common causes of pseudo-resistance, provided more direct estimates of the burden of resistant hypertension, offering insight into an important issue [6]. Resistant hypertension is currently estimated to

P.I. Georgianos, MD, PhD
AHEPA Hospital, Aristotle University of Thessaloniki,
St. Kyriakidi 1, Thessaloniki GR54006, Greece

P.A. Sarafidis, MD, MSc, PhD (✉)
Hippokration Hospital, Aristotle University of Thessaloniki,
Konstantinoupoleos 49, Thessaloniki GR54642, Greece
e-mail: psarafidis11@yahoo.gr

© Springer Science+Business Media New York 2016
A.K. Singh, R. Agarwal (eds.), *Core Concepts in Hypertension in Kidney Disease*, DOI 10.1007/978-1-4939-6436-9_5

affect about 9–12 % of hypertensives in the general population. Furthermore, recent studies on large cohorts of patients with CKD showed that resistant hypertension affects about 20–35 % of people with CKD depending on the stage of the disease [6]. This higher burden of resistant hypertension in the CKD setting may be relevant to specific factors associated with kidney damage per se, such as impaired sodium handling leading to volume overload, excessive activation of the sympathetic nervous system (SNS), accelerated arterial stiffness, and endothelial dysfunction [6–8]. Importantly, a growing body of evidence from prospective observational studies started to shed light on the prognostic implications of resistant hypertension, showing that this entity is a strong and independent predictor of adverse cardiovascular outcomes and progression to end-stage renal disease (ESRD) [9, 10].

This chapter discusses the currently available evidence on the prevalence, incidence, and prognosis of resistant hypertension, offering also insights into factors associated with pseudo-resistance and true resistance to antihypertensive treatment among patients with CKD.

Pseudoresistant Hypertension

Before discussing in detail the pathogenesis and epidemiology of resistant hypertension, it is crucial to distinguish true resistance to therapy from the phenomenon of pseudo-resistance [3]. Pseudo-resistance relates to the appearance of uncontrolled BP under appropriate therapy with at least three antihypertensive agents in patients who have well-controlled hypertension. An important step in diagnostic evaluation of a patient with suspected resistant hypertension is the investigation and exclusion of specific factors giving falsely the impression of drug resistance, such as improper BP measurement technique, heavily calcified arteries that are difficult to compress, inappropriate doses of drugs or prescription of drug classes that are not synergistic in reducing BP, and, most importantly, poor compliance to the prescribed antihypertensive regimen and white-coat hypertension [3].

Non-Adherence to Therapy

Poor compliance to the prescribed antihypertensive therapy is a major factor contributing to pseudo-resistance. It is estimated that approximately 50 % of patients with newly diagnosed hypertension who initiate drug therapy stop following the regimen within the first year of diagnosis [11, 12]. Other studies show significant reductions in the percentage of patients who remain compliant with their antihypertensive regimen in the long-term; 5–10 years after the onset of antihypertensive treatment, only 10–15 % of the originally treated patients are still adherent to their regimen [13]. Prevalence of non-adherence among patients presenting with resistant hypertension is likely to be much higher than originally reported, since recent clinical studies using urinary therapeutic drug monitoring to evaluate drug intake without patients' awareness of the test have shown that the majority of resistant patients were either poorly adherent or totally non-adherent to their drug therapies [14]. Potential factors contributing to poor compliance include drug-related side effects, complicated dosing schedules, poor relationship between physicians and patients, failure to educate the patient on the significance of achieving adequate hypertension control, and high costs of therapy [3].

Drug adherence should be addressed during every follow-up visit, with specific questions that emphasize on the importance of long-term compliance with therapy [15]. Drug adherence monitoring is suggested to be a beneficial approach to distinguish patients with uncontrolled BP who exhibit perfect compliance to the prescribed regimen and are possibly in need of additional diagnostic evaluations and therapeutic interventions from patients who are non-adherent and require interventions aiming to improve long-term acceptance of the need to receive antihypertensive treatment. In an observational study including 41 patients with hypertension resistant to a triple-drug regimen, Burnier and co-workers showed that electronic compliance monitoring over a 2-month period was associated with significant reductions in ambulatory BP by 11 mmHg in systolic and 9 mmHg in diastolic BP. After the 2-month monitoring period, about one third of patients on monitoring adherence normalized their BP, whereas another third of patients improved their BP control without any modification in the background antihypertensive treatment throughout the study [16]. Single-pill antihypertensive combinations were shown to improve patient compliance and can be of particular help to overcome the problem of polypharmacy [17, 18].

White-Coat Effect

The white-coat effect [i.e., an elevation in BP that occurs during clinic visits with normal out-of-office BP recordings obtained either with home or with ambulatory BP monitoring (ABPM)] is another important component of pseudo-resistance [3, 19]. Earlier studies using ABPM in order to confirm the diagnosis of resistant hypertension suggested that approximately 30 % of patients classified as resistant hypertensives on the basis of office BP measurements indeed had normal ambulatory BP values [20, 21]. A more recent analysis of the Spanish Ambulatory Blood Pressure Monitoring Registry incorporating office and ambulatory BP data from 68,045 patients receiving drug treatment for hypertension aimed to clarify the influence of white-coat phenomenon on identification of true drug resistance [22]. In this study, a total of 8295 patients met the definition of resistant hypertension on the basis of conventional office BP recordings (i.e., uncontrolled office BP >140/90 mmHg under treatment with ≥3 antihypertensive drugs, including a diuretic). However, when resistant hypertension status was determined according to the ambulatory BP values, only 5182 of these patients (62.5 %) had truly resistant hypertension, whereas the remaining 3113 patients (37.5 %) had normal ambulatory BP and were classified as white-coat resistant hypertensives [22]. A subsequent analysis from the Spanish ABPM registry showed that the prevalence of white-coat hypertension among patients with CKD is as high as 28.8 %, suggesting that the white-coat phenomenon is also quite common in these patients and should not be neglected in diagnostic approach of a patient with suspected resistant hypertension [23].

Apart from its usefulness in confirmation of the diagnosis of resistant hypertension, performance of ABPM offers several additional advantages in improving cardiovascular risk stratification of the patients [24], particularly in the setting of CKD. In this regard, ABPM provides the ability to record BP during the night-time period and to identify the presence of a "non-dipping" pattern, which is the diminution or reversal of the normal 10–20 % nocturnal fall in BP [24]. A growing body of evidence suggests that elevated night-time BP is stronger predictor of all-cause and cardiovascular mortality than day-time BP, whereas a non-dipping status has been shown to confer a twofold higher risk for cardiovascular morbidity and mortality in comparison with a normal dipping pattern, independently from the presence of hypertension [25–27]. In addition, ABPM enables the identification of masked hypertension, which is defined as abnormally elevated out-of-office BP while BP measurements during clinic visits remain within the normal range [24]. Notably, in a recent observational study, in which 489 outpatients treated for hypertension with stage 2–4 CKD were prospectively followed for a median period of 5.2 years, masked hypertension was associated with 3.17 times higher risk for the occurrence of a composite cardiovascular endpoint consisting of fatal and nonfatal myocardial infarction, congestive heart failure, stroke, revascularization, peripheral vascular disease, and non-traumatic amputation relative to controlled office and ambulatory BP [28]. Masked hypertension was also associated with a threefold greater risk for the combined renal endpoint of initiating dialysis or death. The overall cardio-renal risk attributable to masked hypertension was comparable with that of uncontrolled hypertension [28].

Truly Resistant Hypertension and Its Potential Causes in Chronic Kidney Disease

Renal parenchymal disease is considered as one of the most common medical causes of resistant hypertension. Multiple pathways associated with impaired renal function are likely to contribute to the development of resistance to antihypertensive drug treatment. These mechanistic factors are summarized in Table 5.1 and are discussed in detail below.

Sodium and Volume Overload

A key factor responsible for many cases of resistant hypertension is excessive dietary salt intake leading to chronic volume overload [29]. This is supported by several studies showing that the vast majority of patients with resistant hypertension

Table 5.1 Factors contributing to antihypertensive drug resistance in CKD

Sodium and volume excess
Sympathetic nervous system overactivity
Overactivity of the renin–angiotensin–aldosterone-system
Increased endothelium-derived vasoconstrictors
Decreased endothelium-derived vasodilators
Arterial stiffness
Pre-existing hypertension
Specific medications (cyclosporine, tacrolimus, steroids, erythropoietin)

have expanded plasma volume, which is causally related to a higher salt intake in comparison with the general population [30]. In a pilot, randomized, cross-over study including 12 patients with uncontrolled hypertension despite receiving therapy with an average of 3.4 antihypertensive agents, Pimenta et al. compared the effects of a low (50 mmol/24 h) versus a high (250 mmol/24 h) sodium-containing diet on office and 24-hour ambulatory BP [31]. The mean urinary sodium excretion was significantly lower during the low-sodium than during the high-sodium intake period (46.1±26.8 vs 252.2±64.6 mmol/24 h). Dietary sodium restriction was associated with remarkable reductions in office BP, by 22.7 and 9.1 mmHg in systolic and diastolic BP, respectively. These BP-lowering effects were consistent during the whole 24-hour period [31]. Thus, sodium restrictive diet should be considered as an important part of the therapeutic approach of patients with resistant hypertension, particularly when CKD is present.

The major factor contributing to salt and fluid accumulation in patients with CKD is impaired renal sodium handling and reduced capacity of the kidney to excrete daily sodium intake. Reduced nephron number and the potential excess of multiple sodium-retaining hormones such as aldosterone and endothelin create a sizable barrier to efficient urinary sodium excretion [31–33]. Overactivity of the SNS, particularly when CKD is accompanied by other co-morbid conditions such as diabetes and heart failure, is another factor that may promote sodium retention [34, 35]. Failure to use diuretic agents in appropriate doses adjusted to the level of renal function is another major issue affecting efficient sodium excretion, resulting in antihypertensive drug resistance. In patients with an estimated glomerular filtration rate (eGFR) <40 ml/min/1.73 m², thiazide diuretics are unlikely to be effective, with a possible exception of metolazone, which is probably active down to an eGFR of 20 ml/min/1.73 m², but is not available in many countries. Preliminary data suggest that chlorthalidone may also be effective in advanced renal failure. However, for eGFR of <30 ml/min/1.73 m², loop diuretics are often needed. Use of combinations of loop diuretics with other diuretic compounds may be necessary in selected cases to enhance natriuresis [36].

Sympathetic Overactivity

Activation of the SNS is suggested to play a pivotal role in pathogenesis of hypertension in CKD [8]. The kidney is a richly innervated organ and experimental studies suggest that the kidneys may be modulators of the SNS overactivity; this regulation is mediated through renal afferent nerves connected with integrative nuclei of the SNS in the central nervous system [37]. In animal studies, acute stimulation of these afferent nerves in response to renal ischemia and reperfusion injury was shown to induce a reflex elevation in efferent SNS activity and in BP levels [38, 39]. In experimental models of 5/6 nephrectomized rats, the turnover rate and release of norepinephrine from the posterior hypothalamic nuclei were higher in CKD than in control rats; bilateral dorsal rhizotomy down-regulated the SNS activity and preserved the BP levels within the normal range [40]. In addition, muscle sympathetic nerve activity (MSNA) studies in hemodialysis patients showed that the rate of sympathetic discharge was twice the normal and correlated strongly with the rise in plasma catecholamine levels. In contrast, patients with bilateral nephrectomy manifested lower MSNA, BP, and peripheral vascular resistance as compared with patients with retained native kidneys [41]. Taken together, the studies in animals and in humans support the notion that increased renal sensory impulses originating from the affected kidney and transmitted to the central nervous system activate brain regions involved in the noradrenergic control of BP, resulting in vasoconstriction, sodium retention, and hypertension. However, the exact mechanisms mediating the development of the excessive sympathetic activation within the kidney parenchyma still remain unclear. Other mechanisms potentially responsible for the increase in SNS activity in the CKD setting include decreased central dopaminergic tone, lower baroreceptor sensitivity, elevated plasma β-endorphin and β-lipotropin, increased serum leptin levels, and reduced renalase availability [8, 42].

Overactivity of the Renin–Angiotensin–Aldosterone-System

Excessive activation of the renin–angiotensin–aldosterone-system (RAAS) is suggested to be another major pathway for sustained BP elevation, promotion of end-organ damage, and development of antihypertensive drug resistance, particularly in the setting of CKD. One clear mechanism through which aldosterone excess promotes drug resistance, identified shortly after the discovery of the hormone itself, is its action on the distal nephron of the kidney to regulate intravascular volume and promote sodium reabsorption [43]. The original belief that aldosterone acts solely on specific receptors in epithelial tissues and modulates electrolyte and water balance via a genomic mechanism has been challenged by the identification of mineralocorticoid receptors in non-epithelial tissues, such as heart, vasculature, and the brain, suggesting that aldosterone mediates target-organ damage through non-genomic mechanisms of action [44, 45]. This notion is supported by a number of animal and human studies showing that aldosterone exerts hypertrophic, proliferative, proinflammatory, prothrombotic, and profibrotic actions in target organs beyond the kidney, inducing endothelial dysfunction, vascular inflammation, fibrosis, and necrosis [44, 45]. This pathologic process leads to functional and structural alterations of small and large arteries, leading to sustained BP elevation. Blocking the adverse actions of aldosterone on the vasculature through selective mineralocorticoid receptor antagonists (MRAs), such as spironolactone and eplerenone, has gained renewed interest as a novel therapeutic approach of resistant hypertension in patients with or without CKD. This notion is strongly supported by the results of the Anglo-Scandinavian Cardiac Outcomes Trial-Blood Pressure Lowering Arm (ASCOT-BPLA) [46], in which fourth-line add-on therapy with spironolactone administered at a starting dose of 25 mg/day was accompanied by a mean BP reduction of 21.9/9.5 mmHg over a median treatment duration of 1.3 years. With close monitoring of serum potassium levels, add-on MRA therapy could be an effective and safe therapeutic approach of resistant hypertension even in the CKD setting [47, 48].

Arterial Stiffness

A typical feature of arterial remodeling in CKD is long-term structural alterations in intrinsic elastic properties of the arterial wall. These alterations include fibroelastic intimal thickening, calcification of elastic lamellae, increased extracellular matrix deposition, elastinolysis and elevated collagen along with reduced elastic fiber content [49]. This arteriosclerotic process affects mainly the central arteries, such as the aorta and the carotid artery, where cushioning the stroke volume ejected by the left ventricle is essential in order to transform the pulsatile blood flow oscillations into the continuous flow pattern required for perfusion of organs and tissues [49]. The principal mechanism through which arterial stiffness contributes to BP elevation is that higher arterial stiffness (in other words, the higher velocity of pulse wave transfer across the arterial tree) results in premature arrival of reflected wave from the periphery back to the ascending aorta during the systolic phase of the cardiac cycle [50]. Thus, the forward- and backward-traveling pulse waves are in phase and their overlap during systole rather than diastole generates an amplification effect on systolic and pulse pressures in the aorta [49, 50].

The notion that arterial stiffness makes hypertension more resistant to antihypertensive therapy is strongly supported by a post-hoc analysis of the Preterax in Regression of Arterial Stiffness in a Controlled Double-Blind (REASON) study [51]. In this study, 375 patients with essential hypertension were treated with either perindopril/indapamide combination (20/0.625 mg daily) or atenolol (50 mg daily) for 12 months. The study found that higher baseline aortic PWV was associated with smaller in extent reductions in office BP levels and that baseline aortic PWV was an independent predictor of achievement of BP control after 12 months of therapy [51]. In addition, a prospective analysis from the Framingham cohort study showed that reduced arterial compliance is a strong and independent predictor of a future diagnosis of hypertension over approximately 8 years of follow-up [52].

The reverse phenomenon was not true, since higher BP levels were unable to predict greater changes in arterial stiffness over time. The role of arterial stiffness as predictor of BP response to the antihypertensive therapy was evaluated in a post-hoc analysis of the Hypertension in Hemodialysis patients treated with Atenolol or Lisinopril (HDPAL) trial. In contrast to the observations in the general population, among hypertensive hemodialysis patients, aortic PWV at baseline was not predictor of the treatment-induced improvement in 44-hour interdialytic ambulatory BP over the course of the trial [53].

Endothelial Dysfunction

An imbalance between endothelium-derived vasoconstrictors and vasodilators in favor of the former may be another mechanistic pathway of resistant hypertension in CKD [8]. This is supported by animal studies showing down-regulation of the endothelial and inducible nitric oxide synthase activity in 5/6 nephrectomized rats, an alteration that resulted in sustained BP elevation [54]. Endothelial dysfunction is suggested to be the result of several mechanisms at play when renal function is impaired. One of these mechanisms is the higher circulating levels of asymmetric dimethylarginine (ADMA) in CKD; ADMA is an endogenous nitric oxide synthase inhibitor and its accumulation results in reduced generation of nitric oxide. The higher levels of ADMA result from both a diminished intracellular degradation by desamino-D-argininehydrolase and by reduced renal clearance of ADMA, since this molecule is mainly excreted by the kidney [55]. Apart from promoting endothelial dysfunction, ADMA also acts as a stimulus for increased generation of proinflammatory mediators, such as interleukin-6 and profibrotic molecules such as transforming growth factor-β [56]. Increased production of the potent endogenous vasoconstrictor endothelin-1 in patients with CKD is proposed to be another important player in pathogenesis of resistant hypertension [57]. The pathologic effects of endothelin-1, including vasoconstriction, inflammation, cellular injury and fibrosis, are mainly mediated by the endothelin-A receptors, which have recently become promising targets of therapy in preclinical and clinical studies [58]. Endothelin receptor blockers have been shown to produce significant reduction in BP among patients with resistant hypertension, but their role in treating this entity in patients with CKD has not been specifically investigated.

Epidemiology of Resistant Hypertension

Prevalence

In the past, the exact prevalence of resistant hypertension in the general hypertensive population was not established, since information on the epidemiology of resistant hypertension was derived from indirect sources (i.e., observations on hypertension control from population-based studies, retrospective studies from tertiary hypertension centers, and sub-analyses of large randomized clinical trials in hypertension) [59–63]. Identification of the exact burden of resistant hypertension would ideally require properly designed prospective studies using forced titration of BP-lowering therapy up to maximally tolerated doses of ≥3 agents, including a diuretic; ideally, relevant studies should exclude common causes of pseudo-resistance [3]. Population-based studies with detailed record of the prescribed anti-hypertensive medications would also advance our knowledge; however, such studies would unavoidably suffer from inherent methodological limitations related to common causes of pseudo-resistance (e.g., white-coat effect, non-adherence to therapy, etc.) [3]. More recently, epidemiological studies have been performed to ascertain the prevalence of resistant hypertension. They are summarized in Table 5.2 and discussed in some detail below.

An early retrospective, observational study using electronic medical records of the years 2002–2005 provided the first direct estimate of the prevalence of resistant hypertension in the US hypertensive population [64]. In this analysis, 9.1 % of 29,474 hypertensive participants from an ambulatory care setting (or 12.1 % of drug-treated patients) were classified as having resistant hypertension, according to the definition of uncontrolled BP >140/90 mmHg despite the use of ≥3 antihypertensive medications. Another 6 % of study participants had uncontrolled BP despite receiving ≥4 antihypertensive agents, but not a diuretic. Furthermore, around 29.5 % of participants had uncontrolled BP, without receiving therapy; of these, 10–15 % had resistant hypertension [64].

A subsequent study [65] aimed to determine the prevalence of resistant hypertension in the USA using the 2003–2008 National Health and Nutrition Examination Survey (NHANES) dataset. Resistant hypertension in this survey was defined as BP >140/90 mmHg and reported use of >3 different antihypertensive medications within the previous month or use of ≥4 antihypertensive agents regardless of measured BP. In this analysis, 8.9 % of 5230 participants (or 12.8 % of drug-treated hypertensive participants) met the criteria of resistant hypertension according to the aforementioned definition [65]. Again, another 30.7 % of patients had uncontrolled BP without receiving antihypertensive treatment. Assuming that 10 % of these patients might have had resistant hypertension, the actual prevalence of resistant hypertension might have been another 3 % higher.

Trends in prevalence of uncontrolled hypertension and resistant hypertension during 1988–2008 in the USA were explored in another analysis of 13,375 hypertensive adults participating in the 3 NHANES surveys (1988–1994, 1999–2004, 2005–2008) [66]. Uncontrolled hypertension was defined as BP >140/90 mmHg among drug-treated hypertensives and resistant hypertension was defined as uncontrolled hypertension among treated patients despite the reported use of ≥3 antihypertensive drugs during the previous month. Rates of uncontrolled hypertension declined from 73.2 % in 1988–1994 to 52.5 % in 1999–2004. In contrast, the prevalence of resistant hypertension (expressed as percentage of drug-treated hypertensives) exhibited an increasing trend from 15.9 % in 1988–1994 to 28.0 % in 2005–2008 [66]. When patients with controlled BP treated with ≥4 antihypertensive drugs were also considered as resistant hypertensives, the prevalence of resis-

Table 5.2 Prevalence of resistant hypertension in the general hypertensive population

Study ID	Population characteristics	Definition of resistant hypertension	Prevalence estimates
McAdam-Marx et al. [64] Clin Ther 2009	29,474 US adults with a diagnosis of hypertension in the General Electric Centricity Medical Record	Uncontrolled BP >140/90 mmHg (or >130/80 mmHg for those with diabetes or CKD) with ≥3 antihypertensive drugs, including a thiazide	A total of 2640 out of 29,474 hypertensive patients (9.1 %) were classified as having resistant hypertension
Pershell et al. [65] Hypertension 2011	5230 hypertensive US adults participating in the 2003–2008 NHANES dataset	Uncontrolled BP >140/90 mmHg with ≥3 antihypertensive drugs in the previous month or reported use of ≥4 antihypertensive drugs regardless of BP	A total of 539 out of 5230 hypertensive patients (8.9 %) met the criteria of resistant hypertension
Egan et al. [66] Circulation 2011	13,375 hypertensive US adults from the NHANES datasets in the 3 time-periods (1988–1994, 1999–2004, 2005–08)	Uncontrolled BP >140/90 mmHg with ≥3 antihypertensive drugs in the previous month or reported use of ≥4 antihypertensive drugs regardless of BP	5.5 % of all hypertensives in 1988–1994, 8.5 % of all hypertensives in 1999–2004, and 11.8 % of all hypertensives in 2005–08 had resistant hypertension
Brambilla et al. [68] J Hypertens 2013	1312 drug-treated hypertensive participants of the BP-CARE study	Uncontrolled BP >140/90 mmHg despite the concurrent use of ≥3 antihypertensive medications or use of ≥4 antihypertensive drugs regardless of BP	A total of 255 patients (19.4 % of drug-treated hypertensive patients) were classified as resistant hypertensives
Sim et al. [67] Mayo Clin Proc 2013	470,386 hypertensives participating in the Kaiser Permanente Southern California health system during 2006–2007	Uncontrolled BP >140/90 mmHg despite triple antihypertensive therapy or current use of ≥4 antihypertensive drugs irrespective of BP control	A total of 60,327 participants (12.8 % of all hypertensives) or 15.3 % of those receiving antihypertensive medications fulfilled the diagnostic criteria of resistant hypertension
Weitzman et al. [69] Hypertension 2014	172,432 hypertensive patients belonging to the Maccabi Healthcare System in Israel	Uncontrolled BP >140/90 mmHg despite the treatment with ≥3 antihypertensive drugs at maximally tolerated doses, including a diuretic	0.86 % of the entire hypertensive population (or 2.26 % of hypertensives with uncontrolled BP) had resistant hypertension

US United States, *NAHANES* National Health and Nutrition Examination Survey, *BP* blood pressure, *CKD* chronic kidney disease, *BP-CARE* Blood Pressure control rate and CArdiovascular Risk profilE (BP-CARE) study tant hypertension among all adult US NHANES hypertensive participants was 5.5% in 1988–2004, increased to 8.5% in 1999–2004 and reached 11.8% in the 2005–2008.

The largest cross-sectional survey so far aiming to estimate the burden of resistant hypertension in the USA [67] used data obtained from 470,386 hypertensive patients participating in the Kaiser Permanente Southern California health system during 2006–2007. By defining resistant hypertension as BP >140/90 mmHg despite triple antihypertensive therapy or current use of ≥4 antihypertensive drugs irrespective of BP control, study investigators observed that 12.8% of all hypertensives (or 15.3% of those receiving antihypertensive medications) fulfilled the diagnostic criteria of resistant hypertension [67]. Black race, older age, male gender, obesity, impaired renal function, presence of diabetes, and history of previous cardiovascular disease were the main factors associated with higher risk of resistant hypertension. Paradoxically, rates of adherence to the prescribed antihypertensive regimen were higher among resistant hypertensives than in those with controlled hypertension.

Data on the prevalence of resistant hypertension in Europe were provided by the Blood Pressure control rate and CArdiovascular Risk profilE (BP-CARE) study [68]. Among 1312 drug-treated hypertensive participants, 255 (19.4% of the study cohort) were classified as suffering from resistant hypertension according to the definition of uncontrolled BP >140/90 mmHg despite the concurrent use of ≥3 antihypertensive medications or use of ≥4 antihypertensive drugs regardless of BP levels [68]. Another recent survey in Israel incorporating data from 172,432 hypertensive patients followed in the Maccabi Healthcare System showed that 0.86% of the entire hypertensive population (or 2.26% of hypertensives with uncontrolled BP) had resistant hypertension [69]. Resistant hypertension was defined as uncontrolled BP >140/90 mmHg despite the treatment with ≥3 antihypertensive drugs at maximally tolerated doses, including a diuretic, over the previous month of BP measurement. When analysis was performed taking into account the prescribed antihypertensive medications during the 2 previous months before the BP measurement, instead of the last month, estimated prevalence of resistant hypertension increased to 1.24% of the entire hypertensive population (or to 3.24% of those with uncontrolled BP) [69]. These estimates of the prevalence of resistant hypertension are far lower than previously reported. This may be explained by the fact that patients with controlled hypertension under treatment with ≥4 agents were not classified as resistant hypertensives in this survey. Other factors, such as improved patient compliance, reduced physician inertia or even yearly higher average temperatures in the country of the last study compared to the USA, or North Europe may also apply.

Overt or incipient CKD is long considered as common cause of truly resistant hypertension [6]. As discussed above, several factors closely related to impaired renal function (such as greater difficulty of excreting daily salt intake, increased SNS activity, endothelial dysfunction, higher levels of proinflammatory markers, and arterial stiffness) are likely to contribute to antihypertensive drug resistance in the CKD setting [8]. The phenomenon of resistant hypertension in patients CKD is also increasingly studied in recent years. Large epidemiological studies conducted in the general hypertensive population showed that resistant hypertensives are more likely to have reduced kidney function and micro- or macro-albuminuria, suggesting a higher burden of resistant hypertension in CKD. For example, in the NHANES 2003–2008 dataset, 33.7 % of resistant hypertensives had eGFR <60 ml/min/1.73 m^2 and 12.8 % had albumin-to-creatinine ratio (ACR) >300 mg/g relative to 16.5 and 1.9 % of patients with controlled hypertension, respectively [65]. A retrospective study of 300 patients with hypertension and CKD referred to a nephrology clinic in Italy showed that prevalence of resistant hypertension increased from 26 to 38 % after the first 6 months of standard nephrology care [70]. This observation should not be considered causally related, since simply intensification of antihypertensive therapy may qualify the identification of resistant hypertension, even when BP may be poorly controlled.

Two recent studies with more accurate methodology advanced our knowledge on the prevalence of resistant hypertension in the CKD population (see Table 5.3). The first was an analysis from a population-based sample of US hypertensive adults participating in the Geographic and Racial Differences in Stroke (REGARDS) study during 2003–2007 [71]. Resistant hypertension was defined as uncontrolled BP >140/90 mmHg, despite the current use of >3 antihypertensive drugs or therapy with ≥4 agents regardless of measured BP. Antihypertensive drug use was assessed via pill bottle review of all medications participants reported taking during the previous 2 weeks and BP was measured in the home setting. The original REGARDS study was designed to include 15,277 participants with history of hypertension under treatment with ≥1 antihypertensive drug. In the final cohort of 10,700 patients eligible for determination of their resistant hypertension status, prevalence of resistant hypertension was 15.8 % among those with eGFR ≥60 ml/min/1.73 m^2, but 24.9 % among those with eGFR 45–59 ml/min/1.73 m^2 (Stage 3A CKD) and 33.4 % among those with eGFR <45 ml/min/1.73 m^2 (Stage 3B or more advanced CKD). When participants were classified according to the levels of albuminuria, the prevalence of resistant hypertension was 12.1, 20.8, 27.7, and 48.3 % for ACR <10, 10–29, 30–299, and ≥300 mg/g, respectively [71]. It has to be noted that although the study provided important information, the reported rates of resistant hypertension, even when notably higher than the other reports, may still be an underestimation of the exact prevalence for two reasons: first, at the time of the study, the recommended threshold for BP lowering in CKD was at 130/80 mmHg in the office; second, this study used home BP readings, for which the proposed thresholds for assessment of BP control are lower than the office [72].

Another prospective observational study including 436 patients with hypertension and CKD attending four outpatient nephrology clinics in Italy during 2003–2005 used simultaneously office BP readings and ABPM in order to determine the influence of the white-coat effect on estimation of the prevalence of resistant hypertension [10]. At baseline, study participants were classified into four different categories on the basis of a normal or high ambulatory BP, according to the 125/75 mmHg threshold for mean 24-hour ambulatory BP, and absence or presence of resistant hypertension, defined as office BP >130/80 mmHg despite using ≥3 full-dose antihypertensive drugs, including a diuretic. This study showed that 100 out of 436

Table 5.3 Prevalence of resistant hypertension among patients with chronic kidney disease

Study ID	Population characteristics	Definition of resistant hypertension	Prevalence estimates
Tanner et al. [71] cJASN 2013	10,700 hypertensive US adults participating in the REGARDS study	Uncontrolled BP >140/90 mmHg with ≥3 antihypertensive drugs or use of >4 antihypertensive drugs regardless of BP	15.8 % for eGFR ≥60 ml/min/1.73 m²; 24.9 % for eGFR 45–59 ml/min/1.73 m²; 33.4 % for eGFR ≤45 ml/min/1.73 m²
De Nicola et al. [10] JACC 2013	436 hypertensive CKD patients, defined as office BP >130/80 mmHg and eGFR <60 ml/min/1.73 m² or eGFR between 60–90 ml/min/1.73 m² and albuminuria >300 mg/day	Uncontrolled office BP >130/80 mmHg with ≥3 antihypertensive drugs, including a diuretic, or >4 drugs and ABP >125/75 mmHg	A total of 100 out of 436 patients (22.9 %) were classified as resistant hypertensives

REGARDS Geographic and Racial Differences in Stroke Study, *BP* blood pressure, *CKD* chronic kidney disease, *ABP* ambulatory blood pressure, *eGFR* estimated glomerular filtration rate

study participants (22.9 %) had true resistant hypertension with high ambulatory BP and 31 participants had white-coat pseudoresistant hypertension (7.1 %). Another 187 participants (42.9 %) had sustained hypertension (i.e., high ambulatory BP without resistant hypertension according to the office readings) and 118 patients (27.1 %) had controlled hypertension (i.e., normal office and ambulatory BP) [10]. Presence of diabetes, left ventricular hypertrophy, higher levels of proteinuria, and poor adherence to a sodium restrictive diet were significant determinants of true resistant hypertension in multivariate analysis. Since publication of the Italian study, the threshold of diagnosis of hypertension in CKD has been changed to 140/90 mmHg. Thus, the estimates provided may well be lower if the new thresholds are utilized.

Incidence of Resistant Hypertension

A recent retrospective cohort study aiming to evaluate the incidence of resistant hypertension in people adequately treated studied 205,750 subjects with newly diagnosed hypertension who participated in two health plan programs within the Cardiovascular Health Network registry in USA during 2002–2006 [9]. Over a 1.5-year follow-up, a total of 42,474 patients (20.6 % of the original study cohort) were receiving ≥3 antihypertensive agents for at least 1-month. After excluding those who were non-adherent, on the basis of a >80 % pharmacy refill rate for all prescribed antihypertensive medications, the investigators showed that 1.5 years after treatment initiation, 1 in 50 patients became resistant to therapy on the basis of the American Heart Association (AHA) definition of having uncontrolled BP >140/90 mmHg on three medications or controlled BP on at least four antihypertensive medications.

This accounts to an incidence rate for resistant hypertension of 1.9% with a median follow-up of 1.5 years (0.7 cases per person-year of follow-up) [9]. With more extended follow-up, it is likely that the incidence would have been even higher, as the medications were further titrated for the remaining uncontrolled patients; further, on an even longer observational period, the increasing age and worsening obesity would further aggravate the risk of developing resistance to multiple drug therapy. In the presence of CKD, it could be hypothesized that the incidence rate of resistant hypertension might be even higher. However, there is no study to assess the incidence of resistant hypertension in the CKD setting until now.

A post-hoc analysis of data from 3666 previously untreated hypertensive patients participating in the Anglo-Scandinavian Cardiac Outcome Trial (ASCOT) provided additional evidence on incidence and possible predictors of resistant hypertension [73]. In ASCOT study, 19,257 hypertensive patients with ≥3 other cardiovascular risk factors were randomly assigned to receive atenolol adding a thiazide diuretic or to amlodipine adding perindopril. ASCOT had a 2×2 factorial design and a subgroup of 10,305 patients was further randomized to atorvastatin or placebo in a lipid-lowering study-arm. Definition of uncontrolled BP (>140/90 mmHg) on treatment with ≥3 antihypertensive drugs was used for identification of resistant hypertension. Among previously untreated hypertensive patients, 33% (and among all participants 50%) developed resistant hypertension during a median follow-up of 5.3 and 4.8 years, respectively (incidence rates of 75.2 and 129.7 cases per 1000 person-years, respectively) [73]. Multivariate analysis showed that independent predictors of incident resistant hypertension were raised systolic BP at baseline, diabetes, left ventricular hypertrophy, male gender, obesity, and high alcohol intake. Importantly, patients randomized to receive amlodipine relative to atenolol, those previously administered aspirin and those randomized to atorvastatin relative to placebo were less likely to develop resistant hypertension over the course of the trial [73], suggesting that the initial therapeutic approach after the diagnosis of hypertension may be of relevance for the risk of developing antihypertensive drug resistance.

Prognosis of Resistant Hypertension

In comparison with patients achieving adequate BP control with fewer than three antihypertensive drugs, whether resistant hypertension per se signifies an independent prognostic association with cardiovascular and renal outcomes is an issue that remained unclear until recently. In addition to the cardio-renal risk attributable to the degree of BP elevation [1, 74], several lines of evidence suggest that resistant hypertension is also associated with a combination of other risk factors, which may further aggravate the risk of cardiovascular morbidity and mortality. In this regard, several epidemiological studies provided evidence that more patients with resistant hypertension have target-organ damage, higher number of comorbidities, and higher rates of documented cardiovascular disease than those with controlled hypertension [75–77]. Another source of data supporting the prognostic association of resistant hypertension with cardiovascular and renal outcomes are clinical studies evaluating the patterns of ambulatory BP profile in patients with resistant hypertension; these studies showed that resistant hypertension is associated with higher ambulatory BP values, a non-dipping night-time BP pattern and higher ambulatory arterial stiffness index [26, 78, 79], factors directly linked with increased risk for cardiovascular morbidity and mortality.

Over the past few years, a number of prospective observational studies evaluating "hard" cardiovascular and renal endpoints have provided additional evidence supporting the strong and independent association of resistant hypertension with adverse outcomes. In the aforementioned study of Daugherty et al. [9], after excluding patients with known history of cardiovascular disease, patients who developed resistant hypertension were more likely to reach the prespecified combined outcome of all-cause mortality, myocardial infraction, congestive heart failure or CKD during a mean follow-up of 3.8 years [unadjusted hazard ratio (HR): 1.54; 95 % confidence intervals (CI): 1.40–1.69] [9]. After adjustment for several risk factors, resistant hypertension remained significantly associated with elevated risk of adverse cardiovascular outcomes (adjusted HR: 1.47; 95 % CI: 1.33–1.62). When patients with pre-existing cardiovascular disease were included in a secondary analysis, patients who developed antihypertensive drug resistance were again more likely to experience an adverse cardiovascular outcome at any time-point of follow-up relative to those without incident resistant hypertension (HR: 2.49; 95 % CI: 1.96, 3.15) [9].

The association of resistant hypertension with cardiovascular outcomes was explored in a prospective study of 53,530 hypertensive patients with subclinical or established atherothrombotic disease enrolled in the international Reduction of Atherothrombosis for Continued Health (REACH) registry [80]. In this analysis, patients with resistant hypertension at baseline exhibited an 11 % higher risk of reaching the composite endpoint of cardiovascular death, myocardial infarction, or stroke at 4 years of follow-up (HR: 1.11, 95 % CI: 1.02–1.20; $P=0.017$). Hospitalizations due to congestive heart failure were also higher among resistant hypertensives as compared to those with controlled hypertension [80]. The potential role of resistant hypertension as predictor of kidney injury progression was investigated in a prospective analysis of 9974 hypertensive patients participating in the REGARDS study [81]. During a median follow-up of 6.4 years, the cumulative incidence of ESRD per 1000 person-years for hypertensive participants with and without treatment-resistant hypertension was 8.86 (95 % CI: 7.35–10.68) and 0.88 (95 % CI: 0.65–1.19), respectively. After adjustment for several risk factors, patients with resistant hypertension had 6.3 times higher risk of incident ESRD throughout the study (HR: 6.32; 95 % CI, 4.30–9.30) [81].

Subsequently, the prognostic significance of resistant hypertension on cardiovascular and renal outcomes was investigated in post-hoc analyses of two large-scaled randomized trials in hypertension. The first incorporated data from 14,867 hypertensive patients participating in the Antihypertensive and Lipid-Lowering Treatment to Prevent Heart Attack Trial (ALLHAT) study [82]. Study participants not at goal BP while taking ≥3 classes of antihypertensive medications or taking ≥4 classes of antihypertensive medications with controlled BP during the Year 2 ALLHAT study visit were classified as resistant hypertensives for the purposes of this analysis. After adjustment for several risk factors, patients with resistant hypertension versus those with controlled hypertension had 30 % higher risk of all-cause mortality (HR: 1.30; 95 % CI: 1.11–1.52), 44 % higher risk of coronary heart disease (HR: 1.44; 95 % CI: 1.18–1.76), 57 % higher risk of stroke (HR: 1.57; 95 % CI: 1.18–2.08), 88 % higher risk of congestive heart failure (HR: 1.88; 95 % CI: 1.52–2.34), and 95 % higher risk of developing ESRD (HR: 1.95; 95 % CI: 1.11–3.41) until the study completion [82]. In the second, 17,190 hypertensive patients with coronary artery disease participating in the INternational VErapamil SR-Trandolapril STudy (INVEST) trial were classified as having controlled, uncontrolled, or resistant hypertension according to the in-treatment BP levels achieved at the visit immediately prior to an event or censoring [83]. Resistant hypertension was defined as uncontrolled BP >140/90 mmHg on triple antihypertensive therapy or in any patient receiving at least four antihypertensive medications regardless of BP control. Compared with controlled hypertension, resistant hypertension was independently associated with 27 % higher risk of the composite endpoint of first occurrence of all-cause death, nonfatal myocardial infarction, or nonfatal stroke (HR: 1.27; 95 % CI: 1.13–1.43) [83]. In contrast, occurrence of adverse outcomes, with the exception of nonfatal stroke, was no different between patients with resistant and uncontrolled hypertension.

The long-term prognosis of resistant hypertension in CKD was investigated during a prospective study of 436 hypertensive patients with non-dialysis requiring CKD under standard nephrology care over a mean follow-up period of 52 months [10]. The study had a composite cardiovascular outcome of cardiovascular death or nonfatal cardiovascular event requiring hospitalization (myocardial infarction, congestive heart failure, stroke, revascularization, peripheral vascular disease, and non-traumatic amputation) and a composite renal endpoint of progression to ESRD requiring dialysis or death. Given the fact that elevated BP is a strong mediator of kidney injury progression in CKD, it was no surprise that patients with resistant hypertension had an adjusted twofold increased risk of reaching the composite cardiovascular endpoint (HR: 1.98; 95 % CI: 1.14, 3.13) and an adjusted 2.6 times higher risk of reaching the renal endpoint during follow-up (HR: 2.66; 95 % CI: 1.62, 4.37) in comparison with controlled hypertensives [10]. In contrast to true resistant hypertension, which predicted both cardiovascular and renal endpoints, patients with uncontrolled hypertension shared an adjusted 2.1-fold higher risk of reaching the composite renal outcome (HR: 2.14; 95 % CI: 1.35, 3.40), but had no additional cardiovascular risk as compared to patients who had their BP adequately controlled (adjusted HR: 1.11; 95 % CI: 0.67, 1.84) [10].

Conclusion

Resistant hypertension is a growing clinical problem that based on office readings is estimated to affect about 9–12 % of hypertensives in the general population. Although CKD is for long considered as a major medical cause of resistance to antihypertensive treatment, the epidemiology and pathogenesis of this phenomenon in the CKD was poorly studied until recently. Over the past few years, epidemiological studies highlighted that the prevalence of resistant hypertension is much higher in the CKD than in the general hypertensive population, affecting approximately 20–35 % of people with CKD depending on the stage of the disease. Specific mechanisms associated with impaired renal function, such as greater difficulty in excreting daily sodium intake, excessive SNS and RAAS activation, arterial stiffness and endothelial dysfunction, are proposed to be prominent players in pathogenesis of resistant hypertension in CKD. Furthermore, prospective observational studies over the past few years have demonstrated that resistant hypertension signifies an independent prognostic association with adverse cardiovascular outcomes and kidney injury progression to ESRD. Of importance, before labeling the diagnosis of resistant hypertension, a careful examination for and exclusion of factors related to pseudo-resistance, mainly non-adherence to therapy and white-coat phenomenon, is required. Epidemiologic studies that account for pseudo-resistance are warranted in order to fully elucidate the exact prevalence, incidence, and prognostic significance of truly resistant hypertension in CKD.

References

1. Chobanian AV, Bakris GL, Black HR, Cushman WC, Green LA, Izzo JL, et al. The Seventh Report of the Joint National Committee on Prevention, Detection, Evaluation, and Treatment of High Blood Pressure: the JNC 7 report. JAMA. 2003;289:2560–72.
2. Calhoun DA, Jones D, Textor S, Goff DC, Murphy TP, Toto RD, et al. Resistant hypertension: diagnosis, evaluation, and treatment. A scientific statement from the American Heart Association Professional Education Committee of the Council for High Blood Pressure Research. Hypertension. 2008;51:1403–19.
3. Sarafidis PA, Georgianos P, Bakris GL. Resistant hypertension--its identification and epidemiology. Nat Rev Nephrol. 2013;9:51–8.
4. Pimenta E, Gaddam KK, Oparil S. Mechanisms and treatment of resistant hypertension. J Clin Hypertens (Greenwich). 2008;10:239–44.
5. Sarafidis PA, Bakris GL. State of hypertension management in the United States: confluence of risk factors and the prevalence of resistant hypertension. J Clin Hypertens (Greenwich). 2008;10:130–9.
6. Sarafidis PA, Georgianos PI, Zebekakis PE. Comparative epidemiology of resistant hypertension in chronic kidney disease and the general hypertensive population. Semin Nephrol. 2014;34:483–91.
7. Drexler YR, Bomback AS. Definition, identification and treatment of resistant hypertension in chronic kidney disease patients. Nephrol Dial Transplant. 2014;29:1327–35.
8. Townsend RR. Pathogenesis of drug-resistant hypertension. Semin Nephrol. 2014;34:506–13.
9. Daugherty SL, Powers JD, Magid DJ, Masoudi F, Margolis K, O'Connor P, et al. Incidence and prognosis of resistant hypertension in hypertensive patients. Circulation. 2012;125:1635–42.
10. De Nicola L, Gabbai FB, Agarwal R, Chiodini P, Borrelli S, Bellizzi V, et al. Prevalence and prognostic role of resistant hypertension in chronic kidney disease patients. J Am Coll Cardiol. 2013;61:2461–7.

11. Irvin MR, Shimbo D, Mann DM, Reynolds K, Krousel-Wood M, Limdi NA, et al. Prevalence and correlates of low medication adherence in apparent treatment-resistant hypertension. J Clin Hypertens (Greenwich). 2012;14:694–700.
12. Mazzaglia G, Mantovani LG, Sturkenboom MC, Filippi A, Trifiro G, Cricelli C, et al. Patterns of persistence with antihypertensive medications in newly diagnosed hypertensive patients in Italy: a retrospective cohort study in primary care. J Hypertens. 2005;23:2093–100.
13. Van Wijk BL, Klungel OH, Heerdink ER, de Boer A. Rate and determinants of 10-year persistence with antihypertensive drugs. J Hypertens. 2005;23:2101–7.
14. Jung O, Gechter JL, Wunder C, Paulke A, Bartel C, Geiger H, et al. Resistant hypertension? Assessment of adherence by toxicological urine analysis. J Hypertens. 2013;31(4):766–74.
15. Burnier M, Wuerzner G, Struijker-Boudier H, Urquhart J. Measuring, analyzing, and managing drug adherence in resistant hypertension. Hypertension. 2013;62:218–25.
16. Burnier M, Schneider MP, Chiolero A, Stubi CL, Brunner HR. Electronic compliance monitoring in resistant hypertension: the basis for rational therapeutic decisions. J Hypertens. 2001;19:335–41.
17. Bangalore S, Ley L. Improving treatment adherence to antihypertensive therapy: the role of single-pill combinations. Expert Opin Pharmacother. 2012;13:345–55.
18. Salahuddin A, Mushtaq M, Materson BJ. Combination therapy for hypertension 2013: an update. J Am Soc Hypertens. 2013;7:401–7.
19. Pickering TG, Gerin W, Schwartz AR. What is the white-coat effect and how should it be measured? Blood Press Monit. 2002;7:293–300.
20. Muxfeldt ES, Bloch KV, Nogueira AR, Salles GF. True resistant hypertension: is it possible to be recognized in the office? Am J Hypertens. 2005;18:1534–40.
21. Obara T, Ohkubo T, Mano N, Yaegashi N, Kuriyama S, Imai Y. Subtypes of resistant hypertension based on out-of-office blood pressure measurement. Hypertension. 2011. doi:10.1161/HYPERTENSIONAHA.111.178996.
22. de la Sierra A, Segura J, Banegas JR, Gorostidi M, de la Cruz JJ, Armario P, et al. Clinical features of 8295 patients with resistant hypertension classified on the basis of ambulatory blood pressure monitoring. Hypertension. 2011;57:898–902.
23. Gorostidi M, Sarafidis PA, de la Sierra A, Segura J, de la Cruz JJ, Banegas JR, et al. Differences between office and 24-hour blood pressure control in hypertensive patients with CKD: a 5,693-patient cross-sectional analysis from Spain. Am J Kidney Dis. 2013;62:285–94.
24. Pickering TG, Shimbo D, Haas D. Ambulatory blood-pressure monitoring. N Engl J Med. 2006;354:2368–74.
25. Boggia J, Li Y, Thijs L, Kikuya M, Björklund-Bodegård K, Richart T, et al. Prognostic accuracy of day versus night ambulatory blood pressure: a cohort study. Lancet. 2007;370:1219–29.
26. Muxfeldt ES, Cardoso CR, Salles GF. Prognostic value of nocturnal blood pressure reduction in resistant hypertension. Arch Intern Med. 2009;169:874–80.
27. Ohkubo T, Hozawa A, Yamaguchi J, Kikuya M, Ohmori K, Michimata M, et al. Prognostic significance of the nocturnal decline in blood pressure in individuals with and without high 24-h blood pressure: the Ohasama study. J Hypertens. 2002;20:2183–9.
28. Minutolo R, Gabbai FB, Agarwal R, Chiodini P, Borrelli S, Bellizzi V, et al. Assessment of achieved clinic and ambulatory blood pressure recordings and outcomes during treatment in hypertensive patients with CKD: a multicenter prospective cohort study. Am J Kidney Dis. 2014;64:744–52.
29. Agarwal R. Resistant hypertension and the neglected antihypertensive: sodium restriction. Nephrol Dial Transplant. 2012;27:4041–5.
30. Graves JW, Bloomfield RL, Buckalew VM. Plasma volume in resistant hypertension: guide to pathophysiology and therapy. Am J Med Sci. 1989;298:361–5.
31. Pimenta E, Gaddam KK, Oparil S, Aban I, Husain S, Dell'Italia LJ, et al. Effects of dietary sodium reduction on blood pressure in subjects with resistant hypertension: results from a randomized trial. Hypertension. 2009;54:475–81.
32. Dhaun N, Macintyre IM, Melville V, Lilitkarntakul P, Johnston NR, Goddard J, et al. Blood pressure-independent reduction in proteinuria and arterial stiffness after acute endothelin-a receptor antagonism in chronic kidney disease. Hypertension. 2009;54:113–9.

33. Greene EL, Kren S, Hostetter TH. Role of aldosterone in the remnant kidney model in the rat. J Clin Invest. 1996;98:1063–8.
34. Lang CC, Rahman AR, Balfour DJ, Struthers AD. The differential effects of circulating norepinephrine and neuronally released norepinephrine on sodium excretion in humans. Clin Pharmacol Ther. 1993;54:514–22.
35. Lang CC, Rahman AR, Balfour DJ, Struthers AD. Effect of noradrenaline on renal sodium and water handling in euhydrated and overhydrated man. Clin Sci (Lond). 1993;85:487–94.
36. Sarafidis PA, Georgianos PI, Lasaridis AN. Diuretics in clinical practice. Part I: mechanisms of action, pharmacological effects and clinical indications of diuretic compounds. Expert Opin Drug Saf. 2010;9:243–57.
37. Katholi RE. Renal nerves and hypertension: an update. Fed Proc. 1985;44:2846–50.
38. Calaresu FR, Ciriello J. Renal afferent nerves affect discharge rate of medullary and hypothalamic single units in the cat. J Auton Nerv Syst. 1981;3:311–20.
39. Faber JE, Brody MJ. Afferent renal nerve-dependent hypertension following acute renal artery stenosis in the conscious rat. Circ Res. 1985;57:676–88.
40. Bigazzi R, Kogosov E, Campese VM. Altered norepinephrine turnover in the brain of rats with chronic renal failure. J Am Soc Nephrol. 1994;4:1901–7.
41. Converse RL, Jacobsen TN, Toto RD, Jost CM, Cosentino F, Fouad-Tarazi F, et al. Sympathetic overactivity in patients with chronic renal failure. N Engl J Med. 1992;327:1912–8.
42. Ziakas A, Gossios T, Doumas M, Karali K, Megarisiotou A, Stiliadis I. The pathophysiological basis of renal nerve ablation for the treatment of hypertension. Curr Vasc Pharmacol. 2014;12:23–9.
43. Leutscher JA, Johnson BB. Observations on the sodium-retaining corticoid (aldosterone) in the urine of children and adults in relation to sodium balance and edema. J Clin Invest. 1954;33:1441–6.
44. Duprez DA. Aldosterone and the vasculature: mechanisms mediating resistant hypertension. J Clin Hypertens (Greenwich). 2007;9(1 Suppl 1):13–8.
45. Marney AM, Brown NJ. Aldosterone and end-organ damage. Clin Sci (Lond). 2007;113:267–78.
46. Chapman N, Dobson J, Wilson S, Dahlöf B, Sever PS, Wedel H, et al. Effect of spironolactone on blood pressure in subjects with resistant hypertension. Hypertension. 2007;49:839–45.
47. Khosla N, Kalaitzidis R, Bakris GL. Predictors of hyperkalemia risk following hypertension control with aldosterone blockade. Am J Nephrol. 2009;30:418–24.
48. Pisoni R, Acelajado MC, Cartmill FR, Dudenbostel T, Dell'Italia LJ, Cofield SS, et al. Long-term effects of aldosterone blockade in resistant hypertension associated with chronic kidney disease. J Hum Hypertens. 2012;26:502–6.
49. Georgianos PI, Sarafidis PA, Liakopoulos V. Arterial stiffness: a novel risk factor for kidney injury progression? Am J Hypertens. 2015;28:958–65.
50. Briet M, Boutouyrie P, Laurent S, London GM. Arterial stiffness and pulse pressure in CKD and ESRD. Kidney Int. 2012;82:388–400.
51. Protogerou A, Blacher J, Stergiou GS, Achimastos A, Safar ME. Blood pressure response under chronic antihypertensive drug therapy: the role of aortic stiffness in the REASON (Preterax in Regression of Arterial Stiffness in a Controlled Double-Blind) study. J Am Coll Cardiol. 2009;53:445–51.
52. Kaess BM, Rong J, Larson MG, Hamburg NM, Vita JA, Levy D, et al. Aortic stiffness, blood pressure progression, and incident hypertension. JAMA. 2012;308:875–81.
53. Georgianos PI, Agarwal R. Aortic stiffness, ambulatory blood pressure, and predictors of response to antihypertensive therapy in hemodialysis. Am J Kidney Dis. 2015;66:305–12.
54. Vaziri ND, Ni Z, Wang XQ, Oveisi F, Zhou XJ. Downregulation of nitric oxide synthase in chronic renal insufficiency: role of excess PTH. Am J Physiol. 1998;274:F642–9.
55. Raptis V, Kapoulas S, Grekas D. Role of asymmetrical dimethylarginine in the progression of renal disease. Nephrology (Carlton). 2013;18:11–21.
56. Schepers E, Barreto DV, Liabeuf S, Glorieux G, Eloot S, Barreto FC, et al. Symmetric dimethylarginine as a proinflammatory agent in chronic kidney disease. Clin J Am Soc Nephrol. 2011;6:2374–83.

57. Dhaun N, Goddard J, Webb DJ. The endothelin system and its antagonism in chronic kidney disease. J Am Soc Nephrol. 2006;17:943–55.
58. Laffin LJ, Bakris GL. Endothelin antagonism and hypertension: an evolving target. Semin Nephrol. 2015;35:168–75.
59. Cutler JA, Sorlie PD, Wolz M, Thom T, Fields LE, Roccella EJ. Trends in hypertension prevalence, awareness, treatment, and control rates in United States adults between 1988-1994 and 1999-2004. Hypertension. 2008;52:818–27.
60. Dahlof B, Devereux RB, Kjeldsen SE, Julius S, Beevers G, de Faire U, et al. Cardiovascular morbidity and mortality in the Losartan Intervention For Endpoint reduction in hypertension study (LIFE): a randomised trial against atenolol. Lancet. 2002;359:995–1003.
61. Garg JP, Elliott WJ, Folker A, Izhar M, Black HR. Resistant hypertension revisited: a comparison of two university-based cohorts. Am J Hypertens. 2005;18:619–26.
62. Hajjar I, Kotchen TA. Trends in prevalence, awareness, treatment, and control of hypertension in the United States, 1988-2000. JAMA. 2003;290:199–206.
63. Pepine CJ, Handberg EM, Cooper-DeHoff RM, Marks RG, Kowey P, Messerli FH, et al. A calcium antagonist vs a non-calcium antagonist hypertension treatment strategy for patients with coronary artery disease. The International Verapamil-Trandolapril Study (INVEST): a randomized controlled trial. JAMA. 2003;290:2805–16.
64. McAdam-Marx C, Ye X, Sung JC, Brixner DI, Kahler KH. Results of a retrospective, observational pilot study using electronic medical records to assess the prevalence and characteristics of patients with resistant hypertension in an ambulatory care setting. Clin Ther. 2009;31:1116–23.
65. Persell SD. Prevalence of resistant hypertension in the United States, 2003-2008. Hypertension. 2011;57:1076–80.
66. Egan BM, Zhao Y, Axon RN, Brzezinski WA, Ferdinand KC. Uncontrolled and apparent treatment resistant hypertension in the United States, 1988 to 2008. Circulation. 2011;124:1046–58.
67. Sim JJ, Bhandari SK, Shi J, Liu IL, Calhoun DA, McGlynn EA, et al. Characteristics of resistant hypertension in a large, ethnically diverse hypertension population of an integrated health system. Mayo Clin Proc. 2013;88:1099–107.
68. Brambilla G, Bombelli M, Seravalle G, Cifkova R, Laurent S, Narkiewicz K, et al. Prevalence and clinical characteristics of patients with true resistant hypertension in central and Eastern Europe: data from the BP-CARE study. J Hypertens. 2013;31:2018–24.
69. Weitzman D, Chodick G, Shalev V, Grossman C, Grossman E. Prevalence and factors associated with resistant hypertension in a large health maintenance organization in Israel. Hypertension. 2014;64:501–7.
70. De Nicola L, Borrelli S, Gabbai FB, Chiodini P, Zamboli P, Iodice C, et al. Burden of resistant hypertension in hypertensive patients with non-dialysis chronic kidney disease. Kidney Blood Press Res. 2011;34:58–67.
71. Tanner RM, Calhoun DA, Bell EK, Bowling CB, Gutiérrez OM, Irvin MR, et al. Prevalence of apparent treatment-resistant hypertension among individuals with CKD. Clin J Am Soc Nephrol. 2013;8:1583–90.
72. Parati G, Stergiou GS, Asmar R, Bilo G, de Leeuw P, Imai Y, et al. European Society of Hypertension practice guidelines for home blood pressure monitoring. J Hum Hypertens. 2010;24:779–85.
73. Gupta AK, Nasothimiou EG, Chang CL, Sever PS, Dahlof B, Poulter NR. Baseline predictors of resistant hypertension in the Anglo-Scandinavian Cardiac Outcome Trial (ASCOT): a risk score to identify those at high-risk. J Hypertens. 2011;29:2004–13.
74. Mancia G, Fagard R, Narkiewicz K, Redon J, Zanchetti A, Böhm M, et al. 2013 ESH/ESC Guidelines for the management of arterial hypertension: the Task Force for the management of arterial hypertension of the European Society of Hypertension (ESH) and of the European Society of Cardiology (ESC). J Hypertens. 2013;31:1281–357.

75. Cuspidi C, Macca G, Sampieri L, Michev I, Salerno M, Fusi V, et al. High prevalence of cardiac and extracardiac target organ damage in refractory hypertension. J Hypertens. 2001;19:2063–70.
76. de la Sierra A, Banegas JR, Oliveras A, Gorostidi M, Segura J, de la Cruz JJ, et al. Clinical differences between resistant hypertensives and patients treated and controlled with three or less drugs. J Hypertens. 2012;30:1211–6.
77. Pierdomenico SD, Lapenna D, Bucci A, Di Tommaso R, Di Mascio R, Manente BM, et al. Cardiovascular outcome in treated hypertensive patients with responder, masked, false resistant, and true resistant hypertension. Am J Hypertens. 2005;18:1422–8.
78. Muxfeldt ES, Cardoso CR, Dias VB, Nascimento AC, Salles GF. Prognostic impact of the ambulatory arterial stiffness index in resistant hypertension. J Hypertens. 2010;28:1547–53.
79. Salles GF, Cardoso CR, Muxfeldt ES. Prognostic influence of office and ambulatory blood pressures in resistant hypertension. Arch Intern Med. 2008;168:2340–6.
80. Kumbhani DJ, Steg PG, Cannon CP, Eagle KA, Smith Jr SC, Goto S, et al. Resistant hypertension: a frequent and ominous finding among hypertensive patients with atherothrombosis. Eur Heart J. 2013;34:1204–14.
81. Tanner RM, Calhoun DA, Bell EK, Bowling CB, Gutiérrez OM, Irvin MR, et al. Incident ESRD and treatment-resistant hypertension: the reasons for geographic and racial differences in stroke (REGARDS) study. Am J Kidney Dis. 2014;63:781–8.
82. Muntner P, Davis BR, Cushman WC, Bangalore S, Calhoun DA, Pressel SL, et al. Treatment-resistant hypertension and the incidence of cardiovascular disease and end-stage renal disease: results from the Antihypertensive and Lipid-Lowering Treatment to Prevent Heart Attack Trial (ALLHAT). Hypertension. 2014;64:1012–21.
83. Smith SM, Gong Y, Handberg E, Messerli FH, Bakris GL, Ahmed A, et al. Predictors and outcomes of resistant hypertension among patients with coronary artery disease and hypertension. J Hypertens. 2014;32:635–43.

Chapter 6
Hypertension in Pregnancy

Sharon Maynard

Physiology of Pregnancy

Pregnancy is characterized by marked vascular and hemodynamic changes. Early in pregnancy, systemic vasodilation leads to decreased systemic vascular resistance and increased arterial compliance [1]. These changes are evident by 6 weeks of gestation [2]. These primary vascular changes lead to several other hemodynamic changes. Diastolic blood pressure falls by an average of 5 mmHg by the late second trimester [3]. Sympathetic activity is increased, reflected in a 15 % increase in heart rate [4]. The combination of increased heart rate and decreased afterload leads to a large increase in cardiac output by the early first trimester [5], which peaks at 50 % above pre-pregnancy levels in the third trimester [4, 6].

The renin–aldosterone–angiotensin system is activated in pregnancy [3, 7]. This is driven by several factors, including extrarenal renin secretion by the ovaries and maternal decidua, a stimulatory effect of estrogen on renal renin release, and primary vasodilation. This leads to salt and water retention. Increased renal interstitial compliance may also contribute to volume retention, via an attenuation of the renal pressure natriuretic response [8]. Total body water increases by 6–8 l, leading to both plasma volume and interstitial volume expansion—hence most women have demonstrable clinical edema at some point during pregnancy. There is also cumulative retention of about 1000 mmol of sodium distributed between the maternal extracellular compartments and the fetus [9]. The plasma volume increases out of proportion to the red blood cell mass, leading to mild physiologic anemia.

The mechanism of vasodilatation in pregnancy is not fully understood. The decrease in systemic vascular resistance is only partially attributable to the presence

S. Maynard, MD (✉)
Associate Professor of Medicine, University of South Florida Morsani
College of Medicine, Lehigh Valley Health Network, 1230 South Cedar Crest Blvd.,
Suite 301, Allentown, PA 18103, USA
e-mail: Sharon_e.maynard@lvhn.org

© Springer Science+Business Media New York 2016
A.K. Singh, R. Agarwal (eds.), *Core Concepts in Hypertension in Kidney Disease*, DOI 10.1007/978-1-4939-6436-9_6

of the low-resistance circulation in the pregnant uterus, as blood pressure and systemic vascular resistance are noted to fall before this system is well developed. Reduced vascular responsiveness to vasopressors such as angiotensin 2 and vasopressin is well documented [10–12].

The hormone relaxin contributes to the global vasodilatory response [13]. Relaxin is a 6-kDa peptide hormone, structurally similar to insulin. Relaxin is released predominantly from the corpus luteum, rising early in gestation in response to human chorionic gonadotrophin (hCG). In the renal circulation, relaxin increases endothelin and nitric oxide production, leading to generalized renal vasodilation and decreased renal afferent and efferent arteriolar resistance [14, 15]. This increases both renal blood flow and glomerular filtration rate, despite high levels of sympathetic activity, renin, angiotensin II, and aldosterone.

Classification of Hypertensive Pregnancy

Hypertension in pregnancy is classified into four categories: preeclampsia-eclampsia, chronic hypertension, chronic hypertension with superimposed preeclampsia, and gestational hypertension. Figure 6.1 outlines the clinical approach to diagnostic evaluation of women with hypertension in pregnancy. The diagnosis of chronic hypertension in pregnancy is based on a history of hypertension prior to pregnancy, or a blood pressure above 140/90 mmHg prior to 20 weeks gestation. Gestational hypertension and preeclampsia are characterized by the new onset of hypertension after 20 weeks gestation, and hypertension resolves after delivery in most cases. Distinguishing chronic hypertension from gestational hypertension/preeclampsia based on the gestational age of the first recorded blood pressure elevation can be subject to pitfalls, however. Some women lack consistent pre-pregnancy and prenatal care, and early pregnancy blood pressure readings are not available. The physiologic dip in blood pressure in the second trimester, which nadirs at about 28 weeks gestation [3], can mask the presence of chronic hypertension in mid-pregnancy. In cases of diagnostic uncertainty, the failure of blood pressure to normalize postpartum confirms the diagnosis of chronic hypertension. The section "Diagnosis of Preeclampsia and Superimposed Preeclampsia" includes a detailed discussion of regarding diagnosis of preeclampsia and superimposed preeclampsia.

Chronic Hypertension in Pregnancy

The prevalence of chronic hypertension in pregnancy in the USA is increasing, from 1.0 % in 1995–1996 to 1.76 % in 2007–2008 [16]. Hypertension in pregnancy is more common in women of advanced maternal age and black race [17]. It is associated with several medical comorbidities, including obesity, diabetes mellitus, chronic renal disease, thyroid disease, and collagen vascular disease [16].

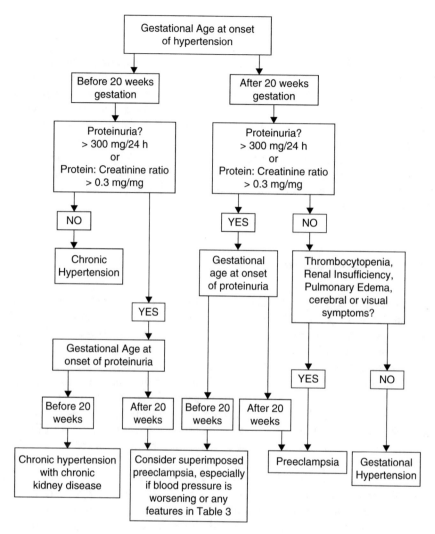

Fig. 6.1 Diagnostic evaluation of hypertension in pregnancy

There are several goals of care in the assessment and management of chronic hypertension in women who are pregnant or planning pregnancy. First, the diagnosis should be established, including assessment for secondary causes of hypertension and end-organ damage. The pregnancy risks (see section "Renovascular Hypertension") should be communicated to the patient. The blood pressure should be managed, including the appropriate use of antihypertensive medications that are safe in pregnancy. Strategies to reduce the risk of preeclampsia, including the use of low-dose aspirin, should be considered. The patient should be monitored for the development of preeclampsia. These goals of care will be reviewed in detail in the following sections.

Secondary Hypertension

The prevalence of secondary causes of hypertension in pregnancy is unknown, but is probably similar to that seen in healthy non-pregnant hypertensive women of childbearing age. In one retrospective study, 25 % of women in whom hypertension failed to resolve 6 months following preeclampsia were found to have a secondary cause of hypertension (primary aldosteronism and renovascular hypertension) [18]. Findings suggestive of a secondary cause of hypertension include severe or refractory hypertension, onset of hypertension at young age (<35 years), absence of family history, and the presence of hypokalemia or palpitations. Secondary hypertension should also be suspected after preeclampsia, when blood pressure fails to resolve following delivery.

Primary Aldosteronism

A population-based study in the USA reported a diagnosis of primary aldosteronism (PA) in 0.02 % of pregnancies with chronic hypertension [16], and fewer than 50 cases of primary aldosteronism in pregnancy have been described in the literature [19]. However, its true incidence is probably much higher, as primary aldosteronism is estimated to affect up to 10 % of non-pregnant patients with chronic hypertension.

Pregnancy is associated with changes in progesterone and the renin–angiotensin–aldosterone system that provide challenges to diagnosis and affect the clinical course of PA. Progesterone, which is increased throughout pregnancy, acts as a competitive antagonist to aldosterone at the mineralocorticoid receptor in the collecting tubule [20]. This mitigates the hypokalemia and hypertension that might be expected from the high plasma aldosterone concentrations of normal pregnancy. For women with primary aldosteronism, the antagonistic effect of progesterone at the mineralocorticoid receptor sometimes leads to improvement in hypertension and hyperkalemia. However, such remission is not universal and women with primary aldosteronism may have a pregnancy-induced exacerbation of hypertension and hypokalemia [21].

The diagnosis of PA should be considered in all hypertensive women who are pregnant or considering pregnancy, particularly if hypokalemia is present. Screening and diagnosis of PA during pregnancy can be challenging owing to the physiologic activation of the renin–angiotensin–aldosterone system in pregnancy. In normal pregnancy, plasma renin activity and aldosterone concentrations are typically five to tenfold higher than in the non-pregnant state [3]. The major indicator of the presence of PA in pregnancy is suppression of the plasma renin activity [19]. The aldosterone–renin ratio is useful when abnormal, however false negatives can occur, primarily due to pregnancy-induced stimulation of renin production [22]. Standard suppression testing with salt loading is not advisable due to potential exacerbation of hypertension, and adrenal vein sampling during pregnancy is not recommended due to the requisite radiation exposure.

Most cases of PA in pregnancy result from an aldosterone-producing adenoma (APA) [23]. Imaging with MRI or ultrasound is safe. Since non-functional adenomas are rare in women under 50, the diagnosis of APA vs. idiopathic adrenal hyperplasia (IAH) can often be made with imaging alone.

For women diagnosed with aldosterone-producing adenoma during pregnancy, there is little data to favor either immediate surgical adrenalectomy versus medical management until after delivery, though case reports have suggested success with both approaches. Conventional wisdom and expert opinion suggest surgical adrenalectomy is the optimal treatment in the first and early second trimesters, while medical management is often favored after fetal viability (23 weeks gestation) [24].

For women with IAH or APA who are managed medically, adequate blood pressure control is important, as most adverse pregnancy outcomes occur when blood pressure is uncontrolled [19]. Although there are several case reports of the use of spironolactone in pregnancy without adverse fetal effects, there is a theoretical risk of feminization and ambiguous genitalia in male fetuses and it is generally avoided in pregnancy. Eplerenone is a selective mineralocorticoid antagonist without clinically significant antiandrogenic effects. Animal studies have not shown any adverse fetal effects, and case reports describe its safe use in humans [24]. Hence, it is generally considered safe in pregnancy. Blood pressure targets are similar to those recommended in women with chronic primary hypertension in pregnancy: between 120/80 and 160/105 for women without evidence of target organ damage, and below 140/90 for women with evidence of target organ damage.

Renovascular Hypertension

Renovascular hypertension, particularly due to fibromuscular dysplasia, occasionally presents in pregnancy. Published experience with renovascular hypertension in pregnancy is limited to case series and case reports. Renovascular hypertension during pregnancy is characterized by extremely high vascular resistance, likely mediated by high circulating angiotensin 2 levels [25]. Unrecognized renovascular hypertension in pregnancy can present as accelerated hypertension, or early or severe preeclampsia [26]. Neonatal complications are common, including iatrogenic preterm delivery, placental abruption, and fetal demise. Computed tomography (CT) is usually avoided in pregnancy due to fetal radiation exposure, but renal ultrasound with Doppler and magnetic resonance (MR) angiography are both safe diagnostic studies.

With regard to treatment, there is little evidence to guide the decision regarding revasularization vs. medical management. ACE inhibitors and angiotensin receptor antagonists are contraindicated in pregnancy. If blood pressure can be controlled medically with agents suitable for pregnancy, intervention can be deferred until after delivery. Successful angioplasty and stent placement in the second and third trimesters of pregnancy has been described in patients with refractory hypertension

[25, 27]. Radiation exposure should be minimized (<5 rad) or avoided, particularly during fetal organogenesis in the first trimester. Surgical repair during pregnancy is not a viable option, as cross clamping of the aorta may result in compromised placental perfusion.

Pheochromocytoma

Although rare, pheochromocytoma can be devastating when it first presents during pregnancy. This syndrome occasionally is unmasked during labor and delivery, when fatal hypertensive crisis can be triggered by labor and spinal anesthesia [28]. Maternal and neonatal morbidity and mortality are as high as 50 % when the diagnosis is made during labor or after delivery, but much lower (less than 15 %) when the diagnosis is made antepartum [29]. Since prenatal diagnosis significantly impacts both perinatal management and fetal and maternal mortality, the clinician needs to have a high level of suspicion for pheochromocytoma despite its low incidence.

Most women diagnosed with pheochromocytoma during pregnancy present in the second or third trimester with hypertension, palpitations, chest pain, pallor, sweating, nausea, or abdominal pain [29]. Paroxysmal, orthostatic, or severe hypertension with complications such as pulmonary edema and heart failure should lead to consideration of pheochromocytoma. Although standard diagnostic testing for pheochromocytoma has not been specifically validated in pregnancy, there are no significant alterations in catecholamine metabolism in pregnancy [23]. Thus, diagnosis is established as with non-pregnant individuals, with the measurement of abnormally high levels of plasma or urine catecholamines. Ultrasound and MRI can be used for imaging and tumor localization.

Once the diagnosis of pheochromocytoma has been established, management options include timely surgical removal or medical management with alpha-blockade until delivery. Among women diagnosed prior to 23 weeks, laparoscopic removal of the tumor during pregnancy appears to result in somewhat better neonatal outcomes in case reports and case series [29]. Alpha-adrenergic blockers such as phenoxybenzamine can be safely used in pregnancy. Beta-blockade, with labetalol or selective beta-blockers such as propranolol, should be initiated only after alpha-blockade is established. Sodium restriction should not be prescribed, especially in the weeks preceding surgical resection, as volume depletion increases the likelihood of postoperative hypotension [23].

If medical management until delivery is elected, labor and vaginal delivery should be avoided, as labor can trigger severe hypertensive crisis. Prenatal consultation should be obtained with an anesthesiologist with expertise in pheochromocytoma. Resection of the pheochromocytoma can be successfully performed at the time of cesarean section, or following delivery [30].

Genetic Causes of Hypertension and Hypokalemia

Glucocorticoid-remediable aldosteronism, or familial hyperaldosteronism type 1 (FH-1), results from a hybrid recombination of the 11beta-hydroxylase and aldosterone synthase genes. This leads to an abnormal aldosterone synthase protein in which aldosterone synthesis is regulated by adrenocorticotropin (ACTH). Most women with FH-1 have stabilization or improvement in their hypertension and hyperkalemia during pregnancy [31]. This may be due to the antagonistic effects of progesterone on the mineralocorticoid receptor, as noted above. Progesterone also appears to directly inhibit both wild-type and chimeric aldosterone synthase genes, which may lead to amelioration of aldosterone production during pregnancy [32].

Geller syndrome is a rare cause of early onset hypertension arising from an activating mutation of the mineralocorticoid receptor. This results in inappropriate receptor activation by progesterone, and affected women develop a marked exacerbation of hypertension and hypokalemia in pregnancy, but without proteinuria or other features of preeclampsia [33]. Geller syndrome clinically resembles primary aldosteronism, but aldosterone levels are low-normal, with a normal aldosterone:renin ratio.

Cushing Syndrome

Hypercortisolism, or Cushing syndrome, is a relatively uncommon cause of hypertension in pregnancy. The clinical clues that usually suggest the diagnosis of Cushing syndrome may not be recognized, as they resemble symptoms of pregnancy itself: weight gain, edema, moon facies, abdominal striae, and glucose intolerance. Diagnosis is challenging, as both serum and urine cortisol are increased in normal pregnancy. The best initial screening test is a 24-hour urine collection for free cortisol, with cortisol excretion greater than 2 times the upper limit of normal strongly suggesting hypercortisolism [34]. Further details on the evaluation and management of Cushing syndrome in pregnancy are reviewed elsewhere [23].

Evaluation for End-Organ Damage

The presence of end-organ damage in women with chronic hypertension in pregnancy may impact the therapeutic blood pressure target (see Pharmacotherapy: Blood Pressure Target). Initial evaluation should always include measurement of a basic metabolic panel and quantification of urine protein. The presence of an elevated serum creatinine concentration or proteinuria can signify chronic kidney disease, which may be both a cause and a consequence of hypertension. If chronic kidney disease is present without apparent cause, renal ultrasound should be performed to evaluate for renal atrophy or polycystic kidneys. Proteinuria in early pregnancy in women with chronic hypertension is associated with an increased risk of intrauterine growth restriction and preterm delivery [35]. The detection of hypokalemia can indicate the presence of other secondary forms of hypertension, such as primary aldosteronism or renovascular hypertension. Early measurement of creatinine and proteinuria establishes a baseline, which can be helpful in the subsequent diagnosis of superimposed preeclampsia. Echocardiogram to evaluate for left ventricular hypertrophy should be considered, particularly in women with severe or longstanding hypertension.

Risk Assessment and Counseling

Women with chronic hypertension in pregnancy have an increased risk of several adverse pregnancy outcomes. Superimposed preeclampsia complicates approximately 25% of these pregnancies [35], and risk is even higher when other preeclampsia risk factors such as diabetes, obesity, or prior preeclampsia are present (see Table 6.1) [36–47]. Hypertension is associated with an increased risk of premature delivery (23–35%), intrauterine growth restriction (13–21%), placental abruption (1–3%), and perinatal mortality (3–5%) [36]. However, most adverse fetal and neonatal outcomes occur in women with uncontrolled hypertension (diastolic blood pressure >110 mmHg), superimposed preeclampsia, or preexisting cardiovascular and renal disease (ACOG practice bulletin 2013) [48]. Although the duration and the severity of hypertension are correlated with perinatal morbidity and preeclampsia risk [49, 50], the treatment of hypertension with medications does not appear to prevent these adverse outcomes (see Sect. 6.3.4.3). Women with mild, uncomplicated chronic hypertension usually have obstetric outcomes comparable to the general population [17]. The presence of baseline proteinuria increases the risk of preterm delivery and IUGR, but not preeclampsia per se [35].

Table 6.1 Risk factors for preeclampsia	
	Prior preeclampsia [37]
	Renal disease [38]
	Chronic hypertension [39]
	Diabetes mellitus [37]
	Primiparity [40]
	Systemic lupus erythematosis [41]
	Antiphospholipid antibody syndrome [37]
	Multiple gestations [42]
	Strong family history of cardiovascular disease [43]
	Obesity (body mass index >30 kg/m^2) [44]
	Family history of preeclampsia [45]
	Advanced maternal age (>40 years) [37, 46]
	Excessive gestational weight gain (>35 lbs) [47]

Management of Chronic Hypertension in Pregnancy

Minimizing Preeclampsia Risk

The most effective measure for reducing preeclampsia risk among high-risk women, including those with chronic hypertension, is the early initiation of low-dose aspirin (pooled relative risk 0.76, 95 % CI, 0.62–0.95) [51]. When started early in pregnancy (before 16 weeks), aspirin may reduce the relative risk of preeclampsia by nearly 50 %[52]. Whether later initiation of aspirin provides benefit is less clear. Early ASA appears to be particularly effective in preventing severe and early onset preeclampsia, and also reduces risk of intrauterine growth restriction [52, 53]. Most trials demonstrating benefit used dosages of 60–100 mg/d [51]. Aspirin is typically held after 36 weeks gestation, to minimize theoretical risk of postpartum hemorrhage.

Daily calcium supplementation (1.5–2.0 g/d) appears to lower preeclampsia risk, particularly in populations with low baseline calcium intake and women at high preeclampsia risk [54]. Low-dose calcium (<1 g/d) may be similarly effective [55].

Other interventions to reduce preeclampsia risk have generally demonstrated little or no beneficial effect. These include vitamin C and vitamin E, bed rest, and dietary sodium restriction. A large randomized controlled trial is currently underway to assess the effect of folic acid supplementation on preeclampsia risk [56]. Vitamin D deficiency is associated with increased preeclampsia risk [57], but trials demonstrating a benefit of vitamin D supplementation are lacking. Neither sodium restriction nor diuretics appear to reduce the risk of preeclampsia [58, 59].

Non-Pharmacologic Interventions for Hypertension Control

In non-pregnant individuals, non-pharmacologic management strategies for hypertension include regular aerobic exercise, weight loss (for overweight and obese individuals), and a diet low in sodium and rich in fruits and vegetables (DASH diet). None of these interventions has been rigorously evaluated in pregnant women with hypertension. A meta-analysis of 15 observational studies found reduced preeclampsia risk with increasing levels of physical activity before and during pregnancy [60]. Hence, regular aerobic exercise is recommended for hypertensive pregnant women, so long as they are accustomed to exercise and their blood pressure is well controlled [61].

Weight loss during pregnancy is not recommended, even in obese individuals. The 2009 Institute of Medicine (IOM) guidelines specifies gestational weight gain targets based on pre-pregnancy body mass index [62]. Normal weight women are advised to gain between 25 and 35 lbs during the course of gestation; obese women (BMI ≥ 30 kg/m²) are advised to gain between 11 and 20 lbs. Weight gain in excess of these amounts is associated with an increased risk of preeclampsia and eclampsia [63]. Although gestational weight gain has not been specifically studied in hypertensive women, avoiding weight gain in excess of the IOM guidelines should be avoided.

Dietary sodium restriction lowers blood pressure and is associated with a decreased risk of cardiovascular disease in non-pregnant individuals [64]. Thus, dietary sodium restriction (<2.0 g/day) is recommended in non-pregnant hypertensive individuals by several major national and international organizations. In pregnancy, dietary sodium restriction could theoretically interfere with the physiologic plasma volume expansion of pregnancy. There are no studies on the effects of dietary sodium restriction in hypertensive pregnant women. The American College of Obstetrics and Gynecology 2013 Task Force suggests that dietary sodium restriction not be used in this setting [65].

Pharmacotherapy: Blood Pressure Target

When hypertension is severe (>160/105 mmHg), antihypertensive therapy is clearly indicated for the prevention of acute stroke and cardiovascular complications [61]. Treatment of mild and moderate hypertension in pregnancy is controversial. The 8th Joint National Commission recommends treating hypertension in members of the general population <60 years to a target blood pressure of less than 140/90 mmHg [66]. However, the strength of recommendation for the 18–29 age group is weak (grade E, expert opinion). Even for women over age 30, the evidence upon which the JNC guidelines are based uniformly excluded pregnant women.

There is little evidence that treatment of mild to moderate hypertension has a short-term benefit for either mother or fetus. Several small clinical trials have evaluated the impact of antihypertensive therapy vs. no treatment in such women, and these have been evaluated in meta-analyses [67–69]. Although antihypertensive therapy lowers the risk of severe hypertension, there is no beneficial effect on the development of preeclampsia, neonatal death, preterm birth, small for gestational age babies, or other adverse outcomes [70].

Potential maternal benefits of antihypertensive treatment need to be balanced against potential adverse fetal effects. Some evidence suggests that aggressive treatment of mild to moderate hypertension in pregnancy may impair fetal growth. Treatment-induced falls in mean arterial pressure are associated with decreased birth weight and fetal growth restriction, presumably as a result of decreased uteroplacental perfusion [71]. For this reason, the American College of Obstetrics and Gynecology Task Force on Hypertension in Pregnancy recommends against antihypertensive medication use in pregnant women with chronic hypertension and BP less than 160/105 mmHg in the absence of evidence of end-organ damage [61]. Similarly, the Seventh Report of the Joint National Committee on Prevention, Detection, Evaluation, and Treatment of High Blood pressure (JNC7) recommends initiating antihypertensive therapy only when maternal blood pressure exceeds 150/100 mmHg [72]. JNC 8 provides no recommendation regarding treatment of hypertension in pregnancy [66]. For women with end-organ damage, such as cardiac hypertrophy or chronic kidney disease, the ACOG Task Force suggests a blood pressure goal of less than 140/90 mmHg [61].

The Control of Hypertension in Pregnancy Study (CHIPS) recently added to the evidence base on this issue [73]. This was an open, multicenter, randomized trial in 987 women with mild to moderate, nonproteinuric gestational or chronic hypertension. Women were randomized to treatment with pharmacotherapy to achieve tight (DBP target <85 mmHg) vs. less-tight (DBP target <100 mmHg) blood pressure control. There were no significant differences in adverse neonatal outcomes (pregnancy loss or need for high-level neonatal care) between treatment groups. However, the less-tight control group had a higher incidence of severe hypertension, thrombocytopenia, elevated AST or ALT with symptoms, and a trend toward a higher incidence of HELLP syndrome. There was no difference between treatment groups in the incidence of IUGR or preeclampsia. The study was not powered to detect a difference in maternal cardiovascular events, and follow-up was short. A major contribution of this trial, the largest and most well designed to date, was the assurance that tight blood pressure control was not associated with intrauterine growth restriction or other adverse neonatal effects. Based on these data, it is reasonable to treat hypertension in pregnancy to a diastolic blood pressure goal of less than 85 mmHg.

Monitoring of Women with Chronic Hypertension in Pregnancy

Close monitoring of blood pressure is important throughout pregnancy. Blood pressure often falls through the first half of pregnancy, and rises in the last trimester, requiring adjustments in medication. After 20 weeks gestation, monitoring for superimposed preeclampsia is required (see section "Diagnosis of Preeclampsia and Superimposed Preeclampsia"). This is accomplished through close blood pressure monitoring, frequent urinalysis for detection of proteinuria, and screening for preeclampsia symptoms. Dipstick testing is routinely used for preeclampsia screening; results ≥1+ should be confirmed with a random urine protein:creatinine ratio or 24-hour urine collection for proteinuria. Women with chronic hypertension in pregnancy should be educated regarding signs and symptoms of preeclampsia, including headache, visual changes, edema, and upper abdominal pain. The use of home blood pressure monitoring using an automated cuff is useful both for ensuring appropriate dosing of antihypertensive medication and for preeclampsia surveillance [61]. Patients should be instructed on proper use of home blood pressure monitors, and instructed to call their provider if they have an increase in blood pressure, particularly when associated with signs or symptoms of preeclampsia. Women with suspected superimposed preeclampsia should be hospitalized for maternal and fetal evaluation and monitoring [61].

Hypertension in pregnancy should be managed by an obstetrician with expertise in high risk pregnancies. Consultation with a maternal–fetal medicine physician is often helpful. Due to the increased risk for intrauterine growth restriction, fetal monitoring with ultrasound and antenatal fetal testing is recommended in women with chronic hypertension.

Intrapartum and Postpartum Care

Oral antihypertensive medications are frequently held during labor and delivery without adverse effects if hypertension is relatively mild. For women with more severe hypertension in pregnancy, intravenous agents can be used in the peripartum period (see section "Intravenous Agents"). Medications should be resumed following delivery, unless blood pressure is low. Blood pressure should be reassessed within 6 weeks postpartum. For women with an indication for an ACE-I or ARB, these medications are safe in breastfeeding and can be safely started immediately following delivery.

Gestational Hypertension and Preeclampsia

Gestational Hypertension

Gestational hypertension is defined as the new onset of hypertension, without proteinuria, after 20 weeks gestation. A subset of women with gestational hypertension have unrecognized preexisting chronic hypertension. In such cases, if the woman presents for medical care during the second-trimester nadir in blood pressure, she may be inappropriately presumed to be previously normotensive. In such a circumstance the diagnosis of chronic hypertension is established postpartum, when blood pressure fails to return to normal.

Gestational hypertension progresses to overt preeclampsia in 10–25 % of cases [74]. When gestational hypertension is severe, it carries similar risks for adverse outcomes as preeclampsia, even in the absence of proteinuria [75]. A renal biopsy study suggests that a significant proportion of women with gestational hypertension have renal glomerular endothelial damage [76]. Hence, gestational hypertension may share the same pathophysiologic underpinnings as preeclampsia, and should be monitored and treated as such. For these reasons, the American College of Obstetric and Gynecology guidelines no longer require proteinuria for the diagnosis of preeclampsia if severe features are present (see Table 6.2).

Preeclampsia

Preeclampsia is a pregnancy-specific syndrome characterized by hypertension and proteinuria, with onset in the second half of pregnancy. Preeclampsia affects 3–5 % of all pregnancies [49]. Although most cases of preeclampsia occur in healthy nulliparous women, several maternal and pregnancy risk factors are associated with a marked increase in preeclampsia risk (Table 6.1). Preeclampsia can lead to the development of severe maternal and fetal/neonatal complications. Maternal complications may include liver failure, hepatic hematoma or rupture, pulmonary edema,

Table 6.2 Features of severe preeclampsia

Feature	Comment
Severe hypertension	SBP ≥160 mmHg or diastolic blood pressure ≥110 mmHg on two occasions at least 4 h apart (lower threshold may be applied if treated with antihypertensive medications). Treat with oral or intravenous agents
Thrombocytopenia	Platelet count less than 100,000/mcl
Microangiopathic hemolytic anemia	Schistocytes on peripheral smear Low haptoglobin, elevated bilirubin, and/or lactate dehydrogenase levels
Impaired liver function	Liver enzymes >2-fold above normal
Severe persistent right upper quadrant pain or epigastric pain	May indicate liver injury
Progressive renal insufficiency	Serum creatinine >1.1 mg/dl or doubling of serum creatinine, in the absence of other reason for renal disease
Dyspnea	Pulmonary edema should be treated with loop diuretics
Persistent and/or severe headache	Can indicate erebral edema
Confusion/encephalopathy	Can indicate erebral edema
Visual disturbances	Blurry vision, scotomata, photophobia
Eclampsia	Seizures should be treated with magnesium sulfate

seizures (eclampsia), hypertensive encephalopathy, intracranial hemorrhage, renal failure, placental abruption, and death. For the fetus, preeclampsia can lead to intrauterine growth restriction, placental abruption, stillbirth, and neonatal death [77, 78]. Severe maternal complications can usually be avoided with careful prenatal monitoring and expedient delivery when severe features emerge. Since delivery is the definitive treatment for preeclampsia, premature delivery for maternal or fetal distress is often required, with consequent neonatal morbidity.

Pathogenesis

The preeclampsia syndrome is characterized by widespread maternal endothelial dysfunction [79]. Inadequate placental vascular development is an early event, particularly in early onset preeclampsia [80]. This early placental vascular insufficiency is incompletely understood, with genetic, immunologic, and environmental factors all playing a role. Preeclampsia is a state of sympathetic overactivity. Maternal vascular reactivity to the vasopressors angiotensin II and norepinephrine is increased [81]. In normal pregnancy, the renin–angiotensin–aldosterone system is activated; in preeclampsia, plasma renin levels are low [82].

The full-blown preeclampsia syndrome culminates in oxidative stress, endothelial damage, and maternal end-organ dysfunction. Maternal diseases characterized by vascular dysfunction, such as diabetes mellitus, chronic hypertension, chronic kidney disease, and obesity, are associated with increased preeclampsia risk. This suggests that maternal susceptibility contributes to pathogenesis. Molecular and cellular pathways linking placental insufficiency to subsequent maternal endothelial dysfunction include angiogenic factors such as sFlt1 (VEGFR1), angiotensin-2 receptor autoantibodies, immunologic factors, and oxidative stress. A full discussion of the pathogenesis of preeclampsia is beyond the scope of this book and is reviewed elsewhere [83].

Diagnosis of Preeclampsia and Superimposed Preeclampsia

The diagnostic criteria for preeclampsia are in evolution. Historically, preeclampsia was defined by the new onset of hypertension (SBP >140 mmHg or DBP >90 mmHg) and proteinuria (>0.3 g/day in a 24-hour collection or random urine protein:creatinine ratio >0.3 mg protein/mg creatinine) after 20 weeks gestation. However, preeclampsia complications are more strongly associated with the severity of hypertension than the presence or severity of proteinuria [75, 84]. Following the lead of other national and international organizations [85–87], the 2013 American College of Obstetrics and Gynecology Task Force on Hypertension in Pregnancy recommended that proteinuria should no longer be required for the diagnosis of preeclampsia (Table 6.3) [61, 88, 89]. These broader criteria allow for the diagnosis of preeclampsia in the absence of proteinuria when one or more other features of endorgan damage are present. In addition, the presence of severe proteinuria (>5 g/day) is no longer considered indicative of severe preeclampsia, as the degree of proteinuria is poorly correlated with adverse outcomes [84]. The HELLP syndrome (hemolytic anemia, elevated liver enzymes, and low platelets) is a severe form of preeclampsia, not a distinct pathologic and clinical entity.

The use of spot urine protein:creatinine ratio to quantify proteinuria in pregnancy has slowly gained broader use in the obstetric community. Suggested cutoffs for the diagnosis of abnormal proteinuria are >0.3 mg protein/mg creatinine, or >30 mg protein/mmol creatinine, ideally performed on a first morning voided sample [88].

The diagnosis of superimposed preeclampsia in the setting of chronic hypertension can be challenging. The presence of preexisting hypertension robs the clinician of preeclampsia's key diagnostic feature. Clinical practice guidelines variably define superimposed preeclampsia as worsening hypertension, resistant hypertension, new or worsening proteinuria, or the presence of one or more systemic features of preeclampsia in a woman with previously diagnosed chronic hypertension [88]. In the absence of baseline proteinuria, the new onset of proteinuria (>300 mg/day), usually with worsening hypertension, may be the most reliable sign of superimposed preeclampsia. When preexisting proteinuria is present, diagnosis is even more difficult. In these cases, a sudden, substantial increase in proteinuria, accompanied by worsening blood pressure, should suggest superimposed preeclampsia. Features of severe preeclampsia such as headache, visual changes, epigastric pain, pulmonary edema,

Table 6.3 Diagnostic criteria for preeclampsia [61, 88]

Preeclampsia	
Hypertension	Systolic BP ≥140 mmHg or diastolic BP ≥90 mmHg after 20 weeks gestation on two occasions at least 4 h apart in a woman with a previously normal blood pressure
And	
Proteinuria	≥300 mg/24 h (or this amount extrapolated from a timed collection) or Protein/Creatinine ratio ≥0.3 mg/mg or ≥30 mg/mmol [85, 89] or Dipstick 1+ (used only if other quantitative methods not available)
Or, in the absence of proteinuria, new onset hypertension with the new onset of any of the following:	
Thrombocytopenia	Platelet count <100,000/ml
Renal insufficiency	Serum creatinine concentration greater than 1.1 mg/dl or a doubling of the serum creatinine concentration in the absence of other renal disease
Impaired liver function	Elevated blood concentrations of liver transaminases to twice normal concentrations
Pulmonary edema	
Cerebral or visual symptoms	
Superimposed Preeclampsia	
Chronic hypertension	Systolic BP ≥140 mmHg or diastolic BP ≥90 mmHg after 20 weeks gestation on two occasions at least 4 h, or the use of antihypertensive medication prior to pregnancy
And	
Worsening hypertension	A sudden increase in blood pressure in a woman with chronic hypertension that was previously well controlled or escalation of antihypertensive medications to control blood pressure
Or	
New or worsening proteinuria	New onset of proteinuria in a woman with chronic hypertension or a sudden increase in proteinuria in a women with known proteinuria before or in early pregnancy
Or	
One or more features of severe preeclampsia (Table 6.2).	

thrombocytopenia, renal insufficiency, and elevated liver enzymes (Table 6.2) should also prompt consideration of superimposed preeclampsia.

Management

The definitive treatment for preeclampsia is delivery. However, early preterm delivery carries a high morbidity for the neonate. Mild preeclampsia remote from term can sometimes be managed for a few weeks with bed rest, antihypertensive medication, and close maternal and fetal monitoring [90]. However, progression to severe preeclampsia over days to weeks is typical. Expectant management of severe preeclampsia leads to a high rate of maternal morbidity and fetal and neonatal mortality [91]. Immediate delivery should be considered with women with uncontrolled severe hypertension or other severe features of preeclampsia (Table 6.2). Delivery is also appropriate in those who develop even mild preeclampsia at or near term [92].

Patients who develop preeclampsia with severe features should be monitored in a hospital setting. Hypertension should be treated with medication when severe (>150–160/100–110) [88]. Intravenous magnesium sulfate prevents the development of seizures in women with preeclampsia [93], and is recommended when severe features are present. Magnesium is also used for the treatment of seizures if eclampsia occurs. Administration of antenatal corticosteroids to enhance fetal lung maturity is recommended prior to 34 weeks gestation [88].

Following delivery, preeclampsia generally remits over a period of days to weeks. Antihypertensive therapy should generally be continued, and tapered as dictated by the maternal blood pressure. Continued monitoring is important, as complications—particularly seizures—can occur in the postpartum period. A spontaneous diuresis usually ensues within days after delivery. Diuretics during this period may hasten improvement in hypertension but do not affect hospital length of stay or adverse outcomes [94].

Postpartum Hypertension and Preeclampsia

Newly recognized hypertension presenting in the postpartum period can be due to either postpartum preeclampsia or the new recognition of chronic hypertension. Since pregnancy itself can lower blood pressure, chronic hypertension is sometimes unmasked and first diagnosed following delivery.

Postpartum preeclampsia can present up to 4 weeks following delivery, and can be severe: up to 1/3rd of eclampsia occurs in the postpartum period [95]. Most women who present with eclampsia or stroke in the postpartum period have prodromal symptoms, which can include headache, visual changes, nausea, vomiting, or epigastric pain [95]. For this reason, it is important that both pregnant women and their providers be informed regarding the signs and symptoms of postpartum preeclampsia. As with antepartum preeclampsia, early recognition and treatment with magnesium sulfate and antihypertensive medications may prevent severe complications.

Long-Term Outcomes After Preeclampsia

In the past, women with preeclampsia were reassured that the disease is cured by delivery, and future risk was limited to the higher probability of preeclampsia in subsequent pregnancies. There is now strong epidemiologic data to show that women with a history of preeclampsia have a substantially increased risk of cardiovascular, cerebrovascular, and renal disease later in life.

Hypertension and proteinuria begin to improve soon after delivery in the majority of women with preeclampsia, and resolve completely an average of 5–6 weeks postpartum. However, up to 20 % of women have persistent hypertension 6 months postpartum [18]. Women who have had preeclampsia are more likely to have physical and biochemical markers of cardiovascular risk, such as obesity, hypercholesterolemia, hypertension, and albuminuria, as compared with women who had normotensive pregnancies [96–98]. Long-term cardiovascular complications, including ischemic heart disease, cerebrovascular disease, and cardiovascular mortality, are increased two to threefold in women with a history of preeclampsia, as compared to women with no such history [99, 100]. Severe preeclampsia, recurrent preeclampsia, preeclampsia with preterm birth, and preeclampsia with intrauterine growth restriction are associated with the highest risk of adverse cardiovascular outcomes. The 2011 American Heart Association Guidelines now include a history of preeclampsia as a risk factor for cardiovascular disease [101].

Preeclampsia, especially in association with low neonatal birth weight, also carries an increased risk of subsequent maternal kidney disease [102]. A Norwegian study using birth and renal registry data on over 570,000 women showed that preeclampsia is associated with a nearly fivefold increase in the risk of subsequent ESRD [103]. Familial aggregation of risk factors does not seem to explain this risk [104].

The mechanism underlying the link between preeclampsia and subsequent cardiovascular and renal disease is unknown. Preeclampsia and cardiovascular disease share many common risk factors, such as chronic hypertension, diabetes, obesity, renal disease, and the metabolic syndrome. Still, the increase in long-term cardiovascular mortality holds even for women who develop preeclampsia in the absence of any overt vascular risk factors. Whether cardiovascular complications in these women result from vascular damage caused by preeclampsia, or simply reflect the common subclinical risk factors shared by preeclampsia and cardiovascular disease, remains speculative. Regardless of etiology, it is recommended that women who with a history of preeclampsia, especially with preterm birth or intrauterine growth restriction, be screened for potentially modifiable cardiovascular and renal disease risk factors (hypertension, diabetes mellitus, hyperlipidemia, obesity) at their postpartum obstetrician visit and yearly thereafter [61, 105].

Antihypertensive Drugs in Pregnancy

Treatment of blood pressure in pregnancy is frequently required for women with chronic hypertension in pregnancy, gestational hypertension, preeclampsia, and superimposed preeclampsia. General principles of treatment are similar for all four disorders. The selection of oral vs. intravenous medications should be driven by the severity of hypertension and presence of end-organ damage, rather than by the underlying etiology of hypertension. Even severe hypertension can frequently be managed with oral agents [106]. Thresholds for initiation of pharmacologic agents and therapeutic targets are discussed in Sects. 6.3.4.3 and "Management".

Oral Agents

Recommended antihypertensive agents in pregnancy are summarized in Table 6.4. The major classes of medication used for treatment of hypertension in pregnancy are calcium channel blockers, beta-blockers, methyldopa, and hydralazine.

Beta-adrenergic antagonists have been used extensively in pregnancy and are effective without known teratogenicity or known adverse fetal effects. Labetalol has found widespread use and acceptance, both as an oral and an intravenous agent [107]. Labetalol is preferred over pure beta-blockers, as the alpha-blocking effect may augment placental perfusion. Some data suggest atenolol is associated with fetal growth restriction, so this agent is usually avoided [108].

There is extensive clinical experience supporting the safety of calcium channel blockers in pregnancy. Long-acting nifedipine is the most well studied, and is both safe and effective [109]. Non-dihydropyridine calcium channel blockers such as verapamil and diltiazem have also been used without apparent adverse effects.

Methyldopa continues to be widely used for the management of hypertension in pregnancy. Methyldopa is a centrally acting alpha-2 adrenergic agonist, now seldom used outside of pregnancy. Of all antihypertensive agents, it has the most extensive safety data and has no apparent adverse fetal effects. Limitations include short duration of action, sedation, and rare adverse effects include elevated liver enzymes and hemolytic anemia. Clonidine appears to be comparable to methyldopa in terms of mechanism and safety, but data are fewer.

Diuretics are usually avoided in preeclampsia, since blood volume is already low. In pregnant women with chronic hypertension, diuretics could theoretically impede the physiologic volume expansion of pregnancy. However, there is no evidence that diuretics are associated with adverse fetal or maternal outcomes. Thus, although not considered first-line, it is reasonable to continue thiazide diuretics when these agents are part of a stable pre-pregnancy antihypertensive regimen [58]. When hypertension in pregnancy or preeclampsia is complicated by pulmonary edema, loop diuretics are appropriate and effective [110]. Aldactone can lead to feminization of male fetuses and are usually avoided. Eplerenone is a more specific antagonist to the mineralocorticoid receptor and theoretically would not lead to anti-androgenic effects. Although experience with eplerenone in pregnancy is limited, case reports have described its successful use in the management of both primary aldosteronism and Gitelman syndrome in pregnancy [24, 111].

Angiotensin-converting enzyme inhibitors (ACE-I) and angiotensin receptor antagonists (ARB) are contraindicated in pregnancy. Exposure during the second and third trimesters leads to major fetal malformations including renal dysgenesis, perinatal renal failure, oligohydramnios, pulmonary hypoplasia, hypocalvaria, and intrauterine growth restriction [112]. Evidence for teratogenicity with first trimester exposure is less compelling. A large population-based study reported congenital malformations of the central nervous and cardiovascular systems were higher among women with first trimester exposure to ACE inhibitors [113]. However, this study has been criticized for the presence of potential confounders and ascertainment bias. Women with a compelling indication for ACE-I or ARB (such as diabetic nephropathy) can probably be continued on these agents while attempting conception, with discontinuation as soon as pregnancy is diagnosed. However, risks and benefits of this strategy should be discussed with the patient, with shared and individualized decision-making. Women inadvertently exposed in early pregnancy can be reassured by a normal mid-trimester ultrasound examination. Fewer data are available on the effects of angiotensin receptor blockers, but a case series strongly suggests fetal effects are similar to ACE-I [114]. The American College of Obstetrics and Gynecology recommends that ACE-I and ARBs be avoided in all women of reproductive age with chronic hypertension unless there is a compelling indication, such as proteinuric chronic kidney disease [61].

Table 6.4 Antihypertensive medications in pregnancy

Medication	Initial dose	Maximum daily dose	Side effects
Long-acting nifedipine (PO)	30 mg once daily	120 mg	Headache, edema
Labetalol (PO)	200 mg twice a day	1200 mg	Bronchospasm, fatigue
Labetalol (IV)	IV bolus: 10–20 mg over 2 min; may administer 40–80 mg at 10-minute intervals IV infusion: 1–2 mg/min, titrate to response	300 mg	Bronchospasm Contraindicated in patients with asthma or acute heart failure
Methyldopa (PO)	250 mg twice a day	1500 mg	Fatigue, sedation
Nicardipine (IV)	IV infusion: 3–5 mg/h	15 mg/h	Headache, edema, tachycardia Suppresses uterine contractions Central line preferred
Hydralazine (PO)	50–100 mg two or three times a day	300 mg	Tachycardia, hypotension
Hydralazine (IV)	5–10 mg IV/IM, may repeat every 20 min	20 mg (IV) 30 mg (IM)	Tachycardia, hypotension, headache, fetal distress. Consider preloading or coadministration of 250–500 ml isotonic crystalloid fluid
Nitroprusside (IV)	0.3–0.5 mcg/kg/min	2 mcg/kg/min, maximum duration 24–48 h	Avoid unless no alternatives are available; risk for fetal cyanide toxicity

PO = oral; IV = intravenous

Intravenous Agents

When hypertension in pregnancy is severe, treatment with intravenous agents is appropriate. This most frequently occurs in the setting of preeclampsia and super-imposed preeclampsia. All intravenous medications commonly used for urgent control of severe hypertension are classified as pregnancy class C by the U.S. Food and Drug Administration (risk not ruled out). Nevertheless, there is extensive clinical experience with several agents, which are widely used with no clinical evidence of adverse effects. Options for intravenous use include labetalol, nicardipine, hydralazine, and diazoxide.

Intravenous labetalol, like oral labetalol, is safe and effective, with the major drawback being its short duration of action. Intravenous nicardipine is also short acting, and requires a continuous infusion treatment of hypertension [115]. The use of oral short-acting nifedipine is controversial due to well-documented adverse effects in the non-pregnant population. However, a recent trial suggests oral short-acting nifedipine is safe in hypertensive emergencies in pregnancy [116], and it may be an option in areas where intravenous agents are unavailable.

Hydralazine has been widely used as a first-line agent for severe hypertension in pregnancy. However, a recent meta-analysis of 21 trials comparing IV hydralazine to either labetalol or nifedipine for acute management of hypertension in pregnancy suggested an increased risk of maternal hypotension, maternal oliguria, placental abruption, and low APGAR scores with hydralazine [117]. Hence, hydralazine should be considered second-line and its use limited. Nitroprusside continues to be used in many low and middle income countries [118], but must be used with great caution due to risks of maternal and fetal cyanide toxicity when used for more than short periods (>4 h).

Diazoxide is a direct vasodilator which appears to be safe and effective in pregnancy for intravenous use to treat severe hypertension [119]. Because it inhibits insulin secretion, diazoxide should be avoided in type 2 diabetics.

Antihypertensive Drugs in Breastfeeding

There are few well-designed studies of the safety of antihypertensive medications in breastfeeding. In general, agents that are considered safe during pregnancy remain so in breastfeeding. Methyldopa, if effective and well tolerated during pregnancy, may be continued. Beta-blockers with high protein binding, such as labetalol and propranolol, are preferred over atenolol and metoprolol, which are concentrated in breast milk [107]. Diuretics may decrease milk production and should be avoided [107]. ACE inhibitors, particularly enalapril and captopril, are poorly excreted in breast milk and generally considered safe in lactating women [120]. Hence, in women with diabetes or proteinuric chronic kidney disease, initiation of ACE inhibitors should be considered immediately after delivery. Specific data on the pharmacokinetics of each medication should be used to guide mothers to time breastfeeding intervals before or well after peak breast milk excretion to avoid significant exposure to the baby. LactMed, a free online database maintained by the National Library of Medicine and the National Institutes of Health, is a useful clinical tool for assessing the safety of specific medications in breastfeeding [121].

References

1. Poppas A, Shroff SG, Korcarz CE, Hibbard JU, Berger DS, Lindheimer MD, et al. Serial assessment of the cardiovascular system in normal pregnancy. Role of arterial compliance and pulsatile arterial load. Circulation. 1997;95(10):2407–15.
2. Chapman AB, Abraham WT, Zamudio S, Coffin C, Merouani A, Young D, et al. Temporal relationships between hormonal and hemodynamic changes in early human pregnancy. Kidney Int. 1998;54(6):2056–63.
3. Wilson M, Morganti AA, Zervoudakis I, Letcher RL, Romney BM, Von Oeyon P, et al. Blood pressure, the renin-aldosterone system and sex steroids throughout normal pregnancy. Am J Med. 1980;68(1):97–104.
4. Desai DK, Moodley J, Naidoo DP. Echocardiographic assessment of cardiovascular hemodynamics in normal pregnancy. Obstet Gynecol. 2004;104(1):20–9.
5. Varga I, Rigo Jr J, Somos P, Joo JG, Nagy B. Analysis of maternal circulation and renal function in physiologic pregnancies; parallel examinations of the changes in the cardiac output and the glomerular filtration rate. J Matern Fetal Med. 2000;9(2):97–104.
6. Thornburg KL, Jacobson SL, Giraud GD, Morton MJ. Hemodynamic changes in pregnancy. Semin Perinatol. 2000;24(1):11–4.
7. Elsheikh A, Creatsas G, Mastorakos G, Milingos S, Loutradis D, Michalas S. The renin-aldosterone system during normal and hypertensive pregnancy. Arch Gynecol Obstet. 2001;264(4):182–5.
8. Khraibi AA. Renal interstitial hydrostatic pressure and sodium excretion in hypertension and pregnancy. J Hypertens Suppl. 2002;20(3):S21–7.
9. Davison JM. Edema in pregnancy. Kidney Int Suppl. 1997;59:S90–6.
10. Paller MS. Decreased pressor responsiveness in pregnancy: studies in experimental animals. Am J Kidney Dis. 1987;9(4):308–11.
11. Gant NF, Chand S, Whalley PJ, MacDonald PC. The nature of pressor responsiveness to angiotensin II in human pregnancy. Obstet Gynecol. 1974;43(6):854.
12. Cunningham FG, Cox K, Gant NF. Further observations on the nature of pressor responsivity to angiotensin II in human pregnancy. Obstet Gynecol. 1975;46(5):581–3.
13. Conrad KP, Jeyabalan A, Danielson LA, Kerchner LJ, Novak J. Role of relaxin in maternal renal vasodilation of pregnancy. Ann N Y Acad Sci. 2005;1041:147–54.
14. Conrad KP. Mechanisms of renal vasodilation and hyperfiltration during pregnancy. J Soc Gynecol Investig. 2004;11(7):438–48.
15. Conrad KP, Davison JM. The renal circulation in normal pregnancy and preeclampsia: is there a place for relaxin? Am J Physiol Renal Physiol. 2014;306(10):F1121–35.
16. Bateman BT, Bansil P, Hernandez-Diaz S, Mhyre JM, Callaghan WM, Kuklina EV. Prevalence, trends, and outcomes of chronic hypertension: a nationwide sample of delivery admissions. Am J Obstet Gynecol. 2012;206(2):134.e1–8.
17. Sibai BM. Treatment of hypertension in pregnant women. N Engl J Med. 1996;335(4):257–65.
18. Podymow T, August P. Postpartum course of gestational hypertension and preeclampsia. Hypertens Pregnancy. 2010;29(3):294–300.

19. Riester A, Reincke M. Progress in primary aldosteronism: mineralocorticoid receptor antagonists and management of primary aldosteronism in pregnancy. Eur J Endocrinol. 2015;172(1):R23–30.
20. Ledoux F, Genest J, Nowaczynski W, Kuchel O, Lebel M. Plasma progesterone and aldosterone in pregnancy. Can Med Assoc J. 1975;112(8):943–7.
21. Wyckoff JA, Seely EW, Hurwitz S, Anderson BF, Lifton RP, Dluhy RG. Glucocorticoid-remediable aldosteronism and pregnancy. Hypertension. 2000;35(2):668–72.
22. Funder JW, Carey RM, Fardella C, Gomez-Sanchez CE, Mantero F, Stowasser M, et al. Case detection, diagnosis, and treatment of patients with primary aldosteronism: an endocrine society clinical practice guideline. J Clin Endocrinol Metab. 2008;93(9):3266–81.
23. Kamoun M, Mnif MF, Charfi N, Kacem FH, Naceur BB, Mnif F, et al. Adrenal diseases during pregnancy: pathophysiology, diagnosis and management strategies. Am J Med Sci. 2014;347(1):64–73.
24. Cabassi A, Rocco R, Berretta R, Regolisti G, Bacchi-Modena A. Eplerenone use in primary aldosteronism during pregnancy. Hypertension. 2012;59(2):e18–9.
25. Easterling TR, Brateng D, Goldman ML, Strandness DE, Zaccardi MJ. Renal vascular hypertension during pregnancy. Obstet Gynecol. 1991;78(5 Pt 2):921–5.
26. Thorsteinsdottir B, Kane GC, Hogan MJ, Watson WJ, Grande JP, Garovic VD. Adverse outcomes of renovascular hypertension during pregnancy. Nat Clin Pract Nephrol. 2006;2(11):651–6.
27. Hayashida M, Watanabe N, Imamura H, Kumazaki S, Kitabayashi H, Takahashi W, et al. Congenital solitary kidney with renovascular hypertension diagnosed by means of captopril-enhanced renography and magnetic resonance angiography. Int Heart J. 2005;46(2):347–53.
28. Del Giudice A, Bisceglia M, D'Errico M, Gatta G, Nardella M, Ciavarella GP, et al. Extra-adrenal functional paraganglioma (phaeochromocytoma) associated with renal-artery stenosis in a pregnant woman. Nephrol Dial Transplant. 1998;13(11):2920–3.
29. Biggar MA, Lennard TW. Systematic review of phaeochromocytoma in pregnancy. Br J Surg. 2013;100(2):182–90.
30. Song Y, Liu J, Li H, Zeng Z, Bian X, Wang S. Outcomes of concurrent Caesarean delivery and pheochromocytoma resection in late pregnancy. Intern Med J. 2013;43(5):588–91.
31. Campino C, Trejo P, Carvajal CA, Vecchiola A, Valdivia C, Fuentes CA, et al. Pregnancy normalized familial hyperaldosteronism type I: a novel role for progesterone? J Hum Hypertens. 2015;29(2):138–9.
32. Vecchiola A, Lagos CF, Fuentes CA, Allende F, Campino C, Valdivia C, et al. Different effects of progesterone and estradiol on chimeric and wild type aldosterone synthase in vitro. Reprod Biol Endocrinol. 2013;11:76.
33. Geller DS, Farhi A, Pinkerton N, Fradley M, Moritz M, Spitzer A, et al. Activating mineralocorticoid receptor mutation in hypertension exacerbated by pregnancy. Science. 2000;289(5476):119–23.
34. Lindsay JR, Jonklaas J, Oldfield EH, Nieman LK. Cushing's syndrome during pregnancy: personal experience and review of the literature. J Clin Endocrinol Metab. 2005;90(5):3077–83.
35. Sibai BM, Lindheimer M, Hauth J, Caritis S, VanDorsten P, Klebanoff M, et al. Risk factors for preeclampsia, abruptio placentae, and adverse neonatal outcomes among women with chronic hypertension. National Institute of Child Health and Human Development Network of Maternal-Fetal Medicine Units. N Engl J Med. 1998;339(10):667–71.
36. Bramham K, Parnell B, Nelson-Piercy C, Seed PT, Poston L, Chappell LC. Chronic hypertension and pregnancy outcomes: systematic review and meta-analysis. BMJ. 2014;348:g2301.
37. Duckitt K, Harrington D. Risk factors for pre-eclampsia at antenatal booking: systematic review of controlled studies. BMJ. 2005;330(7491):565.
38. Mostello D, Catlin TK, Roman L, Holcomb Jr WL, Leet T. Preeclampsia in the parous woman: who is at risk? Am J Obstet Gynecol. 2002;187(2):425–9.
39. Zetterstrom K, Lindeberg SN, Haglund B, Hanson U. Maternal complications in women with chronic hypertension: a population-based cohort study. Acta Obstet Gynecol Scand. 2005;84(5):419–24.

40. Eskenazi B, Fenster L, Sidney S. A multivariate analysis of risk factors for preeclampsia. JAMA. 1991;266(2):237–41.
41. Clowse MEB, Jamison M, Myers E, James AH. A national study of the complications of lupus in pregnancy. Am J Obstet Gynecol. 2008;199(2):127.e1-e6.
42. Krotz S, Fajardo J, Ghandi S, Patel A, Keith LG. Hypertensive disease in twin pregnancies: a review. Twin Res. 2002;5(1):8–14.
43. Ness RB, Markovic N, Bass D, Harger G, Roberts JM. Family history of hypertension, heart disease, and stroke among women who develop hypertension in pregnancy. Obstet Gynecol. 2003;102(6):1366–71.
44. Weiss JL, Malone FD, Emig D, Ball RH, Nyberg DA, Comstock CH, et al. Obesity, obstetric complications and cesarean delivery rate—a population-based screening study. Am J Obstet Gynecol. 2004;190(4):1091–7.
45. Carr DB, Epplein M, Johnson CO, Easterling TR, Critchlow CW. A sister's risk: family history as a predictor of preeclampsia. Am J Obstet Gynecol. 2005;193(3 Suppl 1):965–72.
46. Ananth CV, Keyes KM, Wapner RJ. Pre-eclampsia rates in the United States, 1980–2010: age-period-cohort analysis. BMJ. 2013;347:f6564.
47. Macdonald-Wallis C, Tilling K, Fraser A, Nelson SM, Lawlor DA. Gestational weight gain as a risk factor for hypertensive disorders of pregnancy. Am J Obstet Gynecol. 2013;209(4):327.e1–17.
48. Gynecologists ACoOa. ACOG Practice Bulletin No. 125: chronic hypertension in pregnancy. Obstet Gynecol. 2012;119(2 Pt 1):396–407.
49. August P, Helseth G, Cook EF, Sison C. A prediction model for superimposed preeclampsia in women with chronic hypertension during pregnancy. Am J Obstet Gynecol. 2004;191(5):1666–72.
50. McCowan LM, Buist RG, North RA, Gamble G. Perinatal morbidity in chronic hypertension. Br J Obstet Gynaecol. 1996;103(2):123–9.
51. Henderson JT, Whitlock EP, O'Connor E, Senger CA, Thompson JH, Rowland MG. Low-dose aspirin for prevention of morbidity and mortality from preeclampsia: a systematic evidence review for the U.S. Preventive Services Task Force. Ann Intern Med. 2014;160(10):695–703.
52. Bujold E, Roberge S, Lacasse Y, Bureau M, Audibert F, Marcoux S, et al. Prevention of preeclampsia and intrauterine growth restriction with aspirin started in early pregnancy: a meta-analysis. Obstet Gynecol. 2010;116(2 Pt 1):402–14.
53. Roberge S, Villa P, Nicolaides K, Giguère Y, Vainio M, Bakthi A, et al. Early administration of low-dose aspirin for the prevention of preterm and term preeclampsia: a systematic review and meta-analysis. Fetal Diagn Ther. 2012;31(3):141–6.
54. Hofmeyr G, Duley L, Atallah A. Dietary calcium supplementation for prevention of preeclampsia and related problems: a systematic review and commentary. BJOG. 2007;114(8):933–43.
55. Hofmeyr GJ, Belizán JM, von Dadelszen P. Group CaP-eCS. Low-dose calcium supplementation for preventing pre-eclampsia: a systematic review and commentary. BJOG. 2014;121(8):951–7.
56. Wen SW, Gaudet L, Champagne J, White RR, Rybak N, Walker M. [301-POS]: Effect of folic acid supplementation in pregnancy on preeclampsia—Folic Acid Clinical Trial (FACT). Pregnancy Hypertens. 2015;5(1):149.
57. Tabesh M, Salehi-Abargouei A, Esmaillzadeh A. Maternal vitamin D status and risk of preeclampsia: a systematic review and meta-analysis. J Clin Endocrinol Metab. 2013;98(8):3165–73.
58. Collins R, Yusuf S, Peto R. Overview of randomised trials of diuretics in pregnancy. Br Med J (Clin Res Ed). 1985;290(6461):17–23.
59. Duley L, Henderson-Smart D, Meher S. Altered dietary salt for preventing pre-eclampsia, and its complications. Cochrane Database Syst Rev. 2005;4, CD005548.
60. Aune D, Saugstad OD, Henriksen T, Tonstad S. Physical activity and the risk of preeclampsia: a systematic review and meta-analysis. Epidemiology. 2014;25(3):331–43.

61. Gynecologists ACoOa, Pregnancy TFoHi. Hypertension in pregnancy. Report of the American College of Obstetricians and Gynecologists' Task Force on Hypertension in Pregnancy. Obstet Gynecol. 2013;122(5):1122–31.
62. Weight gain during pregnancy: reexamining the guidelines. Washington: Institute of Medicine; 2009.
63. Truong YN, Yee LM, Caughey AB, Cheng YW. Weight gain in pregnancy: does the Institute of Medicine have it right? Am J Obstet Gynecol. 2015;212(3):362.e1–8.
64. Kotchen TA, Cowley AW, Frohlich ED. Salt in health and disease—a delicate balance. N Engl J Med. 2013;368(26):2531–2.
65. National Heart, Lung, and Blood Institute Task Force Report on Research in Prevention of Cardiovascular Disease 2001.
66. James PA, Oparil S, Carter BL, Cushman WC, Dennison-Himmelfarb C, Handler J, et al. 2014 evidence-based guideline for the management of high blood pressure in adults: report from the panel members appointed to the Eighth Joint National Committee (JNC 8). JAMA. 2014;311(5):507–20.
67. Magee LA, Ornstein MP, von Dadelszen P. Fortnightly review: management of hypertension in pregnancy. BMJ. 1999;318(7194):1332–6.
68. Abalos E, Duley L, Steyn DW, Henderson-Smart DJ. Antihypertensive drug therapy for mild to moderate hypertension during pregnancy. Cochrane Database Syst Rev. 2001;2, CD002252.
69. Ferrer RL, Sibai BM, Mulrow CD, Chiquette E, Stevens KR, Cornell J. Management of mild chronic hypertension during pregnancy: a review. Obstet Gynecol. 2000;96(5 Pt 2):849–60.
70. Abalos E, Duley L, Steyn DW. Antihypertensive drug therapy for mild to moderate hypertension during pregnancy. Cochrane Database Syst Rev. 2014;2, CD002252.
71. von Dadelszen P, Ornstein MP, Bull SB, Logan AG, Koren G, Magee LA. Fall in mean arterial pressure and fetal growth restriction in pregnancy hypertension: a meta-analysis. Lancet. 2000;355(9198):87–92.
72. Chobanian AV, Bakris GL, Black HR, Cushman WC, Green LA, Izzo Jr JL, et al. The Seventh Report of the Joint National Committee on Prevention, Detection, Evaluation, and Treatment of High Blood Pressure: The JNC 7 Report. JAMA. 2003:289.19.2560.
73. Magee LA, von Dadelszen P, Rey E, Ross S, Asztalos E, Murphy KE, et al. Less-tight versus tight control of hypertension in pregnancy. N Engl J Med. 2015;372(5):407–17.
74. Saudan P, Brown MA, Buddle ML, Jones M. Does gestational hypertension become pre-eclampsia? Br J Obstet Gynaecol. 1998;105(11):1177–84.
75. Buchbinder A, Sibai BM, Caritis S, Macpherson C, Hauth J, Lindheimer MD, et al. Adverse perinatal outcomes are significantly higher in severe gestational hypertension than in mild preeclampsia. Am J Obstet Gynecol. 2002;186(1):66–71.
76. Strevens H, Wide-Swensson D, Hansen A, Horn T, Ingemarsson I, Larsen S, et al. Glomerular endotheliosis in normal pregnancy and pre-eclampsia. BJOG. 2003;110(9):831–6.
77. Sibai B, Dekker G, Kupferminc M. Pre-eclampsia. Lancet. 2005;365(9461):785–99.
78. Odegård RA, Vatten LJ, Nilsen ST, Salvesen KA, Austgulen R. Preeclampsia and fetal growth. Obstet Gynecol. 2000;96(6):950–5.
79. Roberts JM, Taylor RN, Goldfien A. Clinical and biochemical evidence of endothelial cell dysfunction in the pregnancy syndrome preeclampsia. Am J Hypertens. 1991;4(8):700–8.
80. Kaufmann P, Black S, Huppertz B. Endovascular trophoblast invasion: implications for the pathogenesis of intrauterine growth retardation and preeclampsia. Biol Reprod. 2003;69(1):1–7.
81. Ashworth JR, Warren AY, Baker PN, Johnson IR. Loss of endothelium-dependent relaxation in myometrial resistance arteries in pre-eclampsia. Br J Obstet Gynaecol. 1997;104(10):1152–8.
82. Brown MA, Wang J, Whitworth JA. The renin-angiotensin-aldosterone system in pre-eclampsia. Clin Exp Hypertens. 1997;19(5–6):713–26.
83. Steegers EA, von Dadelszen P, Duvekot JJ, Pijnenborg R. Pre-eclampsia. Lancet. 2010;376(9741):631–44.

84. Newman MG, Robichaux AG, Stedman CM, Jaekle RK, Fontenot MT, Dotson T, et al. Perinatal outcomes in preeclampsia that is complicated by massive proteinuria. Am J Obstet Gynecol. 2003;188(1):264–8.
85. Magee LA, Pels A, Helewa M, Rey E, von Dadelszen P, Committee SHG. Diagnosis, evaluation, and management of the hypertensive disorders of pregnancy: executive summary. J Obstet Gynaecol Can. 2014;36(7):575–6.
86. HDP CPG Working Group. Association of Ontario Midwives. Hypertensive Disorders of Pregnancy. Clinical Practice Guideline No. 15. Available at: http://www.aom.on.ca/Health_Care_Professionals/Clinical_Practice_Guidelines/2012.
87. Hypertensive Disorders of Pregnancy 2013 [cited 2015 June 10, 2015].
88. Gillon TE, Pels A, von Dadelszen P, MacDonell K, Magee LA. Hypertensive disorders of pregnancy: a systematic review of international clinical practice guidelines. PLoS One. 2014;9(12), e113715.
89. National Institute for Health and Care Excellence (NICE): hypertension in pregnancy: the management of hypertensive disorders during pregnancy 2010 [May 2015]. Available at: http://www.nice.org.uk/guidance/cg107/chapter/1-recommendations.
90. Sibai BM, Mercer BM, Schiff E, Friedman SA. Aggressive versus expectant management of severe preeclampsia at 28 to 32 weeks' gestation: a randomized controlled trial. Am J Obstet Gynecol. 1994;171(3):818–22.
91. Sibai BM, Taslimi M, Abdella TN, Brooks TF, Spinnato JA, Anderson GD. Maternal and perinatal outcome of conservative management of severe preeclampsia in midtrimester. Am J Obstet Gynecol. 1985;152(1):32–7.
92. Koopmans CM, Bijlenga D, Groen H, Vijgen SM, Aarnoudse JG, Bekedam DJ, et al. Induction of labour versus expectant monitoring for gestational hypertension or mild preeclampsia after 36 weeks' gestation (HYPITAT): a multicentre, open-label randomised controlled trial. Lancet. 2009;374(9694):979–88.
93. Altman D, Carroli G, Duley L, Farrell B, Moodley J, Neilson J, et al. Do women with preeclampsia, and their babies, benefit from magnesium sulphate? The Magpie Trial: a randomised placebo-controlled trial. Lancet. 2002;359(9321):1877–90.
94. Ascarelli MH, Johnson V, McCreary H, Cushman J, May WL, Martin JN. Postpartum preeclampsia management with furosemide: a randomized clinical trial. Obstet Gynecol. 2005;105(1):29–33.
95. Chames MC, Livingston JC, Ivester TS, Barton JR, Sibai BM. Late postpartum eclampsia: a preventable disease? Am J Obstet Gynecol. 2002;186(6):1174–7.
96. Smith GN, Walker MC, Liu A, Wen SW, Swansburg M, Ramshaw H, et al. A history of preeclampsia identifies women who have underlying cardiovascular risk factors. Am J Obstet Gynecol. 2009;200(1):58.e1–e8.
97. Edlow AG, Srinivas SK, Elovitz MA. Investigating the risk of hypertension shortly after pregnancies complicated by preeclampsia. Am J Obstet Gynecol. 2009;200(5):e60–2.
98. Nisell H, Lintu H, Lunell NO, Mollerstrom G, Pettersson E. Blood pressure and renal function seven years after pregnancy complicated by hypertension. Br J Obstet Gynaecol. 1995;102(11):876–81.
99. McDonald SD, Malinowski A, Zhou Q, Yusuf S, Devereaux PJ. Cardiovascular sequelae of preeclampsia/eclampsia: a systematic review and meta-analyses. Am Heart J. 2008;156(5): 918–30.
100. Bellamy L, Casas JP, Hingorani AD, Williams DJ. Pre-eclampsia and risk of cardiovascular disease and cancer in later life: systematic review and meta-analysis. BMJ. 2007;335(7627):974.
101. Mosca L, Benjamin EJ, Berra K, Bezanson JL, Dolor RJ, Lloyd-Jones DM, et al. Effectiveness-based guidelines for the prevention of cardiovascular disease in women—2011 update: a guideline from the American Heart Association. J Am Coll Cardiol. 2011;57(12):1404–23.
102. Vikse BE, Irgens LM, Bostad L, Iversen BM. Adverse perinatal outcome and later kidney biopsy in the mother. J Am Soc Nephrol. 2006;17(3):837–45.

103. Vikse BE, Irgens LM, Leivestad T, Skjaerven R, Iversen BM. Preeclampsia and the risk of end-stage renal disease. N Engl J Med. 2008;359(8):800–9.
104. Vikse BE, Irgens LM, Karumanchi SA, Thadhani R, Reisæter AV, Skjærven R. Familial factors in the association between preeclampsia and later ESRD. Clin J Am Soc Nephrol. 2012;7(11):1819–26.
105. Hertig A, Watnick S, Strevens H, Boulanger H, Berkane N, Rondeau E. How should women with pre-eclampsia be followed up? New insights from mechanistic studies. Nat Clin Pract Nephrol. 2008;4(9):503–9.
106. Firoz T, Magee LA, MacDonell K, Payne BA, Gordon R, Vidler M, et al. Oral antihypertensive therapy for severe hypertension in pregnancy and postpartum: a systematic review. BJOG. 2014;121(10):1210–8. discussion 20.
107. Podymow T, August P, Umans JG. Antihypertensive therapy in pregnancy. Semin Nephrol. 2004;24(6):616–25.
108. Magee LA, Duley L. Oral beta-blockers for mild to moderate hypertension during pregnancy. Cochrane Database Syst Rev. 2003;3, CD002863.
109. Smith P, Anthony J, Johanson R. Nifedipine in pregnancy. BJOG. 2000;107(3):299–307.
110. Melchiorre K, Sharma R, Thilaganathan B. Cardiovascular implications in preeclampsia: an overview. Circulation. 2014;130(8):703–14.
111. Morton A, Panitz B, Bush A. Eplerenone for gitelman syndrome in pregnancy. Nephrology (Carlton). 2011;16(3):349.
112. Bullo M, Tschumi S, Bucher BS, Bianchetti MG, Simonetti GD. Pregnancy outcome following exposure to angiotensin-converting enzyme inhibitors or angiotensin receptor antagonists: a systematic review. Hypertension. 2012;60(2):444–50.
113. Cooper WO, Hernandez-Diaz S, Arbogast PG, Dudley JA, Dyer S, Gideon PS, et al. Major congenital malformations after first-trimester exposure to ACE inhibitors. N Engl J Med. 2006;354(23):2443–51.
114. Serreau R, Luton D, Macher MA, Delezoide AL, Garel C, Jacqz-Aigrain E. Developmental toxicity of the angiotensin II type 1 receptor antagonists during human pregnancy: a report of 10 cases. BJOG. 2005;112(6):710–2.
115. Hanff LM, Vulto AG, Bartels PA, Roofthooft DW, Bijvank BN, Steegers EA, et al. Intravenous use of the calcium-channel blocker nicardipine as second-line treatment in severe, early-onset pre-eclamptic patients. J Hypertens. 2005;23(12):2319–26.
116. Raheem IA, Saaid R, Omar SZ, Tan PC. Oral nifedipine versus intravenous labetalol for acute blood pressure control in hypertensive emergencies of pregnancy: a randomised trial. BJOG. 2012;119(1):78–85.
117. Magee LA, Cham C, Waterman EJ, Ohlsson A, von Dadelszen P. Hydralazine for treatment of severe hypertension in pregnancy: meta-analysis. BMJ. 2003;327(7421):955–60.
118. Lalani S, Firoz T, Magee LA, Sawchuck D, Payne B, Gordon R, et al. Pharmacotherapy for preeclampsia in low and middle income countries: an analysis of essential medicines lists. J Obstet Gynaecol Can. 2013;35(3):215–23.
119. Hennessy A, Thornton CE, Makris A, Ogle RF, Henderson-Smart DJ, Gillin AG, et al. A randomised comparison of hydralazine and mini-bolus diazoxide for hypertensive emergencies in pregnancy: the PIVOT trial. Aust N Z J Obstet Gynaecol. 2007;47(4):279–85.
120. Beardmore KS, Morris JM, Gallery ED. Excretion of antihypertensive medication into human breast milk: a systematic review. Hypertens Pregnancy. 2002;21(1):85–95.
121. National Library of Medicine, Drugs and Lactation Database (LactMed) 2015 [6/22/2015]. http://toxnet.nlm.nih.gov/newtoxnet/lactmed.htm.

Chapter 7
Hypertension in the Dialysis Patient

Arjun D. Sinha

Introduction

Hypertension is both a cause and a consequence of the spectrum of chronic kidney disease (CKD) to end stage renal disease (ESRD). Despite steady improvement, mortality remains high in the dialysis population with a 5-year survival rate only at 40 % [1], which compares poorly to some advanced cancers [2]. Cardiovascular events remain the leading cause of death in dialysis [3], with hypertension an important contributor. Thus the diagnosis and management of hypertension in dialysis is a vital topic to all dialysis patients and providers. This chapter will review the epidemiology, diagnosis, treatment, and prognosis of hypertension in the dialysis population.

Epidemiology

Blood pressure in the hemodialysis (HD) patient is a moving target that is influenced by when and where it is measured, complicating diagnosis. The epidemiology of hypertension in HD therefore can vary depending not only on the BP cutoffs employed but also on when and where BP is measured: in the HD clinic before or after dialysis (called peridialytic BP) versus outside the dialysis unit using ambulatory BP monitoring (ABPM) or home BP monitoring during the interdialytic period. Table 7.1 summarizes the various methods of assessing BP in HD.

A.D. Sinha, MD, MS (✉)
Division of Nephrology, Richard L. Roudebush VA Medical Center, University of Indiana
School of Medicine, Indianapolis, IN, USA
e-mail: adsinha@iu.edu

© Springer Science+Business Media New York 2016
A.K. Singh, R. Agarwal (eds.), *Core Concepts in Hypertension in Kidney Disease*, DOI 10.1007/978-1-4939-6436-9_7

Table 7.1 Methods of hemodialysis BP measurement

Method	Description	Comments
Peridialytic BP	Measured both before and after HD	Easily available but highly variable
Intradialytic BP	Median of all BP measures during one HD run	Easily available but needs more study
Ambulatory BP	Measured every 20–30 min over 44 h between HD runs	Gold standard but cumbersome
Home BP	Measured twice daily at home	Correlates well to ambulatory BP and accessible by most patients

Epidemiology Using Peridialytic BP Measurements

Multiple observational studies using peridialytic BP have found a high prevalence of hypertension in HD ranging from 62 to 86 %; notably, these studies used different threshold BP values varying from 140/90 to 160/90 mmHg and variously included antihypertensive drug use in their definitions of hypertension [4–7]. More recent analyses of randomized trials have found similar rates of hypertension.

The Hemodialysis (HEMO) Study was a landmark large multicenter trial of HD dose and dialyzer flux on survival [8] that recruited clinically stable HD patients [9]. An analysis of the baseline characteristics of the first 1238 subjects randomized into the HEMO Study between March 1995 and April 1998 found 72 % of the cohort to be hypertensive, defined as peridialytic BP ≥140/90 mmHg during the baseline HD session [10]. This rate of hypertension was despite 74.2 % of the cohort receiving antihypertensive medications, with a median of 1.0 drug per subject.

The BP data from an even larger randomized double blind and placebo controlled trial of sodium ferric gluconate was examined in detail with similar results [11]. The original trial enrolled 2535 clinically stable HD patients between August 1999 and October 2000 [12]. Using a definition of hypertension as pre-HD BP >150/85 averaged over 1 week or the use of antihypertensive medications, an analysis of baseline data found a prevalence of 86 % for hypertension in this cohort [11]. Within the hypertensive subjects only 30 % were controlled, while 12 % weren't treated pharmacologically and 58 % were treated but still uncontrolled [11], which is similar to previous reports [6].

Epidemiology Using Ambulatory BP Measurements

A recent single center study of 369 prevalent and clinically stable HD patients employed 44 h interdialytic ABPM and found a prevalence for hypertension at 86 % using a definition of hypertension as average ambulatory BP of ≥135/85 mmHg or antihypertensive drug use; [13] this prevalence is similar to prior small studies of ABPM in HD [14]. In the cohort of 369 patients, hypertension was treated with medications in 89 % of patients but was controlled adequately in only 38 % of patients [13].

Epidemiology in Peritoneal Dialysis Patients

It has been suggested that peritoneal dialysis (PD) controls hypertension better than HD, with a single center study of 56 prevalent and clinically stable PD patients finding that only 9 % of the cohort was hypertensive with BP >140/90 mmHg by standardized auscultated BP as compared to a hypertension prevalence of 56 % in the same center's HD unit [15]. Similarly, control of BP was compared in the retrospective Peritoneal Dialysis Core Indicators Study in the mid-1990s that found among the 926 PD patients with BP data only 35 % were hypertensive with BP >150/90 mmHg with the cohort having an average BP of 139/80 as compared to a contemporaneous cohort of HD patients whose average pre-HD BP was 151/79 and post-HD BP 137/74 mmHg [16]. A larger study using United States Renal Data System (USRDS) data from the Dialysis Morbidity and Mortality Wave 2 study in the late 1990s found that from 1034 PD patients 54 % had SBP >140 mmHg while on a mean of 1.6 antihypertensive medications [17].

While the above reported prevalence values for hypertension in PD patients are less than that generally reported for HD, this is not a universal finding. A prospective study of 504 prevalent and clinically stable PD patients found a hypertension prevalence of 88 % defined as BP >140/90 mmHg or use of antihypertensive medications, and of the hypertensive patients only 16 % were adequately controlled [18]. Additionally 24 h ABPM was performed, and of the 414 adequate examinations hypertension was present in 69 % based on BP load >30 %, with load defined as the percent of ambulatory BP readings >140/90 mmHg during the day or >120/80 mmHg at night. Also utilizing ABPM, a study of 22 HD and 24 PD patients that were well matched for major clinical characteristics found no significant difference in either daytime or nighttime BP between the two groups [19]. Thus while there is a suggestion that PD may control hypertension better than HD there is no conclusive evidence that this is the case.

Diagnosis

ABPM is the accepted gold standard for diagnosing hypertension in the general population and in the ESRD population on dialysis [20–23]. ABPM not only permits the diagnosis of nocturnal hypertension, it is also superior to peridialytic BP measurements in correlating end organ damage manifest as left ventricular hypertrophy (LVH) [24] and predicting the outcome of mortality [25]. The proper ABPM technique includes employing a validated monitor [26] to measure BP every 20 min during the day from 6 AM to 10 PM and then every 30 min at night from 10 PM to 6 AM [27]. This prolonged interval of measurement permits observation of the full change in BP during the interdialytic period, where SBP increases an average of 2.5 mmHg every 10 h [28, 29]. Unfortunately, ABPM is also cumbersome to use, especially over 44 continuous hours, so it remains a research technique in ESRD.

As ABPM is not used routinely, more convenient methods of measuring BP and diagnosing hypertension must be employed. Since BP changes both during the HD session and during the interdialytic interval there remains uncertainty about how best to diagnose and manage hypertension in the HD population, which may contribute to both undertreatment [14, 30] and overtreatment of hypertension [31]. Further complicating matters, HD patients have significant seasonal variability in BP with lower BP during the summer and higher during the winter [32], possibly due to temperature mediated vasodilation or sweat induced volume losses.

Classically, the peridialytic BP measures taken before and after an HD session have been used to diagnose and manage hypertension, and while there are no randomized clinical trials to guide goal BP recommendations in ESRD, longstanding professional guidelines have employed peridialytic BP values. The National Kidney Foundation Kidney Disease Outcomes Quality Initiative (NKF KDOQI) guidelines recommend to target pre-HD BP <140/90 mmHg and post-HD BP <130/80 mmHg [33]. Unfortunately, making treatment decisions based on peridialytic BP can be associated with adverse outcomes, as shown by a study of 11 HD units in London, England that found those HD units with more patients reaching the post-HD BP goal had significantly more episodes of symptomatic hypotension requiring saline infusion [34]. Peridialytic BP is highly variable such that the variability within a given patient over time is similar to the variability between patients [35], possibly due in part to these measurements often being made without attention to technique [36]. While peridialytic BP does have a statistically significant relationship to the gold standard interdialytic ambulatory BP [37], it is because of the inherent variability in peridialytic measurements that a meta-analysis of 18 studies comparing peridialytic BP and interdialytic ABPM found very wide limits of agreement between the techniques such that peridialytic BP provides a very imprecise estimate of interdialytic BP [38]. In the meta-analysis the limits of agreement between pre-HD SBP and interdialytic ambulatory SBP ranged from +41.7 mmHg to −25.2 mmHg while the limits of agreement for post-HD SBP were similarly broad, which illustrates the reduced clinical utility of a diagnosis of hypertension or normotension based on peridialytic BP [38].

A readily available alternative to peridialytic BP is to use all the BP measurements made during a single mid-week HD session to calculate a median BP, which is easier to calculate at the bedside compared to mean BP. A study of 150 chronic HD patients found that median intradialytic BP had the best reproducibility and was superior to either pre- or post-HD BP or their average for predicting 44 h interdialytic ambulatory BP [39]. In this study median intradialytic SBP >140 mmHg during a mid-week HD session had an 80 % sensitivity and specificity for diagnosing hypertension by gold standard ABPM [39]. Additionally, median intradialytic BP has been shown to change in response to interventional reduction in dry weight to reduce BP [40], further supporting the clinical usefulness of this measure.

Home BP monitoring is the third alternative to clinically inconvenient gold standard ABPM, as home BP monitoring is the recommended method to routinely diagnose and manage BP in general hypertension populations by both the American Heart Association [41] and the European Society of Hypertension [42] and its use is

Table 7.2 Advantages of home BP monitoring over peridialytic BP

1. Predicts gold standard ambulatory BP
2. Reproducibility
3. Reflects changes in dry weight
4. Correlates to left ventricular hypertrophy
5. Predicts cardiovascular events
6. Predicts mortality
7. Randomized trial evidence for efficacy of BP control
8. Recommended by major professional societies

feasible and practical both in patients with CKD and ESRD [43, 44]. Home BP monitoring is superior to peridialytic BP measurements by every methodological and clinical standard. This includes superior correlation with gold standard ABPM [45], week to week reproducibility [46], the ability to reflect BP changes from interventional probing of dry weight [46], correlation to the end organ damage of LVH [24, 47], and predicting outcomes including cardiovascular events [48] and mortality [48, 49]. Table 7.2 summarizes the advantages of home BP monitoring.

Two small randomized trials have found home BP monitoring to be beneficial versus usual care for management of BP in HD patients. The first randomized 34 patients to home BP monitoring plus usual care versus usual care only over 12 weeks and found that the home BP group had significantly lower BP at the end of the study [50]. A subsequent trial of 65 HD patients randomized participants to usual hypertension care based on pre-HD BP versus open label monthly home BP monitoring for 6 months [51]. At the end of the trial the home BP monitoring group had a significant reduction in ambulatory SBP both from baseline and versus the usual care group, which had no change in ambulatory SBP from baseline. However the primary endpoint of reduction in echocardiographic LVH was no different between groups, possibly due to lack of power and variability in the timing of the echocardiograms relative to the HD schedule [51].

As with ABPM, home BP increases between HD sessions, at an average rate of 4 mmHg every 10 h [52], so it is important to adequately sample home BP at spaced intervals between HD sessions. Randomized trials have used protocols of home BP monitoring performed twice daily over 4–7 days once per month [51, 53], which is a reasonable regimen for routine clinical use and decision making. Measurements performed more than once per month may be needed in more unstable patients including those recently hospitalized. Table 7.3 summarizes the suggested method of home BP monitoring.

There are no randomized trials comparing goal BP levels in the dialysis population using any of the available BP methods including peridialytic BP, intradialytic BP, home BP, or interdialytic ambulatory BP. However, the American Heart Association defines hypertension as home BP >135/85 mmHg on average for the general population [41], so a goal interdialytic home BP target of ≤140/90 mmHg is reasonable [54], as was used in a recent large randomized trial of BP control in HD [53].

Table 7.3 Suggested method for home BP monitoring

1. Check both morning and evening
2. Check for 4–7 consecutive days duration
3. Check once monthly or more often if clinically unstable
4. Goal home BP ≤140/90

Intradialytic Hypertension

While the focus of diagnosis and treatment of hypertension in chronic HD is on interdialytic BP between HD sessions, the case of intradialytic hypertension merits special mention. BP normally declines during the HD, but approximately 5–15 % of chronic HD patients have a paradoxical rise in BP during the HD session [55]. Intradialytic hypertension has been described variously and there is currently no uniformly recognized definition. Definitions have included (1) a change in SBP or mean arterial pressure from pre-HD to post-HD over various thresholds from >0 mmHg to ≥10 mmHg change [56, 57], (2) a positive slope after regression of all intradialytic SBP values [58], or (3) BP increase during or immediately following HD resulting in post-HD BP >130/80 mmHg [55].

Recently it has been recognized that intradialytic hypertension is associated with worse outcomes. Inrig and colleagues performed a secondary analysis of a randomized trial in 443 prevalent HD subjects and found intradialytic hypertension to be significantly associated with greater mortality at 6 months [56]. Similarly, in a subsequent observational study of a cohort of 1748 incident HD patients Inrig and colleagues found 2-year survival to be significantly decreased for each 10 mmHg increase in SBP from pre-HD to post-HD BP, however this relationship was limited to those whose pre-HD SBP was <120 mmHg [59]. Most recently, a prospective cohort study of 115 prevalent HD patients found an average pre-HD to post-HD rise in SBP of >5 mmHg to significantly predict all-cause and cardiovascular mortality [60].

Intradialytic hypertension has been associated with interdialytic hypertension as measured by 44 h ABPM [57, 58], so it is not surprising that the same mechanisms implicated in causing interdialytic hypertension between HD sessions have also been implicated in causing intradialytic hypertension during the HD session [55], but the preponderance of evidence currently points to volume overload and endothelial dysfunction. Markers of volume overload such as increased cardiothoracic ratio have been associated with intradialytic hypertension [60], but most importantly interventional trials have shown volume removal though dry weight reduction improves intradialytic hypertension. An early study from the mid-1990s included seven patients with intradialytic hypertension and found them all to have marked cardiac dilation and to be very hypertensive with mean pre-HD BP 172/99 mmHg despite medications [61]. All subjects had subsequent reduction in dry weight with an average weight loss of 6.7 kg that was associated with an improvement in pre-HD BP by 46/21 mmHg despite discontinuation of all BP meds. More recently a secondary analysis of the Dry Weight Reduction in Hypertensive Hemodialysis Patients (DRIP) trial [62] regressed the intradialytic BP values for the 150 trial subjects and found that the quintile of subjects with the greatest reduction in dry weight, more than 0.94 kg reduction after the first 4 weeks of the trial, also had the most positive BP slope at baseline as they were the only quintile with intradialytic hypertension by this definition [58]. Importantly, after dry weight reduction this same quintile had reduction in BP slopes to finish the trial, meaning their intradialytic hypertension had resolved such that their BP slopes were similar to the other subjects. Thus intradialytic hypertension appears to be a marker of volume overload that is amenable to dry weight reduction.

Additionally, endothelial dysfunction has been identified as an important mediator as there is evidence for both a rise in endothelin-1 levels [63] and a decrease in nitric oxide during HD [64] in patients with intradialytic hypertension. The contribution of endothelial function was investigated in 25 HD patients recruited in an 8-week pilot study with a before–after design using carvedilol [65], which has been shown to block endothelin-1 release in vitro [66]. Subjects were administered carvedilol up to a dose of 50 mg twice a day, and while endothelin-1 levels were unchanged on carvedilol, flow mediated dilation significantly improved [65]. Of clinical importance, the frequency of intradialytic hypertension was significantly reduced from 77 % of HD sessions down to 28 % of sessions and average 44 h interdialytic ambulatory SBP was also reduced from 155 to 148 mmHg with carvedilol treatment.

Thus based on the available evidence, a renewed focus on addressing volume overload should be a priority for those patients with a paradoxical rise in BP on HD, and specifically targeting endothelial dysfunction with agents such as carvedilol can also be considered. The features of intradialytic hypertension are summarized in Table 7.4.

Treatment

As an introduction to the specifics of treating hypertension on dialysis, it's instructive to briefly review the major modifiable causes of hypertension in this population with a focus on those etiologies that can currently be addressed. As both a cause and

Table 7.4 Features of intradialytic hypertension

5–15 % prevalence
No single accepted definition
Associated with increased mortality
Caused by volume overload and endothelial dysfunction
Evidence for improvement with dry weight reduction and carvedilol therapy

Table 7.5 Major treatable causes of hypertension in dialysis

Cause	Treatment
Obstructive sleep apnea	Continuous positive airway pressure
Volume overload	Dry weight reduction
Renin–angiotensin–aldosterone system	ACEi, ARB, and spironolactone
Sympathetic overactivity	Beta-blockers, renal nerve ablation
Erythropoietin	Reduce dose

a consequence of kidney disease, the pathophysiology of hypertension in CKD not only shares commonalities with the general hypertensive population but also has causes that are unique to kidney disease and its treatment. Table 7.5 summarizes the major modifiable causes of hypertension in ESRD.

Risk Factors in Common with the General Population

Patients with CKD often carry a burden of pre-existing primary hypertension prior to the recognition of their kidney disease. Additionally, risk factors in the general hypertensive population are similarly present in the CKD population including obesity, excessive salt intake, alcohol consumption, and physical inactivity. Obstructive sleep apnea (OSA) is an additional comorbidity that is important to consider in more detail.

In the general population OSA frequently coexists with hypertension [67–69], with hypopnea leading to hypoxemia and ultimately to sympathetic activation. OSA is strongly linked with resistant hypertension as the presence of OSA is a risk factor for resistant hypertension and the severity of OSA correlates with the severity of hypertension [70–72]. Given this link it is important to note that OSA is a very common in the setting of CKD with the prevalence increasing with declining renal function [73], culminating in a prevalence over 50% for those patients on dialysis [73, 74]. The association between OSA and resistant hypertension is similarly strong in ESRD as a recent cohort study of subjects with advanced CKD including 75 subjects on HD and 20 on PD found a sevenfold increased risk of resistant hypertension in those dialysis patients with severe OSA [75]. Interestingly, there is a growing recognition that OSA itself is caused or exacerbated by volume overload that leads to parapharyngeal edema, which worsens at bedtime in the recumbent position, both in patients without CKD [69] and in those with ESRD [76, 77].

While most studies of continuous positive airway pressure for OSA in the non-CKD population find significant improvement in BP, this improvement is typically modest compared to medication [78], with CPAP use yielding a 1.7 mmHg improvement in mean 24 h ambulatory BP [79].

Causes of Hypertension Unique to End Stage Renal Disease

The two classic mechanisms felt to be responsible for hypertension in the "renopri-val" state of ESRD are volume overload and an inappropriately activated renin–angiotensin–aldosterone system (RAAS) [80]. Sodium loading has long been clinically recognized as a major and essential contributor to hypertension both in those with normal renal function [81] and in the setting of kidney disease. As the glomerular filtration rate (GFR) declines less sodium is filtered leading to sodium retention and to an expanded extracellular fluid volume. The increased plasma volume leads to increased cardiac output and then to increased total peripheral resistance, whereby normal renal autoregulation would lead to a pressure natriuresis and normalization of BP [82], however this natriuresis is incomplete or absent in advanced CKD and ESRD and the increased total peripheral resistance persists. Randomized trial evidence confirms that ultrafiltration for volume removal improves BP on HD [62].

The other classically recognized contributor is an inappropriately activated RAAS [83], possibly provoked by renal ischemia in patients with renovascular disease or by regional ischemia due to renal fibrosis. Unsurprisingly, angiotensin converting enzyme inhibitor (ACEi) therapy has been shown to be effective at reducing BP in dialysis patients [84, 85].

Among the novel mechanisms of hypertension in advanced kidney disease, sympathetic overactivity is now widely accepted as a contributor. Increased catecholamine levels [86] and increased catecholamine sensitivity [87] in CKD were both demonstrated in the 1980s, and increased catecholamine levels have been shown to predict cardiovascular events and mortality in chronic HD patients [88]. Unidentified uremic toxins were originally thought to provoke this sympathetic overactivity, however Converse and colleagues implicated the diseased kidneys themselves via experiments wherein they measured muscle sympathetic nerve activity in three groups of subjects: those on chronic HD with their native kidneys, those on chronic HD status post bilateral nephrectomy, and normal controls [89]. They found increased sympathetic activity and higher BP in those chronic HD patients still with their native kidneys but those subjects who were surgically anephric have sympathetic nerve activity and BP similar to the normal controls. Uremic toxins don't appear to be the cause of the increased renal afferent nerve signals that increase sympathetic activity, as demonstrated by studies of patients who have normally functioning renal transplants and still retain their native kidneys; [90] but renal ischemia of the native kidneys is a likely contributor [91].

Lastly, medications contribute to hypertension in ESRD. Conventional medications such as over-the-counter nonsteroidal anti-inflammatory drugs and decongestants can exacerbate hypertension, however erythropoiesis stimulating agents (ESA) are commonly prescribed for the anemia of CKD and resultant hypertension has been recognized since the early days of ESA use in ESRD [92]. The incidence of hypertension provoked by ESA administration is associated with the ESA dose but is independent of red blood cell mass or viscosity [93, 94]. While the exact mechanism of how

ESA use causes hypertension is unknown, the current evidence suggests that it is mediated via vasoconstrictor effects, likely through increased levels of endothelin-1 or increased vasoconstrictive response to that peptide [95–97].

Up to 30 % of dialysis patients develop hypertension or require an adjustment in antihypertensive medications with ESA use [98, 99], while the rise in BP with ESA use typically ranges from 5 to 8 mmHg in SBP and 4–6 mmHg in DBP [100]. The rise in BP with ESA administration is more likely in those with baseline hypertension [101] or a family history of hypertension [102]. There is unfortunately a paucity of evidence to guide the prevention of ESA induced hypertension but recommended strategies include changing to subcutaneous administration, reducing the goal hemoglobin level in those who are unresponsive to ESA therapy, minimizing the ESA dose by starting low and increasing slowly, and avoiding ESA use entirely [54].

Volume Control

The focus of nonpharmacologic treatment of hypertension on dialysis is to treat volume overload through complementary strategies both to reduce sodium intake by dietary sodium restriction and individualization of the dialysate sodium while also augmenting sodium removal by dry weight reduction, providing adequate time on dialysis, and considering frequent dialysis. Table 7.6 summarizes the nonpharmacologic treatment of hypertension in dialysis. The archetype for this management of hypertension on dialysis is reported by Charra and colleagues from Tassin, France where patients are dialyzed for extended hours on a low sodium dialysate and low sodium diet is emphasized to the point where low sodium bread is provided to the patients [103]. They report excellent control of BP despite antihypertensive medication use at only 1–2 % [104], as well as low mortality with a 5-year survival rate reported at 87 % [105], which is more than twice the current reported 5-year survival rate in the USA [1]. More recently a trial of low sodium diet and dry weight reduction in 19 hypertensive HD patients with a before–after design found this combined strategy reduced echocardiographic left ventricular hypertrophy [106]. Similar results have been reported in PD from a single center where all 47 of the center's hypertensive patients had their antihypertensive medications withdrawn and BP was subsequently successfully controlled in 37 patients with a combination of strict low sodium diet and added ultrafiltration [107].

Table 7.6 Complementary components of nonpharmacologic treatment of hypertension on dialysis	
	1. Dry weight reduction
	2. Dietary sodium restriction
	3. Dialysate sodium reduction
	4. Adequate time on dialysis
	5. Consideration of frequent dialysis

Dry Weight Reduction

Malignant hypertension was common in ESRD prior to the advent of chronic HD and since those earliest days ultrafiltration has been recognized as an effective means of BP control in ESRD [108], including for the very first chronic HD patient in the USA, Clyde Shields, under the care of Dr. Belding Scribner [109]. Only recently has the randomized controlled DRIP trial of dry weight reduction definitively confirmed those original observations [62]. The DRIP trial recruited 150 chronic and stable HD patients with hypertension confirmed by 44 h interdialytic ABPM despite being on an average of 2.6 antihypertensive medications who were then randomized in a two to one ratio to intervention versus usual care for the 8-week trial. All subjects had their antihypertensive medications and their prescribed time on HD kept stable, and all were visited by a study physician on each HD session during the trial. The intervention group received progressive reduction in dry weight by at least 0.2 kg each HD session until they had symptoms of hypovolemia. Compared to the control group at 8 weeks, the intervention group had 1 kg of weight reduction and average 44 h interdialytic ambulatory BP improved by 6.6/3.3 mmHg [62]. Notably, by design those in the intervention group necessarily had to have symptoms of hypovolemia before dry weight reduction was stopped, but despite this requirement there was no change in any domain of the Kidney Disease Quality of Life questionnaire during the trial.

Management of Dry Weight

Unfortunately there is no single universally accepted definition of dry weight, but a reasonable standard is that used by Sinha and Agarwal who define the dry weight as the lowest tolerated post-HD weight achieved via gradual change in post-HD weight at which there are minimal signs or symptoms of either hypovolemia or hypervolemia [110]. Thus, achieving and maintaining an adequately low dry weight is a hands-on and iterative process that requires attention to details beyond only the prescribed dry weight [111], including adherence to a low sodium diet, minimization of dialysate sodium content, providing adequate time on HD, and consideration of more frequent dialysis.

When deciding whether to adjust the dry weight prescription, the first step is the assessment for volume overload. Unfortunately, while the routine clinical exam performs well at detecting acute or massive volume overload, it performs poorly at detecting subtle and chronic volume overload [110]. This is exemplified by a cross sectional study of 150 chronic HD patients that found the presence of pedal edema to have no correlation with putative objective markers of volume overload including brain natriuretic peptide, echocardiographic inferior vena cava diameter, or relative plasma volume slope [112]. As another example, it is important to consider that all the hypertensive subjects of the DRIP trial were at their clinical dry weight as determined by their primary nephrologist to start the trial, yet the subjects of the intervention group had their dry weight successfully reduced, which resulted in a

Table 7.7 Clinical signs of volume overload on dialysis

1. Elevated interdialytic BP by home or ambulatory monitoring
2. Multiple antihypertensive medications
3. Low interdialytic weight gain
4. Classical signs: peripheral edema, pulmonary congestion, pleural effusion

clinically significant improvement in 44 h ambulatory BP [62]. This further illustrates the difficulty in detecting subtle volume overload that if removed by means of dry weight reduction will improve BP.

A number of experimental objective measures of volume status have been studied including natriuretic peptides, inferior vena cava diameter, relative plasma volume monitoring, and bioelectrical impedance analysis [113]. The latter two have the most supporting evidence with a secondary analysis of the DRIP trial showing that baseline relative plasma volume monitoring identified the most volume overloaded subjects, who subsequently had the largest average reduction in weight at 1.5 kg and the largest improvement in ambulatory SBP at 12.6 mmHg [114]. Most recently, a randomized trial of bioelectrical impedance analysis to guide dry weight management in a cohort of largely normotensive HD subjects found a significant improvement in LVH as well as improvement in peridialytic BP despite reductions in antihypertensive drug use for the intervention group [115].

However, these objective measures of volume status remain investigational and remain to be adequately validated. Therefore the onus is on the treating nephrologist to have a high index of suspicion for occult volume overload. Signs that should prompt consideration for reduction in dry weight include uncontrolled hypertension, especially in those patients who are on multiple medications such as in the DRIP trial where subjects were on an average of 2.6 antihypertensive drugs at baseline [62]. Numerous studies have shown that greater antihypertensive drug use is associated with worse control of hypertension [13, 116], which is plausibly due to inadequately addressed volume overload which could be improved with reduction in dry weight. Table 7.7 summarizes the clinical signs of volume overload.

Another sign to consider reduction in dry weight is a low interdialytic weight gain. This comes from the observation that interdialytic weight gain tends to rise when dry weight is reduced and vice versa [117]. Additionally the secondary analysis of the DRIP trial that employed relative plasma volume monitoring found the flattest relative plasma volume slopes, corresponding to the most volume overload, in the group with the lowest ultrafiltration volume [114]. This is not surprising considering the mechanism of relative plasma volume monitoring, however the ultrafiltration volume generally equals the interdialytic weight gain, and, as noted above, subsequent reduction in dry weight per the trial protocol in the group with the lowest interdialytic weight gain resulted in the greatest weight loss at 1.5 kg and in the greatest reduction in 44 h ambulatory SBP at 12.6 mmHg compared to any of the other groups with higher interdialytic weight gains. Thus low interdialytic weight gain may be a sign of occult volume overload and low interdialytic weight gain should not be considered to be synonymous with euvolemia [118]. As a purely practical matter, a low interdialytic weight gain also makes it easier to challenge the dry weight.

It is important to note that while volume overload is a major contributor to hypertension in ESRD and volume removal is the foundation of hypertension control in ESRD, that hypertension and volume overload are not equivalent. The presence or absence of hypertension doesn't definitively rule volume overload either in or out. This is illustrated by a study of 500 HD patients using bioelectric impedance that found 33 % of the cohort to be euvolemic and normotensive based on peridialytic BP, while 10 % were hypervolemic yet still normotensive, and 13 % were euvolemic but still hypertensive [119]. The distinction is even more important when outcomes are considered. Volume overload has been shown to be independently associated with mortality both when assessed by bioelectrical impedance [120] and by relative plasma volume monitoring [121], even after adjusting for BP in both studies. So while the presence or absence of hypertension is an important finding to guide the clinical assessment of volume status in dialysis, the treating nephrologist must keep an open mind and look for other confirming signs.

The recommended method to reduce dry weight is in decrements as small as 0.2–0.3 kg per HD session based on the recognition that even small changes in dry weight can improve BP, as the DRIP trial had only 1 kg reduction in the dry weight of the intervention group yet found a large change in ambulatory SBP, and other trials of dry weight management have similarly found significant BP reduction with similar changes in dry weight of only 1 kg or less [122, 123]. An added benefit of making small and gradual changes in dry weight is that it builds trust in patients who are often reluctant to permit their dry weight to be lowered for fear of provoking symptoms such as cramping.

There are risks to challenging dry weight including increased risk of clotted vascular access [49], accelerated loss of residual renal function [107], and increased frequency of intradialytic hypotension, which has been associated with myocardial stunning [124] and increased mortality [125]. As the DRIP trial lasted only 8 weeks long-term randomized trials are needed to examine the balance between benefits and risks of dry weight reduction.

Dietary Sodium Restriction

Despite recent observational evidence questioning the benefits of a low sodium diet for the general population [126], there is ample randomized trial evidence supporting the efficacy of low sodium diet to treat resistant hypertension in those without kidney disease [127], to treat hypertension in stage 3–4 CKD [128], and for reduction of proteinuria and albuminuria in diabetic nephropathy [129]. In the HD patient sodium intake provokes increased interdialytic weight gain [130] which also leads to increased ultrafiltration rates, both of which are associated with cardiovascular mortality [131, 132]. Restricting sodium intake reduces interdialytic weight gain, which will also practically improve the ability to achieve an adequately low dry weight with dialysis [133, 134]. However, in the dialysis patient, reducing dietary sodium intake should be followed by probing dry weight to manage hypertension better. In the absence of probing dry weight, the full benefit of restricting dietary sodium intake may not be realized. The American Heart Association recommends <1500 mg (equivalent to 65 mmol) daily intake [135], which is a reasonable prescription for dialysis patients [54]. Notably, except for hyponatremia treatment, there is no rational role for fluid restriction in dialysis patients [130, 136].

Dialysate Sodium Reduction

In the earliest days of chronic HD low dialysate sodium concentrations were used and sodium removal on HD was thus in part due to diffusion in addition to convective removal with ultrafiltration. As the efficiency of dialyzers improved and dialysis times were reduced, higher dialysate sodium concentrations became the norm to reduce hemodynamic instability, cramping, and symptoms of disequilibrium [137] and initial studies suggested that hypertension wasn't a complication [138]. However, more recently it has been recognized that higher dialysate sodium concentrations will reduce or reverse the diffusive removal of sodium on HD, which undermines the effective management of volume control [139]. As an example of the impact of dialysate sodium concentration, in a pilot study that reduced dialysate sodium from 137.8 to 135.6 mmol/L stepwise over 7 weeks, net sodium removal was significantly increased from 383 to 480 mmol per HD session [140].

Numerous studies have shown interdialytic weight gain to be directly related to dialysate sodium concentration with higher dialysate sodium leading to higher intradialytic weight gain [140–142]. Increased interdialytic weight gain is also seen with sodium profiles, also called sodium ramping, where the dialysate sodium concentration generally starts high and then is gradually reduced during the HD session [141, 143, 144]. While higher dialysate sodium concentrations are prescribed to promote hemodynamic stability, the resulting higher interdialytic weight gain can lead to higher ultrafiltration rates which lead to the very hemodynamic instability originally to be avoided. Additionally, more recent studies of higher dialysate sodium concentrations, whether constant or with a profile, have been associated with higher BP in some [143, 144], but not all investigations [142].

An alternative to avoid the vicious cycle above is to individualize the dialysate sodium prescription to the patient's pre-HD serum sodium. The importance of individualization is illustrated by a cross sectional study of 1084 HD patients that examined the difference between the individual dialysate sodium concentration and the patient's pre-HD serum sodium and found that this difference is directly related to interdialytic weight gain, with a higher dialysate sodium concentration relative to the pre-HD serum sodium being associated with greater weight gain [145]. A single-blind crossover study of 27 HD patients illustrated one method of individualizing the dialysate sodium concentration by first dialyzing all patients with a standard 138 mmol/L sodium dialysate for 3 weeks and then on a dialysate sodium concentration set to 0.95 multiplied by the pre-HD serum sodium for 3 weeks [146]. On the low sodium dialysate prescription significant reductions were seen in interdialytic weight gain by 0.6 kg, in the frequency of intradialytic hypotension, and in the pre-HD SBP in the hypertensive subjects. Based on these findings it is reasonable to recommend that dialysate sodium be individualized to avoid being higher than the individual patient's pre-HD serum sodium and possibly as low as 0.95 multiplied by the serum sodium in hypertensive individuals or those with high interdialytic weight gain precluding the achievement of an adequately low dry weight.

A trial in 25 PD patients employed a before–after design to investigate the use of low sodium dialysate over 2 months [147]. All subjects had one exchange per day changed to a low sodium solution, but 10 subjects had the dextrose concentration increased to compensate for reduced osmolality while 15 subjects had no change to their dextrose concentration. The first group had significantly improved BP along with markers of improved volume overload, suggesting that reducing dialysate sodium is only useful if it is accompanied by adequate ultrafiltration.

Adequate Time on Dialysis

Despite reducing dietary sodium intake and the dialysate sodium concentration to reduce interdialytic weight gain, many attempts to reduce dry weight to improve BP will be precluded in many patients due to intradialytic hypotension or symptoms on HD including cramping. In these patients increasing the HD time can make ultrafiltration easier to tolerate thus facilitating the achievement of an adequate dry weight. Shorter HD times have recently been shown in a secondary analysis of the DRIP trial to be associated both with higher BP and slower improvement in BP when dry weight is reduced [148]. A randomized crossover trial of 38 HD patients evaluated time on HD by assigning subjects to 2 weeks of 4 h versus 5 h HD sessions and found significantly less intradialytic hypotension and post-HD orthostatic hypotension during the longer HD runs [149]. An added salutary effect of longer HD time is that for a given amount of interdialytic weight gain, an increased HD time will lead to a lower ultrafiltration rate, which has been associated with mortality [132].

It is for all these reasons that the European Best Practice Guidelines recommend that HD should be delivered at least three times weekly for a total duration of at least 12 h, unless substantial residual renal function remains [150]. However, in the USA a recent cohort study among 32,000 HD patients found that the average single HD session was only 217 min and that one quarter of patients dialyzed less than 3 h and 15 min per session [151]. The lower average treatment times in the USA are likely due to the practice of reducing the prescribed time to achieve a minimum goal Kt/V, however this practice should be avoided on account of the potential deleterious effects that shorter treatment time can have on volume status and hypertension [152].

Frequent Dialysis

An additional strategy to treat patients who cannot achieve an adequately low dry weight on a conventional three times weekly HD schedule is to consider a change in modality to more frequent dialysis. Observational studies have shown frequent

HD to be associated with reductions in BP despite lower antihypertensive drug use [153, 154], as well as with improvements in LVH [154]. More recently randomized trials have confirmed some of these findings with trial of 52 patients that assigned subjects to either conventional 3 times weekly HD versus 6 nights weekly nocturnal HD for 6 months and found significantly improved BP, lower antihypertensive drug use, and improvement left ventricular hypertrophy in the nocturnal HD group [155]. The subsequent Frequent Hemodialysis Network (FHN) Nocturnal trial recruited 87 HD patients and randomized them to 3 times weekly conventional HD versus 6 nights weekly nocturnal HD, and weekly average pre-HD BP was significantly improved in the nocturnal HD group despite a reduction in antihypertensive medication use; however, the trends toward improvement in the primary endpoints including LVH were nonsignificant, possibly due to lack of power from difficultly with subject recruitment [156]. The companion FHN trial of daily HD recruited 245 patients who were randomized to 3 times weekly conventional HD versus 6 days weekly HD for 12 months and this trial did find significantly reduced hazard for both coprimary composite endpoints of death or increase in left ventricular mass and death or decrease in the physical-health composite score [157]. Both weekly average pre-HD SBP and the number of antihypertensive medications for the intervention group were reduced significantly, as well. These improvements in BP and LVH are plausibly due to better control of volume [158], especially when it is recognized that the daily HD group had significantly more ultrafiltration per week at 10.58 L on average compared to 8.99 L for the control group [157].

Pharmacologic Treatment

Patients with ESRD are routinely excluded from drug trials, limiting the evidence base from which to make recommendations for antihypertensive drug therapy. Two meta-analyses of randomized trials employing antihypertensive drugs in dialysis have found significant improvements in the cardiovascular event rates associated with treatment [159, 160], which was particularly pronounced in subjects with hypertension [160]. However, the trials included in these meta-analyses were highly heterogeneous, most trials weren't limited to hypertensive patients, and only two trials targeted a specific BP goal.

Despite the benefits from the use of antihypertensive medication in ESRD, it must be emphasized that greater use of antihypertensive medications is associated with worse control of hypertension [13, 116], which is plausibly due to inadequately treated volume overload in those cases. Thus the first step in treating hypertension in ESRD should be to address volume overload as able. All classes of antihypertensive medications have roles in the treatment of hypertension in ESRD [161], as detailed below.

Diuretics

While published evidence is lacking, diuretics are often used to address hypertension and volume overload in patients with significant residual renal function, which includes those new to HD and nonoliguric patients on PD. In the setting of advanced renal failure higher doses of diuretics will be necessary to be effective [162]. However, in anuric patients even doses of furosemide as high as 250 mg intravenously are ineffective [163]. While some investigators have suggested that thiazide diuretics exert an antihypertensive vasodilator effect [164, 165], the placebo controlled administration of thiazides to anuric dialysis patients has been shown to have no effect on BP [166]. Thus, the role for diuretics in the treatment of hypertension in dialysis is at best limited to the subset of patients with significant residual renal function.

Beta-Blockers

Beta-adrenergic blocking agents have well-established benefits in the non-dialysis population including in the setting of heart failure [167] and coronary artery disease [168]. As cardiovascular events are the leading cause of death in ESRD and increased sympathetic nervous system overactivity is common [89], beta-blockers are an attractive therapy in this population. A retrospective cohort study of PD patients found beta-blocker use to be associated with a significantly reduced risk of new onset heart failure or the composite endpoint of new onset heart failure and cardiac mortality [169]. Cice and colleagues recruited 114 HD patients with reduced left ventricular ejection fraction <35% and randomized them to carvedilol versus placebo and reported significantly improved 2-year survival in the carvedilol group [170].

Despite these encouraging findings, enthusiasm for beta-blockers as first line pharmacological treatment for hypertension in dialysis is tempered by the non-dialysis experience where beta-blockers are not recommended for initial monotherapy of hypertension [171, 172], consequently ACEi medications are often instead recommended for initial therapy of hypertension [173]. While head to head studies of antihypertensives are few, a recent randomized controlled trial in HD comparing lisinopril to atenolol begins to address the question of which medication to prescribe first for hypertension in HD.

The Hypertension in Hemodialysis Patients Treated with Atenolol or Lisinopril (HDPAL) trial recruited 200 chronic HD patients with hypertension confirmed by 44 h interdialytic ABPM and echocardiographic LVH and randomized them to lisinopril or atenolol based therapy for 12 months to determine which drug is superior for reduction of LVH [53]. All patients were treated to target goal home BP ≤140/90 mmHg checked monthly, first by maximizing the study drug, then by addition of other drugs, sodium restriction, and reduction in dry weight. The trial was terminated early by an independent data safety monitoring board for cardiovascular safety because of significantly more serious adverse cardiovascular events in the lisinopril group, which had 43 events in 28 subjects compared to only 20 events in

16 subjects in the atenolol group (incidence rate ratio 2.36, $P=0.001$). Similarly, the combined serious adverse events of myocardial infarction, stroke, hospitalization for heart failure, or cardiovascular death occurred 23 times in 17 subjects in the lisinopril group compared to only 11 events in 10 subjects in the atenolol group (incidence rate ratio 2.29, $P=0.002$). LVH improved in both groups but no differences between drug groups were found.

While 44 h ambulatory BP improved similarly in both groups measured at baseline, 3 months, 6 months, and 12 months, the monthly home BP was consistently lower in the atenolol group despite significantly more antihypertensive medications and greater dry weight reduction in the lisinopril group [53]. Thus atenolol appears to be superior to lisinopril in terms of cardiovascular event rates and BP reduction. Based on the findings of this head to head comparison of atenolol and lisinopril in HD patients it is recommended that beta-blockers be the first line therapy for hypertension. Table 7.8 summarizes the recommendations for pharmacologic therapy for hypertension in dialysis. Atenolol in particular may be practically useful as it can be dosed just 3 times per week after HD, as was the protocol in the HDPAL trial, and this schedule has been previously shown to significantly reduce 44 h interdialytic ambulatory BP [174]. Three times weekly dosing permits the possibility of directly observed administration of atenolol in the HD unit to improve compliance with the antihypertensive regimen.

Angiotensin Converting Enzyme Inhibitors and Angiotensin Receptor Blockers

It cannot be concluded from the HDPAL trial that ACEi medications are harmful because there was no placebo controlled group in the study [53]. Indeed, ACEi and angiotensin receptor blocker (ARB) drugs are mainstays of therapy in pre-dialysis CKD [175] and in cardiovascular disease [176, 177]. Both ACEi [84, 85, 178] and ARB medications [179] have been shown to improve BP in ESRD. As with atenolol, both lisinopril [84] and trandolapril [178] have been shown to be effective at lowering BP when dosed only three times weekly after HD.

Three randomized clinical trials have examined ACEi or ARB therapy in HD patients with cardiovascular events as the primary endpoint, and they warrant more detailed mention. The only randomized clinical trial investigating an ACEi and cardiovascular events in HD patients is the Fosinopril in Dialysis Study (FOSIDIAL) [85], which recruited 397 chronic HD patients with LVH who were followed for a 2-week run-in period on fosinopril, and those who tolerated the therapy were randomized to fosinopril or placebo and treated to goal peridialytic <160/90 mmHg for 24 months [180]. No benefit was found for fosinopril in decreasing cardiovascular events [85].

Two randomized controlled trials have investigated ARB use in HD and found a benefit for cardiovascular events. The first enrolled 80 HD patients who were randomized to candesartan or open label usual care for a planned 3 years [181]. The trial was stopped early on account of an interim analysis that found significant and substantial benefit for candesartan for the primary endpoint of cardiovascular events

Table 7.8 Suggested approach to pharmacologic therapy for hypertension in dialysis

Medication Class	Comments
Beta-blockers	First line therapy, superior in trial vs. ACEi
ACEi or ARB	Second line therapy, superior to calcium channel blockers
Calcium channel blockers	Third line therapy
Centrally acting alpha agonists	Clonidine patch or guanfacine preferred
Direct vasodilators	Minoxidil preferred to hydralazine
Mineralocorticoid receptor antagonists	Emerging evidence of efficacy and mortality benefit
Loop and thiazide diuretics	Role limited only to those with substantial residual renal function

as well as for mortality with zero deaths in the candesartan group and 18.9 % mortality in the control group [181]. The second trial included 360 HD patients randomized to open label ARB therapy with losartan, valsartan, or candesartan versus usual care with goal peridialytic SBP <150 mmHg over 3 years [182]. ARB treatment significantly reduced the primary endpoint of cardiovascular events with a 49 % reduction in risk of cardiovascular event ($HR=0.51$, $P=0.002$).

In the setting of the divergent outcomes for the three randomized clinical trials using ACEi or ARB drugs above, a recent meta-analysis examined the pooled results for cardiovascular events in the 837 total subjects in these trials and found a trend toward benefit with a relative risk for cardiovascular events at 0.66, but this did not reach statistical significance (95 % confidence interval 0.35 to 1.25, $P=0.20$) [183]. Each trial had different definitions for cardiovascular events, and not surprisingly significant heterogeneity was found. Similarly, a systematic review of ACEi and ARB therapy in PD patients included three randomized clinical trials and found no improvement in cardiovascular events for the intervention groups [184].

As ACEi and ARB therapy has been shown to delay progression of pre-dialysis chronic kidney disease [185], these agents may be effective at preserving residual renal function in dialysis patients, which is emerging as an important goal for both PD and HD patients [186]. Two randomized controlled open label trials in PD, one investigating ramipril in 60 subjects [187] and the other studying valsartan in 34 subjects [188], both found active treatments reduced the rate of decline in GFR, while a meta-analysis pooled the difference between the intervention groups and the control groups at 12 months and found a clinically and statistically significant benefit of 0.9 mL/min/1.73 m^2 in favor of the intervention groups [184]. In HD however, a recent randomized placebo controlled trial of irbesartan over 1 year in 82 nonoliguric HD patients found no benefit for irbesartan in decline of GFR or development of anuria [189].

The risk of hyperkalemia with ACEi or ARB use in dialysis appears low based on the evidence from the aforementioned randomized controlled trials in both HD [85, 181, 182] and PD [187]. ACEi or ARB agents are a reasonable second choice after beta-blockers for an antihypertensive medication in dialysis based on their tolerability, the evidence of benefit in the non-dialysis population, and the randomized trial evidence of benefit on intermediate end points such as reduction in LVH [183].

Calcium Channel Blockers

Amlodipine has been shown to be effective versus placebo in improving BP in a randomized trial of 251 hypertensive HD patients where the primary endpoint of cardiovascular events showed no improvement for active treatment [190]. Calcium channel blockers have the practical benefits of being well tolerated and requiring only once a day dosing, however ACEi or ARB therapy is preferred before calcium blockers based on head to head trials showing calcium channel blockers to be significantly inferior for regression of LVH [191, 192].

Centrally Acting Alpha Agonists

These medications are typically reserved only for those patients whose BP is uncontrolled on the combination of beta-blocker, ACEi or ARB, plus calcium channel blocker. To minimize pill burden and dosing schedule, it is recommended to avoid oral clonidine and to instead use the long acting clonidine patch, which can be administered once a week at the dialysis unit as directly observed therapy. As the clonidine patch can be expensive, a cheaper alternative is oral guanfacine, dosed only once daily at bedtime to minimize the impact of dose related drowsiness.

Vasodilators

Direct vasodilator agents are usually reserved as last line therapy for hypertension in ESRD. However, hydralazine use is becoming more common based on trial evidence of benefit for heart failure in the African-American population in combination with isosorbide dinitrate [193], but it is important to recognize that this combination of medications has not been studied in ESRD. Furthermore the pill burden and requirement of three times daily dosing of hydralazine makes it less attractive for use in ESRD. It is for that reason that minoxidil is usually preferable to hydralazine on account of its antihypertensive effectiveness with only once daily dosing in the setting of CKD.

Mineralocorticoid Receptor Antagonists

Mineralocorticoid receptor antagonists have well-established roles in the non-dialysis population for treatment of resistant hypertension [194] and heart failure [195, 196]. In the dialysis population spironolactone has been shown to significantly reduce 24 h ambulatory BP by 10.9/5.8 mmHg in a randomized controlled double blind trial of 76 hypertensive dialysis patients on HD or PD treated with spironolactone 25–50 mg daily versus placebo over 12 weeks [197]. Recently the

Dialysis Outcomes Heart Failure Aldosterone Study (DOHAS) clinical trial randomized 309 HD patients to spironolactone 25 mg daily versus open label usual care for 3 years and found both cardiovascular death and hospitalizations and all-cause mortality were significantly improved in the spironolactone group [198]. Importantly, spironolactone therapy was discontinued for hyperkalemia in only three patients during the trial. While the results of the DOHAS trial are very promising, they require confirmation in future blinded randomized trials to balance the risk of hyperkalemia with the potential benefits before the routine use of spironolactone for hypertension in HD can be recommended.

Invasive Treatment

The history of invasive treatments for hypertension dates back at least to the 1930s when surgical sympathectomy was employed for essential hypertension [199]. As efficacious oral antihypertensive agents with tolerable side effect profiles were discovered, surgery fell out of favor as a treatment for simple hypertension. However, in the early era of chronic HD in the 1960s and 1970s it was recognized that a subset of patients with ESRD didn't achieve adequate control of hypertension despite ultrafiltration on HD and the use of the antihypertensive medications of the day [80]. As high renin levels were common in these cases, bilateral nephrectomy was advocated as an effective means to reduce renin levels and BP, though it was recognized even then that other mechanisms likely were responsible for the improved BP after nephrectomy [80]. With the introduction of ACEi drugs bilateral nephrectomy too became much less common.

However, Converse and colleagues demonstrated that sympathetic overactivity from renal afferent nerves are a major source of hypertension in ESRD [89], and with the invention of a radiofrequency catheter based approach to target the renal nerves there has been renewed interest in renal sympathectomy via the endovascular approach [91]. A pilot study of renal denervation by radiofrequency ablation was performed in 12 chronic HD patients with uncontrolled hypertension and office BP was reduced in the 9 patients who had the procedure versus unchanged BP in those 3 patients whose atrophic renal arteries precluded the endovascular denervation procedure [200]. However, enthusiasm for renal denervation must be tempered by the experience with renal denervation in the resistant hypertension population without CKD where initial trials showed promise [201] but when a randomized, sham placebo controlled, and blinded trial was performed there was no BP reduction for the intervention [202]. While ESRD patients are an ideal group who may benefit from this therapy, it remains to be seen whether the disappointing result from the randomized controlled trial of endovascular renal denervation will preclude further development of this technique.

Prognosis

Despite a strong and direct relationship between hypertension and cardiovascular and all-cause mortality [203] and copious evidence of benefit for treatment of hypertension in the non-dialysis population [175], the relationship between BP and outcomes in dialysis patients remains a topic of controversial [204, 205]. Various studies have found an association between peridialytic hypertension and strokes [206], heart failure [207], arrhythmias [208], cardiovascular events [209], and all-cause mortality [210]. However, other studies suggest that peridialytic hypertension is protective and lower BP is associated with worse mortality [4, 211–213], and the risk of normotensive BP is magnified when BP is considered as a time dependent co-variate [211, 213]. This paradoxical relationship between BP and mortality has been termed the "reverse epidemiology" of hypertension [205] and has raised concern that treatment of hypertension may be harmful [214].

When examining the prognostic value of hypertension in dialysis it is important to additionally consider severity of illness and dialysis vintage as well. This is illustrated by a retrospective cohort study of 2770 prevalent PD patients where a fully adjusted analysis found higher SBP, DBP, mean arterial pressure, and pulse pressure to be associated with decreased mortality during the first year on dialysis [215]. However, higher SBP and pulse pressure were associated with increased mortality for those patients on dialysis ≥6 years. Similar findings have been shown in a cohort of 16,959 HD patients where SBP <120 mmHg was associated with increased mortality within the first 2 years of starting dialysis, but SBP >150 mmHg was associated with increased mortality among those that survived at least 3 years [216]. These findings suggest lower BP may be an indicator of more severe illness in those patients new to dialysis who are likely to have advanced chronic but unstable systemic comorbidities that recently culminated in ESRD, whereas in the survivors that have been on dialysis for at least 6 years have a more normal relationship between hypertension and outcomes because they are less acutely ill. This explanation is further bolstered by the subgroup in the PD cohort who were listed for transplant within 6 months of starting dialysis, as in this healthier subgroup higher SBP, DBP, mean arterial pressure, and pulse pressure were not associated with improved mortality during the first year of dialysis [215].

The technique of BP measurement also contributes to the controversial relationship between BP and outcomes as the reverse epidemiology of hypertension is primarily a phenomenon of peridialytic BP values. However, ambulatory BP has a strong relationship with mortality on HD, first demonstrated by Amar and colleagues in a study of 57 HD patients [217]. Agarwal and colleagues have confirmed the relationship between ambulatory BP and mortality in a cohort of 150 HD patients, and in the same cohort they also demonstrated home BP to similarly have a strong relationship with mortality [49]. In an expanded cohort of 326 HD patients followed for a mean of 32 months Agarwal subsequently has shown increased mortality at the extremes of ambulatory and home BP, and that mortality was best at a home SBP 120–130 mmHg and ambulatory SBP 110–120 mmHg, while peridialytic BP had no relationship with mortality in this cohort [25]. Most recently an analysis of the Chronic Renal Insufficiency Cohort (CRIC) study compared pre-HD SBP and out of HD unit SBP for prediction of mortality in the 403 subjects who started HD since the start of the study [218]. There were 98 deaths over a mean follow-up of 2.7 years and pre-HD SBP showed a U-shaped relationship to mortality consistent with reverse epidemiology of hypertension. However, in the 326 subjects who had BP checked out of the HD unit in a standardized manner during a research visit, there was a significant and direct linear relationship between BP and mortality with hazard ratio 1.26 for every 10 mmHg rise in SBP, which further emphasizes the importance of BP measurement technique when considering prognosis [218].

Thus while there is concern for reverse epidemiology of hypertension when analyzing peridialytic BP, which would suggest that lowering BP would be harmful in HD patients, the evidence from ambulatory and home BP studies doesn't support those conclusions, nor does the evidence from two meta-analyses of randomized clinical trials of antihypertensive medication use in HD which find cardiovascular benefit rather than harm with active treatment [159, 160].

References

1. Saran R, Li Y, Robinson B, Ayanian J, Balkrishnan R, Bragg-Gresham J, et al. US Renal Data System 2014 Annual Data Report: Epidemiology of kidney disease in the United States. Am J Kidney Dis. 2015;65(6 Suppl 1):A7.
2. O'Connell JB, Maggard MA, Ko CY. Colon cancer survival rates with the new American Joint Committee on Cancer sixth edition staging. J Natl Cancer Inst. 2004;96(19):1420–5.
3. U.S. Renal Data System, USRDS 2013 Annual Data Report: Atlas of chronic kidney disease and end-stage renal disease in the United States, National Institutes of Health, National Institute of Diabetes and Digestive and Kidney Diseases, Bethesda, MD, 2013.
4. Salem MM. Hypertension in the hemodialysis population: a survey of 649 patients. Am J Kidney Dis. 1995;26(3):461–8.
5. Mittal SK, Kowalski E, Trenkle J, McDonough B, Halinski D, Devlin K, et al. Prevalence of hypertension in a hemodialysis population. Clin Nephrol. 1999;51(2):77–82.
6. Rahman M, Dixit A, Donley V, Gupta S, Hanslik T, Lacson E, et al. Factors associated with inadequate blood pressure control in hypertensive hemodialysis patients. Am J Kidney Dis. 1999;33(3):498–506.
7. Rahman M, Fu P, Sehgal AR, Smith MC. Interdialytic weight gain, compliance with dialysis regimen, and age are independent predictors of blood pressure in hemodialysis patients. Am J Kidney Dis. 2000;35(2):257–65.
8. Eknoyan G, Beck GJ, Cheung AK, Daugirdas JT, Greene T, Kusek JW, et al. Effect of dialysis dose and membrane flux in maintenance hemodialysis. N Engl J Med. 2002;347(25):2010–9.
9. Greene T, Beck GJ, Gassman JJ, Gotch FA, Kusek JW, Levey AS, et al. Design and statistical issues of the hemodialysis (HEMO) study. Control Clin Trials. 2000;21(5):502–25.
10. Rocco MV, Yan G, Heyka RJ, Benz R, Cheung AK. Risk factors for hypertension in chronic hemodialysis patients: baseline data from the HEMO study. Am J Nephrol. 2001;21(4):280–8.
11. Agarwal R, Nissenson AR, Batlle D, Coyne DW, Trout JR, Warnock DG. Prevalence, treatment, and control of hypertension in chronic hemodialysis patients in the United States. Am J Med. 2003;115(4):291–7.

12. Michael B, Coyne DW, Fishbane S, Folkert V, Lynn R, Nissenson AR, et al. Sodium ferric gluconate complex in hemodialysis patients: adverse reactions compared to placebo and iron dextran. Kidney Int. 2002;61(5):1830–9.

13. Agarwal R. Epidemiology of interdialytic ambulatory hypertension and the role of volume excess. Am J Nephrol. 2011;34(4):381–90.

14. Cheigh JS, Milite C, Sullivan JF, Rubin AL, Stenzel KH. Hypertension is not adequately controlled in hemodialysis patients. Am J Kidney Dis. 1992;19(5):453–9.

15. Boudville NC, Cordy P, Millman K, Fairbairn L, Sharma A, Lindsay R, et al. Blood pressure, volume, and sodium control in an automated peritoneal dialysis population. Perit Dial Int. 2007;27(5):537–43.

16. Rocco MV, Flanigan MJ, Beaver S, Frederick P, Gentile DE, McClellan WM, et al. Report from the 1995 Core Indicators for Peritoneal Dialysis Study Group. Am J Kidney Dis. 1997;30(2):165–73.

17. Goldfarb-Rumyantzev AS, Baird BC, Leypoldt JK, Cheung AK. The association between BP and mortality in patients on chronic peritoneal dialysis. Nephrol Dial Transplant. 2005;20(8):1693–701.

18. Cocchi R, Degli EE, Fabbri A, Lucatello A, Sturani A, Quarello F, et al. Prevalence of hypertension in patients on peritoneal dialysis: results of an Italian multicentre study. Nephrol Dial Transplant. 1999;14(6):1536–40.

19. Tonbul Z, Altintepe L, Sozlu C, Yeksan M, Yildiz A, Turk S. Ambulatory blood pressure monitoring in haemodialysis and continuous ambulatory peritoneal dialysis (CAPD) patients. J Hum Hypertens. 2002;16(8):585–9.

20. Townsend RR, Ford V. Ambulatory blood pressure monitoring: coming of age in nephrology. J Am Soc Nephrol. 1996;7(11):2279–87.

21. Mansoor GA, White WB. Ambulatory blood pressure monitoring is a useful clinical tool in nephrology. Am J Kidney Dis. 1997;30(5):591–605.

22. Peixoto AJ, Santos SF, Mendes RB, Crowley ST, Maldonado R, Orias M, et al. Reproducibility of ambulatory blood pressure monitoring in hemodialysis patients. Am J Kidney Dis. 2000;36(5):983–90.

23. Thompson AM, Pickering TG. The role of ambulatory blood pressure monitoring in chronic and end-stage renal disease. Kidney Int. 2006;70(6):1000–7.

24. Agarwal R, Brim NJ, Mahenthiran J, Andersen MJ, Saha C. Out-of-hemodialysis-unit blood pressure is a superior determinant of left ventricular hypertrophy. Hypertension. 2006;47(1):62–8.

25. Agarwal R. Blood pressure and mortality among hemodialysis patients. Hypertension. 2010;55(3):762–8.

26. Peixoto AJ, Gray TA, Crowley ST. Validation of the SpaceLabs 90207 ambulatory blood pressure device for hemodialysis patients. Blood Press Monit. 1999;4(5):217–21.

27. Agarwal R, Lewis RR. Prediction of hypertension in chronic hemodialysis patients. Kidney Int. 2001;60(5):1982–9.

28. Agarwal R, Light RP. Arterial stiffness and interdialytic weight gain influence ambulatory blood pressure patterns in hemodialysis patients. Am J Physiol Renal Physiol. 2008;294(2):F303–8.

29. Kelley K, Light RP, Agarwal R. Trended cosinor change model for analyzing hemodynamic rhythm patterns in hemodialysis patients. Hypertension. 2007;50(1):143–50.

30. Cannella G, Paoletti E, Ravera G, Cassottana P, Araghi P, Mulas D, et al. Inadequate diagnosis and therapy of arterial hypertension as causes of left ventricular hypertrophy in uremic dialysis patients. Kidney Int. 2000;58(1):260–8.

31. Bishu K, Gricz KM, Chewaka S, Agarwal R. Appropriateness of antihypertensive drug therapy in hemodialysis patients. Clin J Am Soc Nephrol. 2006;1(4):820–4.

32. Argiles A, Mourad G, Mion C. Seasonal changes in blood pressure in patients with end-stage renal disease treated with hemodialysis. N Engl J Med. 1998;339(19):1364–70.

33. K/DOQI Workgroup: K/DOQI clinical practice guidelines for cardiovascular disease in dialysis patients. Am J Kidney Dis. 2005;45(4 Suppl 3):S1–153.

34. Davenport A, Cox C, Thuraisingham R. Achieving blood pressure targets during dialysis improves control but increases intradialytic hypotension. Kidney Int. 2008;73(6):759–64.
35. Rohrscheib MR, Myers OB, Servilla KS, Adams CD, Miskulin D, Bedrick EJ, et al. Age-related blood pressure patterns and blood pressure variability among hemodialysis patients. Clin J Am Soc Nephrol. 2008;3(5):1407–14.
36. Rahman M, Griffin V, Kumar A, Manzoor F, Wright Jr JT, Smith MC. A comparison of standardized versus "usual" blood pressure measurements in hemodialysis patients. Am J Kidney Dis. 2002;39(6):1226–30.
37. Conion PJ, Walshe JJ, Heinle SK, Minda S, Krucoff M, Schwab SJ. Predialysis systolic blood pressure correlates strongly with mean 24-hour systolic blood pressure and left ventricular mass in stable hemodialysis patients. J Am Soc Nephrol. 1996;7(12):2658–63.
38. Agarwal R, Peixoto AJ, Santos SF, Zoccali C. Pre- and postdialysis blood pressures are imprecise estimates of interdialytic ambulatory blood pressure. Clin J Am Soc Nephrol. 2006;1(3):389–98.
39. Agarwal R, Metiku T, Tegegne GG, Light RP, Bunaye Z, Bekele DM, et al. Diagnosing hypertension by intradialytic blood pressure recordings. Clin J Am Soc Nephrol. 2008;3(5):1364–72.
40. Agarwal R, Light RP. Median intradialytic blood pressure can track changes evoked by probing dry-weight. Clin J Am Soc Nephrol. 2010;5(5):897–904.
41. Pickering TG, Miller NH, Ogedegbe G, Krakoff LR, Artinian NT, Goff D. Call to action on use and reimbursement for home blood pressure monitoring: a joint scientific statement from the American Heart Association, American Society Of Hypertension, and Preventive Cardiovascular Nurses Association. Hypertension. 2008;52(1):10–29.
42. Parati G, Stergiou GS, Asmar R, de Leeuw P, Imai Y, Imai Y, et al. European Society of Hypertension guidelines for blood pressure monitoring at home: a summary report of the Second International Consensus Conference on Home Blood Pressure Monitoring. J Hypertens. 2008;26(8):1505–26.
43. Agarwal R. Role of home blood pressure monitoring in hemodialysis patients. Am J Kidney Dis. 1999;33(4):682–7.
44. Agarwal R, Peixoto AJ, Santos SF, Zoccali C. Out-of-office blood pressure monitoring in chronic kidney disease. Blood Press Monit. 2009;14(1):2–11.
45. Agarwal R, Andersen MJ, Bishu K, Saha C. Home blood pressure monitoring improves the diagnosis of hypertension in hemodialysis patients. Kidney Int. 2006;69(5):900–6.
46. Agarwal R, Satyan S, Alborzi P, Light RP, Tegegne GG, Mazengia HS, et al. Home blood pressure measurements for managing hypertension in hemodialysis patients. Am J Nephrol. 2009;30(2):126–34.
47. Moriya H, Ohtake T, Kobayashi S. Aortic stiffness, left ventricular hypertrophy and weekly averaged blood pressure (WAB) in patients on haemodialysis. Nephrol Dial Transplant. 2007;22(4):1198–204.
48. Moriya H, Oka M, Maesato K, Mano T, Ikee R, Ohtake T, et al. Weekly averaged blood pressure is more important than a single-point blood pressure measurement in the risk stratification of dialysis patients. Clin J Am Soc Nephrol. 2008;3(2):416–22.
49. Alborzi P, Patel N, Agarwal R. Home blood pressures are of greater prognostic value than hemodialysis unit recordings. Clin J Am Soc Nephrol. 2007;2(6):1228–34.
50. Kauric-Klein Z, Artinian N. Improving blood pressure control in hypertensive hemodialysis patients. CANNT J. 2007;17(4):24–6.
51. da Silva GV, de Barros S, Abensur H, Ortega KC, Mion Jr D. Home blood pressure monitoring in blood pressure control among haemodialysis patients: an open randomized clinical trial. Nephrol Dial Transplant. 2009;24(12):3805–11.
52. Agarwal R, Light RP. Chronobiology of arterial hypertension in hemodialysis patients: implications for home blood pressure monitoring. Am J Kidney Dis. 2009;54(4):693–701.
53. Agarwal R, Sinha AD, Pappas MK, Abraham TN, Tegegne GG. Hypertension in hemodialysis patients treated with atenolol or lisinopril: a randomized controlled trial. Nephrol Dial Transplant. 2014;29(3):672–81.

54. Agarwal R, Flynn J, Pogue V, Rahman M, Reisin E, Weir MR. Assessment and management of hypertension in patients on dialysis. J Am Soc Nephrol. 2014;25(8):1630–46.

55. Inrig JK. Intradialytic hypertension: a less-recognized cardiovascular complication of hemodialysis. Am J Kidney Dis. 2010;55(3):580–9.

56. Inrig JK, Oddone EZ, Hasselblad V, Gillespie B, Patel UD, Reddan D, et al. Association of intradialytic blood pressure changes with hospitalization and mortality rates in prevalent ESRD patients. Kidney Int. 2007;71(5):454–61.

57. Van Buren PN, Kim C, Toto R, Inrig JK. Intradialytic hypertension and the association with interdialytic ambulatory blood pressure. Clin J Am Soc Nephrol. 2011;6(7):1684–91.

58. Agarwal R, Light RP. Intradialytic hypertension is a marker of volume excess. Nephrol Dial Transplant. 2010;25(10):3355–61.

59. Inrig JK, Patel UD, Toto RD, Szczech LA. Association of blood pressure increases during hemodialysis with 2-year mortality in incident hemodialysis patients: a secondary analysis of the Dialysis Morbidity and Mortality Wave 2 Study. Am J Kidney Dis. 2009;54(5):881–90.

60. Yang CY, Yang WC, Lin YP. Postdialysis blood pressure rise predicts long-term outcomes in chronic hemodialysis patients: a four-year prospective observational cohort study. BMC Nephrol. 2012;13:12.

61. Cirit M, Akcicek F, Terzioglu E, Soydas C, Ok E, Ozbasli CF, et al. 'Paradoxical' rise in blood pressure during ultrafiltration in dialysis patients. Nephrol Dial Transplant. 1995;10(8):1417–20.

62. Agarwal R, Alborzi P, Satyan S, Light RP. Dry-weight reduction in hypertensive hemodialysis patients (DRIP): a randomized, controlled trial. Hypertension. 2009;53(3):500–7.

63. El-Shafey EM, El-Nagar GF, Selim MF, El-Sorogy HA, Sabry AA. Is there a role for endothelin-1 in the hemodynamic changes during hemodialysis? Clin Exp Nephrol. 2008;12(5):370–5.

64. Chou KJ, Lee PT, Chen CL, Chiou CW, Hsu CY, Chung HM, et al. Physiological changes during hemodialysis in patients with intradialysis hypertension. Kidney Int. 2006;69(10):1833–8.

65. Inrig JK, Van BP, Kim C, Vongpatanasin W, Povsic TJ, Toto R. Probing the mechanisms of intradialytic hypertension: a pilot study targeting endothelial cell dysfunction. Clin J Am Soc Nephrol. 2012;7(8):1300–9.

66. Saijonmaa O, Metsarinne K, Fyhrquist F. Carvedilol and its metabolites suppress endothelin-1 production in human endothelial cell culture. Blood Press. 1997;6(1):24–8.

67. Goodfriend TL, Calhoun DA. Resistant hypertension, obesity, sleep apnea, and aldosterone: theory and therapy. Hypertension. 2004;43(3):518–24.

68. Drager LF, Diegues-Silva L, Diniz PM, Bortolotto LA, Pedrosa RP, Couto RB, et al. Obstructive sleep apnea, masked hypertension, and arterial stiffness in men. Am J Hypertens. 2010;23(3):249–54.

69. Dudenbostel T, Calhoun DA. Resistant hypertension, obstructive sleep apnoea and aldosterone. J Hum Hypertens. 2012;26(5):281–7.

70. Goncalves SC, Martinez D, Gus M, de Abreu-Silva EO, Bertoluci C, Dutra I, et al. Obstructive sleep apnea and resistant hypertension: a case–control study. Chest. 2007;132(6):1858–62.

71. Pedrosa RP, Drager LF, Gonzaga CC, Sousa MG, de Paula LK, Amaro AC, et al. Obstructive sleep apnea: the most common secondary cause of hypertension associated with resistant hypertension. Hypertension. 2011;58(5):811–7.

72. Ruttanaumpawan P, Nopmaneejumruslers C, Logan AG, Lazarescu A, Qian I, Bradley TD. Association between refractory hypertension and obstructive sleep apnea. J Hypertens. 2009;27(7):1439–45.

73. Nicholl DD, Ahmed SB, Loewen AH, Hemmelgarn BR, Sola DY, Beecroft JM, et al. Declining kidney function increases the prevalence of sleep apnea and nocturnal hypoxia. Chest. 2012;141(6):1422–30.

74. Forni OV, Ogna A, Pruijm M, Bassi I, Zuercher E, Halabi G, et al. Prevalence and diagnostic approach to sleep apnea in hemodialysis patients: a population study. Biomed Res Int. 2015;2015:103686.

75. Abdel-Kader K, Dohar S, Shah N, Jhamb M, Reis SE, Strollo P, et al. Resistant hypertension and obstructive sleep apnea in the setting of kidney disease. J Hypertens. 2012;30(5):960–6.
76. Tada T, Kusano KF, Ogawa A, Iwasaki J, Sakuragi S, Kusano I, et al. The predictors of central and obstructive sleep apnoea in haemodialysis patients. Nephrol Dial Transplant. 2007;22(4):1190–7.
77. Park J, Campese VM. Resistant hypertension and obstructive sleep apnea in end-stage renal disease. J Hypertens. 2012;30(5):880–1.
78. Pepin JL, Tamisier R, Barone-Rochette G, Launois SH, Levy P, Baguet JP. Comparison of continuous positive airway pressure and valsartan in hypertensive patients with sleep apnea. Am J Respir Crit Care Med. 2010;182(7):954–60.
79. Haentjens P, Van MA, Moscariello A, De WS, Poppe K, Dupont A, et al. The impact of continuous positive airway pressure on blood pressure in patients with obstructive sleep apnea syndrome: evidence from a meta-analysis of placebo-controlled randomized trials. Arch Intern Med. 2007;167(8):757–64.
80. Lazarus JM, Hampers C, Merrill JP. Hypertension in chronic renal failure. Treatment with hemodialysis and nephrectomy. Arch Intern Med. 1974;133(6):1059–66.
81. Murphy RJ. The effect of "rice diet" on plasma volume and extracellular fluid space in hypertensive subjects. J Clin Invest. 1950;29(7):912–7.
82. Guyton AC, Coleman TG, Cowley Jr AV, Scheel KW, Manning Jr RD, Norman Jr RA. Arterial pressure regulation. Overriding dominance of the kidneys in long-term regulation and in hypertension. Am J Med. 1972;52(5):584–94.
83. Schalekamp MA, Beevers DG, Briggs JD, Brown JJ, Davies DL, Fraser R, et al. Hypertension in chronic renal failure. An abnormal relation between sodium and the renin-angiotensin system. Am J Med. 1973;55(3):379–90.
84. Agarwal R, Lewis R, Davis JL, Becker B. Lisinopril therapy for hemodialysis hypertension: hemodynamic and endocrine responses. Am J Kidney Dis. 2001;38(6):1245–50.
85. Zannad F, Kessler M, Lehert P, Grunfeld JP, Thuilliez C, Leizorovicz A, et al. Prevention of cardiovascular events in end-stage renal disease: results of a randomized trial of fosinopril and implications for future studies. Kidney Int. 2006;70(7):1318–24.
86. Ishii M, Ikeda T, Takagi M, Sugimoto T, Atarashi K, Igari T, et al. Elevated plasma catecholamines in hypertensives with primary glomerular diseases. Hypertension. 1983;5(4):545–51.
87. Beretta-Piccoli C, Weidmann P, Schiffl H, Cottier C, Reubi FC. Enhanced cardiovascular pressor reactivity to norepinephrine in mild renal parenchymal disease. Kidney Int. 1982;22(3):297–303.
88. Zoccali C, Mallamaci F, Parlongo S, Cutrupi S, Benedetto FA, Tripepi G, et al. Plasma norepinephrine predicts survival and incident cardiovascular events in patients with end-stage renal disease. Circulation. 2002;105(11):1354–9.
89. Converse Jr RL, Jacobsen TN, Toto RD, Jost CM, Cosentino F, Fouad-Tarazi F, et al. Sympathetic overactivity in patients with chronic renal failure. N Engl J Med. 1992;327(27):1912–8.
90. Hausberg M, Kosch M, Harmelink P, Barenbrock M, Hohage H, Kisters K, et al. Sympathetic nerve activity in end-stage renal disease. Circulation. 2002;106(15):1974–9.
91. Schlaich MP, Socratous F, Hennebry S, Eikelis N, Lambert EA, Straznicky N, et al. Sympathetic activation in chronic renal failure. J Am Soc Nephrol. 2009;20(5):933–9.
92. Buckner FS, Eschbach JW, Haley NR, Davidson RC, Adamson JW. Hypertension following erythropoietin therapy in anemic hemodialysis patients. Am J Hypertens. 1990;3(12 Pt 1):947–55.
93. Abraham PA, Macres MG. Blood pressure in hemodialysis patients during amelioration of anemia with erythropoietin. J Am Soc Nephrol. 1991;2(4):927–36.
94. Kaupke CJ, Kim S, Vaziri ND. Effect of erythrocyte mass on arterial blood pressure in dialysis patients receiving maintenance erythropoietin therapy. J Am Soc Nephrol. 1994;4(11):1874–8.
95. Carlini R, Obialo CI, Rothstein M. Intravenous erythropoietin (rHuEPO) administration increases plasma endothelin and blood pressure in hemodialysis patients. Am J Hypertens. 1993;6(2):103–7.

96. Carlini RG, Dusso AS, Obialo CI, Alvarez UM, Rothstein M. Recombinant human erythro-poietin (rHuEPO) increases endothelin-1 release by endothelial cells. Kidney Int. 1993;43(5):1010-4.

97. Bode-Boger SM, Boger RH, Kuhn M, Radermacher J, Frolich JC. Recombinant human erythropoietin enhances vasoconstrictor tone via endothelin-1 and constrictor prostanoids. Kidney Int. 1996;50(4):1255-61.

98. Eschbach JW, Abdulhadi MH, Browne JK, Delano BG, Downing MR, Egrie JC, et al. Recombinant human erythropoietin in anemic patients with end-stage renal disease. Results of a phase III multicenter clinical trial. Ann Intern Med. 1989;111(12):992-1000.

99. Eschbach JW, Kelly MR, Haley NR, Abels RI, Adamson JW. Treatment of the anemia of progressive renal failure with recombinant human erythropoietin. N Engl J Med. 1989;321(3):158-63.

100. Krapf R, Hulter HN. Arterial hypertension induced by erythropoietin and erythropoiesis-stimulating agents (ESA). Clin J Am Soc Nephrol. 2009;4(2):470-80.

101. Lebel M, Kingma I, Grose JH, Langlois S. Effect of recombinant human erythropoietin ther-apy on ambulatory blood pressure in normotensive and in untreated borderline hypertensive hemodialysis patients. Am J Hypertens. 1995;8(6):545-51.

102. Ishimitsu T, Tsukada H, Ogawa Y, Numabe A, Yagi S. Genetic predisposition to hypertension facilitates blood pressure elevation in hemodialysis patients treated with erythropoietin. Am J Med. 1993;94(4):401-6.

103. Charra B. Control of blood pressure in long slow hemodialysis. Blood Purif. 1994;12(4-5):252-8.

104. Chazot C, Charra B, Laurent G, Didier C, Vo VC, Terrat JC, et al. Interdialysis blood pressure control by long haemodialysis sessions. Nephrol Dial Transplant. 1995;10(6):831-7.

105. Charra B, Calemard E, Ruffet M, Chazot C, Terrat JC, Vanel T, et al. Survival as an index of adequacy of dialysis. Kidney Int. 1992;41(5):1286-91.

106. Ozkahya M, Toz H, Qzerkan F, Duman S, Ok E, Basci A, et al. Impact of volume control on left ventricular hypertrophy in dialysis patients. J Nephrol. 2002;15(6):655-60.

107. Gunal AI, Duman S, Ozkahya M, Toz H, Asci G, Akcicek F, et al. Strict volume control nor-malizes hypertension in peritoneal dialysis patients. Am J Kidney Dis. 2001;37(3):588-93.

108. Vertes V, Cangiano JL, Berman LB, Gould A. Hypertension in end-stage renal disease. N Engl J Med. 1969;280(18):978-81.

109. Scribner BH. A personalized history of chronic hemodialysis. Am J Kidney Dis. 1990;16(6):511-9.

110. Sinha AD, Agarwal R. Can chronic volume overload be recognized and prevented in hemo-dialysis patients? Semin Dial. 2009;22:480.

111. Agarwal R, Weir MR. Dry-weight: a concept revisited in an effort to avoid medication-directed approaches for blood pressure control in hemodialysis patients. Clin J Am Soc Nephrol. 2010;5(7):1255-60.

112. Agarwal R, Andersen MJ, Pratt JH. On the importance of pedal edema in hemodialysis patients. Clin J Am Soc Nephrol. 2008;3(1):153-8.

113. Jaeger JQ, Mehta RL. Assessment of dry weight in hemodialysis: an overview. J Am Soc Nephrol. 1999;10(2):392-403.

114. Sinha AD, Light RP, Agarwal R. Relative plasma volume monitoring during hemodialysis aids the assessment of dry weight. Hypertension. 2010;55(2):305-11.

115. Hur E, Usta M, Toz H, Asci G, Wabel P, Kahvecioglu S, et al. Effect of fluid management guided by bioimpedance spectroscopy on cardiovascular parameters in hemodialysis patients: a randomized controlled trial. Am J Kidney Dis. 2013;61(6):957-65.

116. Grekas D, Bamichas G, Bacharaki D, Goutzaridis N, Kasimatis E, Tourkantonis A. Hypertension in chronic hemodialysis patients: current view on pathophysiology and treatment. Clin Nephrol. 2000;53(3):164-8.

117. Sinha AD, Agarwal R. What are the causes of the ill effects of chronic hemodialysis? The fallacy of low interdialytic weight gain and low ultrafiltration rate: lower is not always better. Semin Dial. 2014;27(1):11-3.

118. Hecking M, Karaboyas A, Antlanger M, Saran R, Wizemann V, Chazot C, et al. Significance of interdialytic weight gain versus chronic volume overload: consensus opinion. Am J Nephrol. 2013;38(1):78–90.

119. Wabel P, Moissl U, Chamney P, Jirka T, Machek P, Ponce P, et al. Towards improved cardiovascular management: the necessity of combining blood pressure and fluid overload. Nephrol Dial Transplant. 2008;23(9):2965–71.

120. Wizemann V, Wabel P, Chamney P, Zaluska W, Moissl U, Rode C, et al. The mortality risk of overhydration in haemodialysis patients. Nephrol Dial Transplant. 2009;24(5):1574–9.

121. Agarwal R. Hypervolemia is associated with increased mortality among hemodialysis patients. Hypertension. 2010;56(3):512–7.

122. Zhu F, Kuhlmann MK, Sarkar S, Kaitwatcharachai C, Khilnani R, Leonard EF, et al. Adjustment of dry weight in hemodialysis patients using intradialytic continuous multifrequency bioimpedance of the calf. Int J Artif Organs. 2004;27(2):104–9.

123. Zhou YL, Liu J, Sun F, Ma LJ, Han B, Shen Y, et al. Calf bioimpedance ratio improves dry weight assessment and blood pressure control in hemodialysis patients. Am J Nephrol. 2010;32(2):109–16.

124. Burton JO, Jefferies HJ, Selby NM, McIntyre CW. Hemodialysis-induced cardiac injury: determinants and associated outcomes. Clin J Am Soc Nephrol. 2009;4(5):914–20.

125. Shoji T, Tsubakihara Y, Fujii M, Imai E. Hemodialysis-associated hypotension as an independent risk factor for two-year mortality in hemodialysis patients. Kidney Int. 2004;66(3):1212–20.

126. O'Donnell M, Mente A, Rangarajan S, McQueen MJ, Wang X, Liu L, et al. Urinary sodium and potassium excretion, mortality, and cardiovascular events. N Engl J Med. 2014;371(7):612–23.

127. Pimenta E, Gaddam KK, Oparil S, Aban I, Husain S, Dell'Italia LJ, et al. Effects of dietary sodium reduction on blood pressure in subjects with resistant hypertension: results from a randomized trial. Hypertension. 2009;54(3):475–81.

128. McMahon EJ, Bauer JD, Hawley CM, Isbel NM, Stowasser M, Johnson DW, et al. A randomized trial of dietary sodium restriction in CKD. J Am Soc Nephrol. 2013;24(12):2096–103.

129. Suckling RJ, He FJ, Macgregor GA. Altered dietary salt intake for preventing and treating diabetic kidney disease. Cochrane Database Syst Rev. 2010;12, CD006763.

130. Ramdeen G, Tzamaloukas AH, Malhotra D, Leger A, Murata GH. Estimates of interdialytic sodium and water intake based on the balance principle: differences between nondiabetic and diabetic subjects on hemodialysis. ASAIO J. 1998;44(6):812–7.

131. Kalantar-Zadeh K, Regidor DL, Kovesdy CP, Van WD, Bunnapradist S, Horwich TB, et al. Fluid retention is associated with cardiovascular mortality in patients undergoing long-term hemodialysis. Circulation. 2009;119(5):671–9.

132. Flythe JE, Kimmel SE, Brunelli SM. Rapid fluid removal during dialysis is associated with cardiovascular morbidity and mortality. Kidney Int. 2011;79(2):250–7.

133. Krautzig S, Janssen U, Koch KM, Granolleras C, Shaldon S. Dietary salt restriction and reduction of dialysate sodium to control hypertension in maintenance haemodialysis patients. Nephrol Dial Transplant. 1998;13(3):552–3.

134. Charra B. Fluid balance, dry weight, and blood pressure in dialysis. Hemodial Int. 2007;11(1):21–31.

135. Appel LJ, Frohlich ED, Hall JE, Pearson TA, Sacco RL, Seals DR, et al. The importance of population-wide sodium reduction as a means to prevent cardiovascular disease and stroke: a call to action from the American Heart Association. Circulation. 2011;123(10):1138–43.

136. Tomson CR. Advising dialysis patients to restrict fluid intake without restricting sodium intake is not based on evidence and is a waste of time. Nephrol Dial Transplant. 2001;16(8):1538–42.

137. Ogden DA. A double blind crossover comparison of high and low sodium dialysis. Proc Clin Dial Transplant Forum. 1978;8:157–65.

138. Cybulsky AV, Matni A, Hollomby DJ. Effects of high sodium dialysate during maintenance hemodialysis. Nephron. 1985;41(1):57–61.

139. Santos SF, Peixoto AJ. Revisiting the dialysate sodium prescription as a tool for better blood pressure and interdialytic weight gain management in hemodialysis patients. Clin J Am Soc Nephrol. 2008;3(2):522–30.
140. Manlucu J, Gallo K, Heidenheim PA, Lindsay RM. Lowering postdialysis plasma sodium (conductivity) to increase sodium removal in volume-expanded hemodialysis patients: a pilot study using a biofeedback software system. Am J Kidney Dis. 2010;56(1):69–76.
141. Daugirdas JT, Al-Kudsi RR, Ing TS, Norusis MJ. A double-blind evaluation of sodium gradient hemodialysis. Am J Nephrol. 1985;5(3):163–8.
142. Barre PE, Brunelle G, Gascon-Barre M. A randomized double blind trial of dialysate sodiums of 145 mEq/L, 150 mEq/L, and 155 mEq/L. ASAIO Trans. 1988;34(3):338–41.
143. Sang GL, Kovithavongs C, Ulan R, Kjellstrand CM. Sodium ramping in hemodialysis: a study of beneficial and adverse effects. Am J Kidney Dis. 1997;29(5):669–77.
144. Song JH, Lee SW, Suh CK, Kim MJ. Time-averaged concentration of dialysate sodium relates with sodium load and interdialytic weight gain during sodium-profiling hemodialysis. Am J Kidney Dis. 2002;40(2):291–301.
145. Munoz MJ, Sun S, Chertow GM, Moran J, Doss S, Schiller B. Dialysate sodium and sodium gradient in maintenance hemodialysis: a neglected sodium restriction approach? Nephrol Dial Transplant. 2011;26(4):1281–7.
146. de Paula FM, Peixoto AJ, Pinto LV, Dorigo D, Patricio PJ, Santos SF. Clinical consequences of an individualized dialysate sodium prescription in hemodialysis patients. Kidney Int. 2004;66(3):1232–8.
147. Davies S, Carlsson O, Simonsen O, Johansson AC, Venturoli D, Ledebo I, et al. The effects of low-sodium peritoneal dialysis fluids on blood pressure, thirst and volume status. Nephrol Dial Transplant. 2009;24(5):1609–17.
148. Tandon T, Sinha AD, Agarwal R. Shorter delivered dialysis times associate with a higher and more difficult to treat blood pressure. Nephrol Dial Transplant. 2013;28(6):1562–8.
149. Brunet P, Saingra Y, Leonetti F, Vacher-Coponat H, Ramananarivo P, Berland Y. Tolerance of haemodialysis: a randomized cross-over trial of 5-h versus 4-h treatment time. Nephrol Dial Transplant. 1996;11 Suppl 8:46–51.
150. Tattersall J, Martin-Malo A, Pedrini L, Basci A, Canaud B, Fouque D, et al. EBPG guideline on dialysis strategies. Nephrol Dial Transplant 2007;22 Suppl 2:ii5–21.
151. Foley RN, Gilbertson DT, Murray T, Collins AJ. Long interdialytic interval and mortality among patients receiving hemodialysis. N Engl J Med. 2011;365(12):1099–107.
152. Twardowski ZJ. Treatment time and ultrafiltration rate are more important in dialysis prescription than small molecule clearance. Blood Purif. 2007;25(1):90–8.
153. Woods JD, Port FK, Orzol S, Buoncristiani U, Young E, Wolfe RA, et al. Clinical and biochemical correlates of starting "daily" hemodialysis. Kidney Int. 1999;55(6):2467–76.
154. Chan CT, Floras JS, Miller JA, Richardson RM, Pierratos A. Regression of left ventricular hypertrophy after conversion to nocturnal hemodialysis. Kidney Int. 2002;61(6):2235–9.
155. Culleton BF, Walsh M, Klarenbach SW, Mortis G, Scott-Douglas N, Quinn RR, et al. Effect of frequent nocturnal hemodialysis vs conventional hemodialysis on left ventricular mass and quality of life: a randomized controlled trial. JAMA. 2007;298(11):1291–9.
156. Rocco MV, Lockridge Jr RS, Beck GJ, Eggers PW, Gassman JJ, Greene T, et al. The effects of frequent nocturnal home hemodialysis: the Frequent Hemodialysis Network Nocturnal Trial. Kidney Int. 2011;80(10):1080–91.
157. Chertow GM, Levin NW, Beck GJ, Depner TA, Eggers PW, Gassman JJ, et al. In-center hemodialysis six times per week versus three times per week. N Engl J Med. 2010;363(24):2287–300.
158. Agarwal R. Frequent versus standard hemodialysis. N Engl J Med. 2011;364(10):975–6.
159. Heerspink HJ, Ninomiya T, Zoungas S, de Zeeuw D, Grobbee DE, Jardine MJ, et al. Effect of lowering blood pressure on cardiovascular events and mortality in patients on dialysis: a systematic review and meta-analysis of randomised controlled trials. Lancet. 2009;373(9668):1009–15.

160. Agarwal R, Sinha AD. Cardiovascular protection with antihypertensive drugs in dialysis patients: systematic review and meta-analysis. Hypertension. 2009;53(5):860–6.
161. Levin NW, Kotanko P, Eckardt KU, Kasiske BL, Chazot C, Cheung AK, et al. Blood pressure in chronic kidney disease stage 5D-report from a kidney disease: improving global outcomes controversies conference. Kidney Int. 2010;77(4):273–84.
162. Brater DC. Diuretic therapy. N Engl J Med. 1998;339(6):387–95.
163. Hayashi SY, Seeberger A, Lind B, Gunnes S, Alvestrand A, do Nascimento MM, et al. Acute effects of low and high intravenous doses of furosemide on myocardial function in anuric haemodialysis patients: a tissue Doppler study. Nephrol Dial Transplant. 2008;23(4):1355–61.
164. Pickkers P, Hughes AD, Russel FG, Thien T, Smits P. Thiazide-induced vasodilation in humans is mediated by potassium channel activation. Hypertension. 1998;32(6):1071–6.
165. Eladari D, Chambrey R. Identification of a novel target of thiazide diuretics. J Nephrol. 2011;24(4):391–4.
166. Bennett WM, McDonald WJ, Kuehnel E, Hartnett MN, Porter GA. Do diuretics have antihypertensive properties independent of natriuresis? Clin Pharmacol Ther. 1977;22(5 Pt 1):499–504.
167. Foody JM, Farrell MH, Krumholz HM. beta-Blocker therapy in heart failure: scientific review. JAMA. 2002;287(7):883–9.
168. Teo KK, Yusuf S, Furberg CD. Effects of prophylactic antiarrhythmic drug therapy in acute myocardial infarction. An overview of results from randomized controlled trials. JAMA. 1993;270(13):1589–95.
169. Abbott KC, Trespalacios FC, Agodoa LY, Taylor AJ, Bakris GL. beta-Blocker use in long-term dialysis patients: association with hospitalized heart failure and mortality. Arch Intern Med. 2004;164(22):2465–71.
170. Cice G, Ferrara L, D'Andrea A, D'Isa S, Di BA, Cittadini A, et al. Carvedilol increases two-year survivalin dialysis patients with dilated cardiomyopathy: a prospective, placebo-controlled trial. J Am Coll Cardiol. 2003;41(9):1438–44.
171. Mancia G, De BG, Dominiczak A, Cifkova R, Fagard R, Germano G, et al. 2007 Guidelines for the management of arterial hypertension: the task force for the management of arterial hypertension of the European Society of Hypertension (ESH) and of the European Society of Cardiology (ESC). J Hypertens. 2007;25(6):1105–87.
172. Wiysonge CS, Bradley HA, Volmink J, Mayosi BM, Mbewu A, Opie LH. Beta-blockers for hypertension. Cochrane Database Syst Rev. 2012;11, CD002003.
173. Denker MG, Cohen DL. Antihypertensive medications in end-stage renal disease. Semin Dial. 2015;28(4):330–6.
174. Agarwal R. Supervised atenolol therapy in the management of hemodialysis hypertension. Kidney Int. 1999;55(4):1528–35.
175. James PA, Oparil S, Carter BL, Cushman WC, Dennison-Himmelfarb C, Handler J, et al. 2014 evidence-based guideline for the management of high blood pressure in adults: report from the panel members appointed to the Eighth Joint National Committee (JNC 8). JAMA. 2014;311(5):507–20.
176. Pfeffer MA, Braunwald E, Moye LA, Basta L, Brown Jr EJ, Cuddy TE, et al. Effect of captopril on mortality and morbidity in patients with left ventricular dysfunction after myocardial infarction. Results of the survival and ventricular enlargement trial. The SAVE Investigators. N Engl J Med. 1992;327(10):669–77.
177. Pfeffer MA, McMurray JJ, Velazquez EJ, Rouleau JL, Kober L, Maggioni AP, et al. Valsartan, captopril, or both in myocardial infarction complicated by heart failure, left ventricular dysfunction, or both. N Engl J Med. 2003;349(20):1893–906.
178. Zheng S, Nath V, Coyne DW. ACE inhibitor-based, directly observed therapy for hypertension in hemodialysis patients. Am J Nephrol. 2007;27(5):522–9.
179. Saracho R, Martin-Malo A, Martinez I, Aljama P, Montenegro J. Evaluation of the Losartan in Hemodialysis (ELHE) Study. Kidney Int Suppl. 1998;68:S125–9.
180. Zannad F, Kessler M, Grunfeld JP, Thuilliez C. FOSIDIAL: a randomised placebo controlled trial of the effects of fosinopril on cardiovascular morbidity and mortality in haemodialysis

patients. Study design and patients' baseline characteristics. Fundam Clin Pharmacol. 2002;16(5):353–60.

181. Takahashi A, Takase H, Toriyama T, Sugiura T, Kurita Y, Ueda R, et al. Candesartan, an angiotensin II type-1 receptor blocker, reduces cardiovascular events in patients on chronic haemodialysis--a randomized study. Nephrol Dial Transplant. 2006;21(9):2507–12.

182. Suzuki H, Kanno Y, Sugahara S, Ikeda N, Shoda J, Takenaka T, et al. Effect of angiotensin receptor blockers on cardiovascular events in patients undergoing hemodialysis: an open-label randomized controlled trial. Am J Kidney Dis. 2008;52(3):501–6.

183. Tai DJ, Lim TW, James MT, Manns BJ, Tonelli M, Hemmelgarn BR. Cardiovascular effects of Angiotensin converting enzyme inhibition or Angiotensin receptor blockade in hemodialysis: a meta-analysis. Clin J Am Soc Nephrol. 2010;5(4):623–30.

184. Akbari A, Knoll G, Ferguson D, McCormick B, Davis A, Biyani M. Angiotensin-converting enzyme inhibitors and angiotensin receptor blockers in peritoneal dialysis: systematic review and meta-analysis of randomized controlled trials. Perit Dial Int. 2009;29(5):554–61.

185. Jafar TH, Stark PC, Schmid CH, Landa M, Maschio G, de Jong PE, et al. Progression of chronic kidney disease: the role of blood pressure control, proteinuria, and angiotensin-converting enzyme inhibition: a patient-level meta-analysis. Ann Intern Med. 2003;139(4):244–52.

186. Krediet RT. How to preserve residual renal function in patients with chronic kidney disease and on dialysis? Nephrol Dial Transplant. 2006;21 Suppl 2:ii42–ii6.

187. Li PK, Chow KM, Wong TY, Leung CB, Szeto CC. Effects of an angiotensin-converting enzyme inhibitor on residual renal function in patients receiving peritoneal dialysis. A randomized, controlled study. Ann Intern Med. 2003;139(2):105–12.

188. Suzuki H, Kanno Y, Sugahara S, Okada H, Nakamoto H. Effects of an angiotensin II receptor blocker, valsartan, on residual renal function in patients on CAPD. Am J Kidney Dis. 2004;43(6):1056–64.

189. Kjaergaard KD, Peters CD, Jespersen B, Tietze IN, Madsen JK, Pedersen BB, et al. Angiotensin blockade and progressive loss of kidney function in hemodialysis patients: a randomized controlled trial. Am J Kidney Dis. 2014;64(6):892–901.

190. Tepel M, Hopfenmueller W, Scholze A, Maier A, Zidek W. Effect of amlodipine on cardiovascular events in hypertensive haemodialysis patients. Nephrol Dial Transplant. 2008;23(11):3605–12.

191. London GM, Pannier B, Guerin AP, Marchais SJ, Safar ME, Cuche JL. Cardiac hypertrophy, aortic compliance, peripheral resistance, and wave reflection in end-stage renal disease. Comparative effects of ACE inhibition and calcium channel blockade. Circulation. 1994;90(6):2786–96.

192. Shibasaki Y, Masaki H, Nishiue T, Nishikawa M, Matsubara H, Iwasaka T. Angiotensin II type 1 receptor antagonist, losartan, causes regression of left ventricular hypertrophy in end-stage renal disease. Nephron. 2002;90(3):256–61.

193. Taylor AL, Ziesche S, Yancy C, Carson P, D'Agostino Jr R, Ferdinand K, et al. Combination of isosorbide dinitrate and hydralazine in blacks with heart failure. N Engl J Med. 2004;351(20):2049–57.

194. Chapman N, Dobson J, Wilson S, Dahlof B, Sever PS, Wedel H, et al. Effect of spironolactone on blood pressure in subjects with resistant hypertension. Hypertension. 2007;49(4):839–45.

195. Pitt B, Zannad F, Remme WJ, Cody R, Castaigne A, Perez A, et al. The effect of spironolactone on morbidity and mortality in patients with severe heart failure. Randomized Aldactone Evaluation Study Investigators. N Engl J Med. 1999;341(10):709–17.

196. Pitt B, Williams G, Remme W, Martinez F, Lopez-Sendon J, Zannad F, et al. The EPHESUS trial: eplerenone in patients with heart failure due to systolic dysfunction complicating acute myocardial infarction. Eplerenone Post-AMI Heart Failure Efficacy and Survival Study. Cardiovasc Drugs Ther. 2001;15(1):79–87.

197. Ni X, Zhang J, Zhang P, Wu F, Xia M, Ying G, et al. Effects of spironolactone on dialysis patients with refractory hypertension: a randomized controlled study. J Clin Hypertens (Greenwich). 2014;16(9):658–63.
198. Matsumoto Y, Mori Y, Kageyama S, Arihara K, Sugiyama T, Ohmura H, et al. Spironolactone reduces cardiovascular and cerebrovascular morbidity and mortality in hemodialysis patients. J Am Coll Cardiol. 2014;63(6):528–36.
199. Allen EV. Sympathectomy for essential hypertension. Circulation. 1952;6(1):131–40.
200. Schlaich MP, Bart B, Hering D, Walton A, Marusic P, Mahfoud F, et al. Feasibility of catheter-based renal nerve ablation and effects on sympathetic nerve activity and blood pressure in patients with end-stage renal disease. Int J Cardiol. 2013;168(3):2214–20.
201. Krum H, Schlaich M, Whitbourn R, Sobotka PA, Sadowski J, Bartus K, et al. Catheter-based renal sympathetic denervation for resistant hypertension: a multicentre safety and proof-of-principle cohort study. Lancet. 2009;373(9671):1275–81.
202. Bhatt DL, Kandzari DE, O'Neill WW, D'Agostino R, Flack JM, Katzen BT, et al. A controlled trial of renal denervation for resistant hypertension. N Engl J Med. 2014;370(15):1393–401.
203. Lewington S, Clarke R, Qizilbash N, Peto R, Collins R. Age-specific relevance of usual blood pressure to vascular mortality: a meta-analysis of individual data for one million adults in 61 prospective studies. Lancet. 2002;360(9349):1903–13.
204. Dorhout Mees EJ. Hypertension in haemodialysis patients: who cares? Nephrol Dial Transplant. 1999;14(1):28–30.
205. Kalantar-Zadeh K, Kilpatrick RD, McAllister CJ, Greenland S, Kopple JD. Reverse epidemiology of hypertension and cardiovascular death in the hemodialysis population: the 58th annual fall conference and scientific sessions. Hypertension. 2005;45(4):811–7.
206. Kawamura M, Fijimoto S, Hisanaga S, Yamamoto Y, Eto T. Incidence, outcome, and risk factors of cerebrovascular events in patients undergoing maintenance hemodialysis. Am J Kidney Dis. 1998;31(6):991–6.
207. Foley RN, Parfrey PS, Harnett JD, Kent GM, Murray DC, Barre PE. Impact of hypertension on cardiomyopathy, morbidity and mortality in end-stage renal disease. Kidney Int. 1996;49(5):1379–85.
208. De Lima JJ, Lopes HF, Grupi CJ, Abensur H, Giorgi MC, Krieger EM, et al. Blood pressure influences the occurrence of complex ventricular arrhythmia in hemodialysis patients. Hypertension. 1995;26(6 Pt 2):1200–3.
209. Takeda A, Toda T, Fujii T, Shinohara S, Sasaki S, Matsui N. Discordance of influence of hypertension on mortality and cardiovascular risk in hemodialysis patients. Am J Kidney Dis. 2005;45(1):112–8.
210. Tomita J, Kimura G, Inoue T, Inenaga T, Sanai T, Kawano Y, et al. Role of systolic blood pressure in determining prognosis of hemodialyzed patients. Am J Kidney Dis. 1995;25(3):405–12.
211. Zager PG, Nikolic J, Brown RH, Campbell MA, Hunt WC, Peterson D, et al. "U" curve association of blood pressure and mortality in hemodialysis patients. Medical Directors of Dialysis Clinic, Inc. Kidney Int. 1998;54(2):561–9.
212. Port FK, Hulbert-Shearon TE, Wolfe RA, Bloembergen WE, Golper TA, Agodoa LY, et al. Predialysis blood pressure and mortality risk in a national sample of maintenance hemodialysis patients. Am J Kidney Dis. 1999;33(3):507–17.
213. Li Z, Lacson Jr E, Lowrie EG, Ofsthun NJ, Kuhlmann MK, Lazarus JM, et al. The epidemiology of systolic blood pressure and death risk in hemodialysis patients. Am J Kidney Dis. 2006;48(4):606–15.
214. Lacson Jr E, Lazarus JM. The association between blood pressure and mortality in ESRD-not different from the general population? Semin Dial. 2007;20(6):510–7.
215. Udayaraj UP, Steenkamp R, Caskey FJ, Rogers C, Nitsch D, Ansell D, et al. Blood pressure and mortality risk on peritoneal dialysis. Am J Kidney Dis. 2009;53(1):70–8.

216. Stidley CA, Hunt WC, Tentori F, Schmidt D, Rohrscheib M, Paine S, et al. Changing rela-
     tionship of blood pressure with mortality over time among hemodialysis patients. J Am Soc
     Nephrol. 2006;17(2):513–20.
217. Amar J, Vernier I, Rossignol E, Bongard V, Arnaud C, Conte JJ, et al. Nocturnal blood pres-
     sure and 24-hour pulse pressure are potent indicators of mortality in hemodialysis patients.
     Kidney Int. 2000;57(6):2485–91.
218. Bansal N, McCulloch CE, Rahman M, Kusek JW, Anderson AH, Xie D, et al. Blood pressure
     and risk of all-cause mortality in advanced chronic kidney disease and hemodialysis: the
     chronic renal insufficiency cohort study. Hypertension. 2015;65(1):93–100.

Chapter 8
Hypertension in the Kidney Transplant Recipient

Sebastian Varas and John Vella

Introduction

The year 1954 ushered the fulfillment of a breakthrough achievement in the management of irreversible kidney disease. Building on a program of preclinical research, the surgical team at the Peter Bent Brigham Hospital in Boston performed the first successful transplant. The kidney recipient was a 23-year-old man with end-stage renal disease (ESRD) due to chronic glomerulonephritis complicated by severe hypertension. The donor was his identical twin-brother. In a world before the development of effective immunosuppression and antihypertensives, the team provided proof of concept that a vascularized solid organ could be transplanted successfully. Pertinent to this chapter, the recipient battled hypertension before and after transplantation and died of myocardial infarction with a functioning allograft 8 years later [1]. Since then, kidney transplantation has prolonged the lives of hundreds of thousands ESRD patients [2–5], improved quality of life and is cost-effective compared with dialysis [6–10].

Before the approval of cyclosporine in 1983 by the United States Food and Drug Administration (FDA), nearly half of all transplant recipients were hypertensive [11]. Currently, more than 90 % of kidney transplant recipients taking calcineurin inhibitor-based therapy are hypertensive [12–14]. Conversely, in a 2003–2005 ($n=94$) cohort reported by Paoletti et al., only 5 % of kidney allograft recipients were normotensive as defined by ambulatory blood pressure monitoring (ABPM) of less than 130/80 mmHg without treatment [15]. This change in the reported

S. Varas, MD
Division of Nephrology, Maine Medical Center, 22 Bramhall St., Portland, ME 04102, USA

J. Vella, MD, FRCP, FACP, FASN (✉)
Maine Transplant Program, Maine Medical Center, 19 West St., Portland, ME 04102, USA
e-mail: vellajp@mmc.org

© Springer Science+Business Media New York 2016
A.K. Singh, R. Agarwal (eds.), *Core Concepts in Hypertension in Kidney Disease*, DOI 10.1007/978-1-4939-6436-9_8

incidence of HTN may partly reflect changing definitions of high blood pressure (BP) over time; thus, direct comparisons may be misleading.

Kidney transplant recipients are at increased risk of cardiovascular disease (CVD) and death compared to the general population [16, 17]. Hypertension is an important independent traditional risk factor for the development of CVD, allograft dysfunction, and death with a functioning allograft [18, 19]. Opelz and coworkers, from the Collaborative Transplant Study group, were among the first to confirm not only a strong and graded relationship between post-transplant blood pressure and kidney allograft failure, but also demonstrated improved long-term outcomes when blood pressure was controlled (see Management). In Opelz's landmark multi-national study published in 1998, a cohort of 29,751 kidney transplant recipients followed for 7 years indicated that HTN was a major predictor of subsequent allograft failure. Opelz and colleagues also demonstrated that the association of elevated BP and allograft survival was independent of prior episodes of transplant rejection; a concept that was later confirmed by Mange and others [19–22]. It should be noted that most data pertaining to hypertension after kidney transplantation have accrued from clinical trials that focused on immunotherapeutic regimens, as well as analyses of registry databases, rather than studies focusing primarily on hypertension as an end-point [23].

Definitions and Diagnosis

According to the World Health Organization, approximately 1.5 billion people worldwide have hypertension (25 % of estimated global adult population), and the proportion of individuals whose hypertension is controlled with medication remains low [24, 25]. According to the 2012 NHANES analysis, 25.5 % of American adults are hypertensive [26].

Several groups have developed guidelines to define, diagnose, and treat elevated blood pressure levels in different populations, more recently with particular reference to elderly, diabetic (DM), chronic kidney disease (CKD) patients and kidney transplant recipients (see Table 8.1) [27].

The 8th Joint National Committee guidelines (JNC 8) published in 2014 redefined hypertension treatment targets. In adults with CKD and/or DM, pharmacologic therapy is recommended when blood pressure exceeds 140/90 mmHg [28]. This relaxation of targets for the CKD/DM population is a major change from the JNC 7 guidelines. Inasmuch as JNC 8 extensively reviewed published evidence, there were no specific recommendations regarding patients with proteinuria, hypertension, kidney transplantation, or living kidney donors. The JNC 8 guidelines are similar to those of the European Society of Hypertension/European Society of Cardiology (ESH/ESC) published in 2013 [29]. In the latter, two aspects were highlighted: target diastolic BP for diabetics was set at less than 85 mmHg, and an emphasis placed on ABPM as a valuable diagnostic tool to assist in the BP

Table 8.1 Blood pressure goals

Guideline	Population	Goal BP (mmHg)
JNC 8	General, age ≥60 years	<150/90
	General, age <60 years	<140/90
	DM or CKD	<140/90
JNC 7	General, any age	<140/90
	DM or CKD	<130/80
KDIGO 2012 & ERBP	CKD without proteinuria	<140/90
	CKD with proteinuria	≤130/80
	Kidney transplant recipient	≤130/80

BP blood pressure, *CKD* chronic kidney disease, *DM* diabetes mellitus, *ERBP* European Renal Best Practice, *JNC* Joint National Committee, *KDIGO* Kidney Disease: Improving Global Outcomes. Adapted from Rossi AP, Vella JP. Hypertension, Living Kidney Donors, and Transplantation: Where Are We Today? Advances in chronic kidney disease. 2015;22(2):154–64; used with permission [27]

Table 8.2 Definition of hypertension by method of blood pressure measurement

Category	ESH/ESC (BP mmHg)	JNC 7 (BP mmHg)
Office BP	≥140/90	≥140/90
Ambulatory BP		
Daytime	≥135/85	≥135/85
Nighttime	≥120/70	≥120/75
24-h (mean)	≥130/80	
Home BP	≥135/85	≥135/85

BP blood pressure, *ESC* European Society of Cardiology, *ESH* European Society of Hypertension, *JNC* Joint National Committee. Adapted from: Rossi A. and Vella J. [27]

management-decision-making process, compared to office blood pressure measurements (see Table 8.2) [27].

Current Kidney Disease: Improving Global Outcomes (KDIGO) guidelines published in 2012 recommend for adult kidney transplant recipients a goal BP of less than or equal to 130/80 mmHg irrespective of albuminuria level [30], and in 2014 the European Renal Best Practice (ERBP) guidelines endorsed the above target BP and included definitions for HTN based on the method used for its measurement (see Table 8.2) [27, 31].

In 2015, the Systolic Blood Pressure Intervention Trial (SPRINT) [32] determined that for patients at high risk for cardiovascular events but without diabetes mellitus, targeting a systolic BP of less than 120 mmHg, as compared with less than 140 mmHg, resulted in lower rates of fatal and nonfatal major cardiovascular events and death from any cause, although significantly higher rates of some adverse events were observed in the intensive-treatment group. The applicability of these conclusions to the post-transplant population remains unclear as such patients were not included in the study groups.

Table 8.3 Post-transplantation hypertension categories, prevalence, and risk factors

Category	Prevalence (%)	Potential risk factors
Masked hypertension	18–39	
Nocturnal hypertension	29–79	
Non-dippers	25–82	
Reverse-dippers [36]	31–39	Pre-transplant HTN Increased BMI CNI-based immunotherapy
Resistant hypertension [54, 55]	7–24	Male Age >59 DM Worse CV profile Poor eGFR Increased 24-h proteinuria Steroid immunotherapy

BMI body mass index, *CNI* calcineurin inhibitor, *CV* cardiovascular, *DM* diabetes mellitus, *eGFR* estimated glomerular filtration rate, *HTN* hypertension

Nocturnal and Masked Hypertension

Blood pressure can be measured in different ways: office-based (OBPM), home or self-based (SBPM), and ambulatory 24-h (ABPM) measurement (see Table 8.3). In kidney transplant recipients, Prasad et al. found that OBPM may be elevated by 3–4 mmHg more than the daily average BP [33]. Stenehjem et al. studying 49 kidney recipients determined that ABPM was the most sensitive diagnostic method, detecting 84 % of uncontrolled hypertension, followed by 71 % with SBPM and 47 % with OBPM. In this analysis, they also found non-dipping nocturnal hypertension in 82 % and reverse-dipping (i.e., nocturnal BP increase from daytime systolic BP by ABPM night-day BP ratio >0.1) in 39 % of the cohort [34, 35]. Ibernon et al. found reverse-dipping nocturnal hypertension in 31 % of a prospective cohort of 126 kidney transplant recipients that was associated with increased risk of CV events or allograft failure. They also described associations between the reverse-dipping pattern and the presence of: pre-transplantation DM, increasing BMI, and the use of calcineurin inhibitor immunosuppressive drugs [36].

The prevalence of nocturnal hypertension after kidney transplantation has been reported between 29 % [15] and 79 % [27, 37]. In the CKD population, nocturnal hypertension has been associated with increased mortality and left ventricular hypertrophy (LVH) [38–40]. LVH is known to be an independent marker of CV mortality as described in the Framingham study [41]. Wadei et al. have further described the negative impact of nocturnal hypertension in kidney recipients 1 year after transplant, reporting that for every 10 % increase in nocturnal systolic BP there was an associated decline in GFR by an average of 4.6 ml/min/1.73 m^2 ($p < 0.04$) [42]. In a later sub-cohort from this study, reduced GFR at 3 years post-transplant correlated with abnormal circadian BP pattern at 1-year ($p \leq 0.03$), suggesting causation [43].

In the general population, masked hypertension (MHT) is predictor of worsened CV outcomes as Fagard et al. demonstrated in a 2006 analysis that indicated the relative risk of mortality was twofold higher compared with normotensives [44]. In the kidney transplant population, the prevalence of MHT was found to be at 18–39% [45]. Kayrak and coworkers reported its prevalence in a cohort of 114 kidney transplant recipients, to be at 39% (average daytime BP≥135/85 mmHg, compared to OBPM previously deemed normal at <140/90 mmHg). Interestingly, the incidence of MHT was 40% in deceased-donor recipients versus 19% in living-donor recipients [46].

To further acknowledge and address the relationship between HTN and LVH in the kidney transplant population, Lipkin et al. analyzed data from a small observational cohort of normotensive kidney transplant recipients ($n=28$; previous OBPM <140/90 mmHg) not taking antihypertensive medications. All patients were more than 12-months post-transplantation with stable kidney function (creatinine clearance of 70 ± 4 ml/min) and without anemia or valvular heart disease. Several important findings were described: elevated left ventricular mass index (LVMI) was present in 25% of the cohort and was more commonly found in the cyclosporine-treated recipients. When comparing ABPM versus OBPM, LVMI was more closely correlated with systolic BP than diastolic BP. 25% were non-dippers and they also showed statistically significant higher LVMI compared to dippers, a finding consistent with that of the general population [40, 47]. These associations have been re-validated in most recent times by a cross-sectional investigation by Sezer et al. who studied a non-diabetic cohort of kidney transplant recipients ($n=98$) more than 12-months post-transplant, and examined the relationship between LVMI, ABPM, and renal resistive index (RRI; a sonographic measurement of renal arterial disease [48]). They described an association between RRI with mean systolic OBPM, and mean systolic diurnal and nighttime ABPM. After multiple logistic regression analysis, mean nighttime systolic BP and RRI were independent risk factors for increased LVMI [49].

Resistant Hypertension

Resistant hypertension (RH) is defined as a blood pressure >140/90 mmHg, or ≥130/80 in CKD or DM patients, while taking three or more full-dose antihypertensives from different classes, one of which being a diuretic [28, 50, 51]. Persell et al. analyzed NHANES 2003–2008 data, and described the prevalence of RH in the USA at 12.8% (roughly 50% of the adult hypertensive population) [52]. Similarly, de la Sierra et al. reported the prevalence of RH in a Spanish population to be 12.2% (OBPM-based) [53].

In the kidney transplant population, data about RH is limited. Gago-Fraile et al. performed a cross-sectional analysis of 529 patients with a functioning allograft over 11.4 ± 6.5 years. Hypertension was prevalent in 85% of patients, with RH in 6.8% of them. This subgroup tended to be older, diabetic, had inferior kidney function (eGFR MDRD of 36.2 ± 20.4 ml/min per 1.73 m²; more proteinuria [mean

2.55±2.61 g/d]), and were steroid maintained [54]. Similarly, reporting for the RETENAL group (Control of Resistant Hypertension in Renal Transplant), Arias-Rodriguez et al. highlighted the current prevalence and potential implications of RH on kidney transplant patient's CVD risk, patient and allograft survival. In this Spanish multi-center cross-sectional observational study, they described RH prevalence to be at 23.5% (OBPM-based), citing as risk factors: men, older age, and worse CV risk profile [55].

In summary, ABPM use in the kidney transplant recipient population is a valuable tool to diagnose and classify hypertensive patients [56–58]. Masked and nocturnal HTN with its different categories are highly prevalent and associated with inferior allograft and patient outcomes (see Table 8.3).

Epidemiology

The leading cause of kidney allograft failure is death with a functioning graft, and the leading cause of death after kidney transplantation is cardiovascular disease, with an annual risk of 3.5–5%, this being a 50-fold higher than the general population [16, 17, 59]. Traditional risk factors for coronary heart disease (CHD) in the general population are the same for kidney transplant recipients, with the caveat that risk-prediction calculations validated and used in the general population underestimate CHD risk in the latter group (see Fig. 8.1) [27, 60, 61].

Pathogenesis

The pathogenesis of hypertension after kidney transplantation is complex, variable, and multifactorial. Initially, hypertension can be attributed to ESRD with concomitant salt and water retention. As allograft function leads to auto-diuresis, blood pressure often improves although with persistent dysregulation in salt, water, and use of immunotherapy with vaso-active consequence. This is superimposed on the recipient's underlying CVD continuum that includes genetics, pre-transplant comorbidities, vascular calcification, left ventricular hypertrophy as well as factors that relate to immunosuppression. Furthermore, Opelz et al. theorized that hypertension may trigger mechanical injury that amplifies immunologically induced processes [21]. This premise would be in harmony with Luft and Haller's general finding that high blood pressure activates inflammatory effector mechanisms in the renal tissue, that manifest themselves as tubulointerstitial inflammation, with perivascular monocyte and macrophage infiltration, fibroblast proliferation, and increased interstitial matrix deposition, all yielding a not surprising fibrotic process [62]. In the early days of transplantation, chronic rejection and failure to remove the native kidneys were considered to be the most common causes of hypertension after transplantation [63]. More recently, chronic rejection seems to have been replaced by CNI-induced nephrotoxicity leading to hypertension as a more common issue [64].

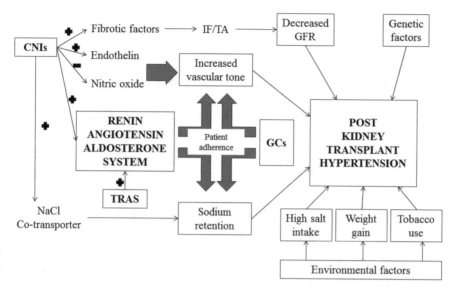

Fig. 8.1 Pathophysiology of post-kidney transplant hypertension. *CNI* calcineurin inhibitor, *GC* glucocorticoid, *GFR* glomerular filtration rate, *IF/TA* interstitial fibrosis and tubular atrophy, *NaCl* sodium chloride, *TRAS* transplant renal artery stenosis. Adapted from: Rossi AP, Vella JP. Hypertension, Living Kidney Donors, and Transplantation: Where Are We Today? Advances in chronic kidney disease. 2015;22(2):154–64

Risk Factors

Multiple factors influence hypertension after kidney transplantation including pre-transplant HTN[65], increased body mass index (BMI), primary kidney disease, quality of the donor kidney, delayed graft function, acute rejection, immunosuppressive medications, transplant renal artery stenosis, and chronic allograft nephropathy (see Fig. 8.1) [27]. It is useful to consider such elements as being those that derive from the donor, the recipient, and those related to the transplant itself (see Table 8.4) [27, 66, 67].

Donor Characteristics

Non-modifiable factors such as donor age, gender, nephron mass, personal and family history of HTN have all been associated with post-transplant hypertension. Ducloux et al. performed a retrospective cohort of 321 kidney recipients, and found by multivariate analysis that donor age was associated with post-transplant HTN risk by 28 % per each 10-year increase in donor age (RR 1.28, 95 % CI 1.05–1.59) [68]. It is known that recipients from expanded-criteria kidney donors (i.e., death from stroke; age >60; or age 50–59 with 2 of the following: HTN or serum

Table 8.4 Factors contributing to hypertension after kidney transplantation

Recipient	Donor	Transplant continuum
Pre-existing hypertension	Age [68, 70]	Delayed graft function
Native kidney disease	Gender	*Immunotherapy*
Chronic kidney disease	Hypertension	CNI (CsA>Tac)
Obesity	Nephron mass	Corticosteroids
Genetics	Genetics	mTORi/CNI combination
		Allograft dysfunction
		Acute rejection
		Chronic allograft nephropathy
		Thrombotic microangiopathy
		Recurrent or de novo glomerulopathy
		Surgical complications
		TRAS
		Page kidney
		Ureteric stenosis
		Lymphocele

CNI calcineurin inhibitor, *CsA* cyclosporine, *mTORi* mammalian target of rapamycin inhibitor; Page kidney is a rare entity caused by extrinsic compression of the renal parenchyma from a hematoma or a mass; about 130 cases have been reported up to 2009 [66, 67]; *Tac* tacrolimus, *TRAS* transplant renal artery stenosis. Adapted from: Rossi A. and Vella J. [27]

creatinine ≥1.5 mg/dl) are associated with hypertension and reduced patient survival compared to recipients from standard-criteria donors [69]. Delahousse et al. described a longitudinal cohort of 78 first deceased-donor kidney recipients in which donor age was associated with the development of recipient aortic stiffness (estimated via carotid-femoral pulse wave velocity Doppler measurement) [70]. Aortic stiffness has been previously well established as an independent predictive marker for total and CV mortality both in the general and ESRD populations. This concept has been validated in the transplant community when evaluating carotid artery pulse wave velocity [71], predicting the occurrence of CV events and decreased allograft function [72].

In terms of gender, in the same evaluation from Ducloux et al., they only described a trend towards the prevalence of post-transplant HTN in male recipients who received a kidney from a female donor (RR 1.06, 95 % CI 0.99–1.14, $p=0.07$).

Guidi et al., in a prospective observational study of 85 renal transplant recipients with stable kidney function not on cyclosporine, found that those without a family history of HTN engrafted with a kidney obtained from a donor with a positive family history of HTN were more likely to be hypertensive compared to recipients whose allografts were procured from donors without a positive HTN family history. This effect was not found when the recipient had a family history of HTN [73]. It was found in follow-up that higher diastolic BP and greater degrees of acute kidney injury during acute rejection occurred more frequently on those recipients whose allograft came from hypertensive families, compared to kidneys from normotensive ones [74].

Role of Immunosuppressive Medications

As summarized in the recent 2013 OPTN/SRTR annual report, immunosuppressive protocols for kidney transplantation have not changed significantly since 2008. There has been a steady trend towards providing induction with the use of T-cell depleting antibodies (anti-thymocyte globulin—55.7 %) compared to interleukin-2 receptor antagonists (basiliximab—36.8 %); for maintenance: among the CNIs, there has been a larger proportion of tacrolimus usage compared to cyclosporine; among the anti-metabolites, mycophenolate mofetil has triumphed compared to the mammalian target of rapamycin inhibitors ([mTOR inhibitors]: sirolimus, everolimus), and less than 40 % of recipients used a glucocorticoid-free protocol [75].

Glucocorticoids

The estimated incidence of glucocorticoid-associated HTN is approximately 15 % [76]. This result is greatest in kidney recipients with pre-transplant HTN and is more commonly seen when daily doses exceed 20 mg [77, 78].

Glucocorticoid-associated HTN is mediated by mineralocorticoid-induced sodium retention, increased responsiveness to vasoconstrictors, and decreased vasodilator production. Surprisingly, steroid-free or early withdrawal immunosuppressive regimens have not shown benefit in terms of BP control, albeit findings of lower CV risk surrogates such as lesser use of anti-lipemic medications and new-onset diabetes after transplantation (see Table 8.5). In the FREEDOM trial, a 12-month open-label, international multi-center study ($n=337$), in which de novo kidney transplant recipients were randomized to receive no steroids, steroids for 7 days post-transplant (steroid withdrawal), or standard steroid maintenance regimen, all in combination with: CsA, enteric-coated mycophenolate sodium, and basiliximab induction. No differences were observed in regard to systolic or diastolic BP between groups. Mean systolic BP at study end was 133 ± 20, 135 ± 8, and 132 ± 16 mmHg in each group, respectively. There was a significantly higher rejection incidence in the first two groups, but more interesting there was no difference in patient or allograft survival at 12-months [79]. Kramer et al. compared the long-term efficacy and safety of two steroid-free regimens (Basiliximab induction for all, then tacrolimus [Tac] monotherapy, and Tac/MMF, against a triple immunosuppressive therapy [Tac/MMF/steroids]) in a randomized multi-center cohort of 421 kidney transplant recipients. They concluded that despite a higher rate of acute rejection in the first 6 months with the steroid-free regimens, the long-term patient and allograft survival was no different between groups. There was a non-significant statistical trend towards a more promising CV risk by metabolic profiles with the Tac/Bas regimen compared to others, though no changes in BP among all groups [80–82]. Finally, to understand the rationale of the present state of practice in regard to steroid maintenance protocols in kidney transplantation, the work from Woodle et al. in a randomized, double-blind, placebo-controlled multi-center trial ($n=386$)

Table 8.5 Summary of steroid withdrawal trials and post-transplant hypertension

Trials/Published	Follow-up	Study groups	Induction + maintenance immunotherapy	Size (n)	Outcomes
FREEDOM [79] 2008	12-months	No GC GC only 7-days post-transplant Standard GC regimen	Basiliximab + MPA, CsA	337	No intergroup BP change No difference in patient or graft survival
ATLAS [80–82] 2005–2012	36-months	Tac Tac/MMF Tac/MMF/GC	Basiliximab	421	No intergroup BP change No difference in patient or graft survival
Woodle et al. [83] 2008	60-months	Early GC-withdrawal (7-day) Standard GC regimen	Bas or Dac or ATG + MMF, Tac	386	No intergroup BP change No difference in patient or graft survival

ATG anti-thymocyte globulin, *Bas* basiliximab, *CsA* cyclosporine, *Dac* daclizumab, *GC* glucocorticoid, *MMF* mycophenolate mofetil, *MPA* mycophenolic acid, *Tac* tacrolimus

comparing early GC-withdrawal (7 day, $n = 191$; 97 % prevalent HTN) versus long-term low-dose prednisone (5 mg/daily, $n = 195$; 94 % prevalent HTN), after 5 years of follow-up, found that there were no differences: in the proportion of patients experiencing the primary end-point (i.e., composite of death, allograft loss, or moderate/severe acute rejection), patient death, death-censored allograft-loss, biopsy-confirmed acute rejection (BCAR), and moderate/severe acute rejection. Kaplan Meier analysis revealed a higher incidence of BCAR with the early withdrawal regimen without differences between groups in allograft function ($p = 0.04$). Similarly, no significant changes were found among both groups in systolic or diastolic BP, as well as on the number of antihypertensives needed (see Fig. 8.2) [83].

In summary, it seems that low-dose prednisone therapy has a minimal effect on post-transplant HTN. This, concept was strengthened by a post-hoc analysis from Knight et al., of their 2010 published meta-analysis results of steroid avoidance/withdrawal regimens and outcomes in kidney transplantation [84, 85], as well as confirmed by Opelz and Döhler sub-analysis of the Collaborative Transplant Study (CTS), where from a cohort of 41,953 deceased-donor kidney transplant recipientswas studied. They concluded that, 1-year post-transplant systolic BP associated with higher dose steroids, but during years 2–5 the association with de novo occurrence of DM or HTN was not present [86].

Calcineurin Inhibitors

Since FDA approval in 1983, cyclosporine (CsA) has been known to cause or exacerbate hypertension after transplantation [12, 87–90]. Calcineurin inhibitors induce endothelial dysfunction via upregulation of endothelin and inhibition of inducible nitric oxide [91–93], increased vascular resistance accompanied by failed

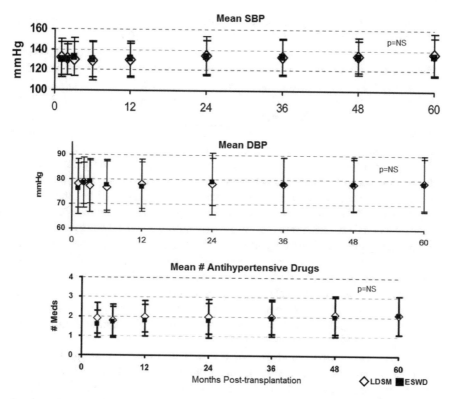

Fig. 8.2 Absence of HTN benefits in early steroid withdrawal versus low-dose maintenance regimens. Absence of changes in the mean of: systolic blood pressure (SBP), diastolic blood pressure (DBP), and in the number of antihypertensive drugs used, in a comparison between low-dose steroid maintenance (LDSM) versus early steroid withdrawal (ESWD) regimens. Adapted from: Woodle E., et al. [83]

endothelium-dependent vasodilation [94, 95], and sodium retention via activation of the renin–angiotensin–aldosterone (RAAS) system [96–98]. Cyclosporine-induced sympathetic nerve system activation generally only lasts 2 weeks after exposure. It seems there is little enhancement of sympathetic tone with tacrolimus [99]. Independent of the hemodynamic effect, CNIs may induce development of interstitial fibrosis and tubular atrophy (IFTA) via transforming growth factor-β[beta], FGF-1, and osteopontin upregulation [100]. In a recent histopathology study, Singh et al. described finding chronic CsA changes in a pediatric cohort with idiopathic nephrotic syndrome. Protocol biopsies after 1 year of therapy revealed: upregulation of immunohistochemical markers for endothelial injury, oxidative stress, and fibrogenic cytokines, along with histological evidence of significant glomerulosclerosis, IFTA, and arteriolar hyalinosis [101]. Lastly, there is evidence indicating tacrolimus induces direct activation of the tubular sodium chloride co-transporter leading to hypertension via a mechanism similar to pseudohyperaldosteronism type II (also known as Gordon syndrome) that is accompanied by hyperkalemia. In this study, a sodium-chloride channel blocking drug, hydrochloro-thiazide, reversed tacrolimus-induced hypertension [102, 103].

As previously reviewed by several authors, the hypertensive and nephrotoxic effects of CNIs have been observed in different organ transplant cohorts, including bone marrow and cardiac recipients, in whom the incidence of HTN increased from less than 10 % overall to 70–90 %, after the introduction of cyclosporine [12, 23, 27, 104, 105]. Despite the observations linking CNIs with hypertension, withdrawal studies have been plagued by higher degrees of acute rejection and/or kidney allograft loss, especially for early CNI withdrawal [106, 107]. Tacrolimus was FDA-approved in 1994 initially for liver and later for kidney transplantation. It is also associated with hypertension though to a lesser extent than cyclosporine [63, 64, 108]. In a head-to-head comparison, Margreiter et al. reported that the effect of tacrolimus on BP is 5 % lower than that of cyclosporine [109]. Bolin et al. reported the results of the OPTIMA study, a prospective multi-center analysis ($n = 328$; stable kidney transplant recipients on CsA) that randomized patients to one of the three arms (i.e., continue CsA, convert to "reduced" Tac [serum target trough level 3.0–5.9 ng/ml], or "standard" Tac [serum level 6.0–8.9 ng/ml]), in order to ascertain optimal tacrolimus trough levels to minimize adverse effects. Results at 12-months showed favorable eGFR improvements for the "reduced-Tac" group compared to CsA, improved lipids in the tacrolimus treated patients although with little difference in blood pressure between groups [110].

The concept of CNI withdrawal as a means of prolonging allograft survival has been investigated. Mourer et al. found that late CNI withdrawal was significantly associated with lowering of ambulatory day- and nighttime BP [111–113]. Nevertheless, such improvements may not necessarily translate into improved outcomes such as reduced death from CVD. Roodnat et al. performed a 15-year follow-up analysis ($n = 212$) [114] from a previous randomized multi-center cohort [115] and concluded that in CsA/MMF/Steroid treated patients, there was no benefit of CNI withdrawal regarding allograft and patient survival, or concerning prevalence of or death by comorbidities. However, rejection shortly after CNI withdrawal was associated with decreased allograft survival. And most recently, in an attempt to find a more suitable kidney transplant recipient cohort that might truly benefit from this strategy, the prospective Clinical Trials in Organ Transplantation-09 trial (CTOT-09) by Hricik et al., randomized 21 non-sensitized primary living-donor recipients (i.e., "immunologically quiescent") at 6-months of stable post-transplantation state, to either continuation or Tac withdrawal (after having received the current standard-of-care immunosuppressive therapy: rabbit ATG induction, and maintenance with Tac, MMF, Prednisone). The study was terminated prematurely due to unacceptable rates of acute rejection and/or de novo donor-specific antibodies [116]. In summary, CNI withdrawal for management of hypertension in most patients seems most unwise.

Belatacept

Belatacept is a novel co-stimulation blocker that binds CD80/CD86 on antigen-presenting cells to prevent T cell activation [117]. It is generally used in conjunction with mycophenolate and steroids. Vincenti et al. analyzed the safety and efficacy of belatacept compared to cyclosporine finding that 86% of patients in the belatacept arm and 89% in the cyclosporine arm were receiving antihypertensive medications [118]. However, long-term follow-up of the BENEFIT and BENEFIT-EXT trials showed that subjects in the belatacept arms had an SBP approximately 8 mmHg lower and a DBP approximately 4 mmHg lower than subjects in the cyclosporine arm [119, 120]. Additionally, in the BENEFIT trial, 82% of patients in the belatacept group and 96% of patients in the cyclosporine group were receiving at least one antihypertensive [119]. Thus it appears that belatacept based immunosuppressive regimens are associated with less hypertension compared with cyclosporine based regimens.

Role of the Native kidneys

In an era before effective antihypertensive agents were broadly available, bilateral native nephrectomy was a treatment option for dialysis or transplant patients with refractory hypertension. Fortunately, such procedures are rarely necessary at present. Nevertheless, important information about the role of the native kidneys in the genesis of hypertension is available. Curtis et al. had described a 24% prevalence of HTN in a cohort of kidney transplant recipients that were following an alternate-day prednisone protocol. In a sub-cohort analysis, they found that among 32 patients who had undergone bilateral native nephrectomies, only 6% were hypertensive [121]. Remnant native kidneys have the potential to promote HTN via sympathetic nervous system (SNS) activation and/or through renin secretion. Their role in the kidney transplant recipient population, and pre- or post-transplant uni- or bilateral nephrectomy, has not yet been clearly delineated, as several small studies have revealed confounding results [122]. In 2002, Hausberg et al. hypothesized that improved blood pressure control after successful kidney transplantation may be associated with reduced sympathetic nervous system activation as seen in uremic patients. They found that muscle sympathetic nerve activity (MSNA) in kidney transplant recipients was no different compared with hemodialysis patients. However, among allograft recipients who had undergone bilateral nephrectomy post-transplantation, MSNA was significantly lower and comparable to healthy controls (see Fig. 8.3) [123, 124].

Transplant Renal Artery Stenosis

Transplant renal artery stenosis (TRAS) has been variably reported to develop in 1–23% of recipients, accounting for about 1–5% of post-transplantation HTN cases [125, 126]. Based on 2000–2005 USRDS registry data, Hurst et al. described the

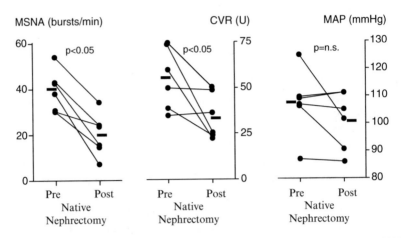

Fig. 8.3 Potential implications of sympathetic nerve activation in native-nephrectomized kidney transplant recipients. Mean values of MSNA, CVR, and MAP, from 6 kidney transplant recipients studied pre- and 3 months post-nephrectomy of second native kidney. *CVR* calf vascular resistance, *MAP* mean arterial blood pressure, *MSNA* muscle sympathetic nerve activity. Adapted from: Hausberg M., et al. [123]

overall incidence of TRAS at 8.3 cases per 1000 patients-years (95 % CI 7.8–8.9). In addition, they found TRAS to be strongly associated with an increased risk for allograft loss including death (adjusted hazard ratio 2.84, 95 % CI 1.70–4.72) [127]. TRAS is often diagnosed between 3 and 24 months after surgery, with the highest frequency in the first 6-month period, though it can present at any time. Early TRAS (0–3 months) is most likely related to donor vessel surgical trauma (at procurement, or implantation), suture technique, or malposition of the allograft [128, 129]. Risk factors associated with late TRAS (after 3-months post-transplantation) include: CMV infection [130], delayed graft function [131], acute rejection [131], prolonged ischemia time [132], multiple renal arteries implanted on a common aortic patch [133], and pediatric donor source [134]. TRAS was previously considered to be a more frequent complication in living-donor recipients compared to deceased donors, based on the observation that the living donor's artery was anastomosed using an end-to-side technique to the recipient's iliac artery compared to the use of the deceased donor's aortic cuff or aortic patch. This association has been refuted, however; evidence comparing end-to-side versus end-to-end vascular anastomosis with TRAS has yielded variable conclusions [135–138]. It has been suggested that late stenosis may be more likely associated with atherosclerotic disease of either the allograft artery or the proximal iliac artery [139]. Diffuse stenosis may reflect immune-mediated endothelial damage, as it was described in a case-series of deceased-donor kidney recipients by Porter et al. [140]. De novo donor-specific antibody generation was found to be more common in post-anastomotic TRAS, as described in a study by Willicombe et al. (hazard ratio (HR): 4.41 [2.0–9.73], $p < 0.001$), as well as to more likely have had "rejection with arteritis" (odds ratio (OR): 4.83 [1.47–15.87], $p = 0.0095$) [141]. Lastly, case reports have described malignant HTN from TRAS secondary to mechanical extrinsic compression by: an enlarged native polycystic kidney [142], or a compressive main donor artery pseudoaneurysm [126].

Clinically, TRAS presents with worsening or refractory HTN, fluid retention, flash pulmonary edema ("Pickering Syndrome" [143, 144]), and acute kidney injury ([AKI], that may or may not be associated with either angiotensin-converting enzyme inhibitor [ACE-i] or angiotensin II-receptor blocker [ARB] initiation). The presence of a bruit over the kidney allograft suggests this diagnosis although such a finding is both insensitive and non-specific [145]. Severe stenosis can also be present without an audible bruit [27, 126, 135].

The "gold standard" diagnostic test for TRAS is allograft arteriography, though considering its invasive nature and risk for contrast-induced AKI, other imaging techniques have been studied. Kidney ultrasonography with Doppler has been reported to be useful for diagnosis of TRAS by several centers [125, 146–148]. Doppler criteria for TRAS include kidney allograft artery blood flow velocity above 200 cm/s, a proximal to distal stenosis segment gradient of at least 2:1, and a parvus-tardus wave-form [147]. The resistive index (RI) is not a useful parameter for the diagnosis of TRAS [149, 150]. Gadolinium-enhanced magnetic resonance angiography (MRA) has also been reported as efficacious in some series (sensitivity and specificity of 100 %) [151, 152]. The caveats are that surgical clips often obscure the origin of the kidney allograft vasculature (leading to "clip artifact"), and exposure to gadolinium is contraindicated when eGFR is less than 30 ml/min because of the increased risk for nephrogenic systemic fibrosis [153].

Once TRAS is suspected, obtaining allograft histology may be an important management step to define and grade the occurrence of co-morbid entities that could independently impact allograft prognosis [132, 134]. When the allograft is deemed viable, revascularization options include: medical therapy combined with either percutaneous transluminal angioplasty (PTA) ± stenting, or surgical revascularization. Initial medical therapy is aimed at controlling HTN, preserving allograft viability, and mitigating risk of flash pulmonary edema and acute decompensated heart failure. Thus, use of loop diuretics is often necessary. Although the use of ACE-i/ARB medications may counteract the RAAS activation, they potentially can induce acute kidney injury, thus need to be used with caution [125].

Data comparing PTA alone or with stenting have yielded variable results in terms of allograft function, blood pressure control, and rate of re-stenosis. Touma et al. performed a retrospective cohort of 17 kidney transplant recipients with angiography-proven TRAS (median follow-up of 19.6 months), and all with end-to-side anastomosis to the external iliac artery. Five (29 %) underwent balloon-PTA alone versus 12 who had a bare metal stent (BMS) placed. Their technical success rate was 88.2 %, with eGFR correction, however, without significant improvement in hypertension control. In the early post-intervention period, there were 4 re-stenoses (1 from PTA alone and 3 from BMS group; 25 % incidence) [154]. Reported re-stenosis rates vary between endovascular intervention (EVI) modality (i.e., PTA alone, bare metal stent [BMS], or drug-eluting stent [DES]). Post-PTA alone have ranged from 20 to 60 %[132, 134, 155], although it should be noted that PTA is often used as the initial intervention, with the use of either bare metal or drug eluting stents reserved for lesions that recur. Marini et al. described a retrospective analysis of 62 TRAS cases that underwent PTA±stent, achieving 90% procedural success rate, significant HTN control, and preserved allograft function up to 97% in year-1 and 85% in year-10 post-procedure [156]. When comparing drug eluting stents with bare metal stents and angioplasty alone, Biederman et al. described a technical success rate of 98% with improved blood pressure control, and reduced requirement for antihypertensives at 30-day pre-EVI across all sub-groups, although this finding didn't persist to the 180–360 days ($p=0.1$) [157]. Surgical revascularization is technically challenging and is used mostly as the last resort for patients with recurrent disease after EVIs, or for those with lesions considered not suitable for EVIs. Its success rate seems to be similar to PTA with stenting, albeit an associated higher rate of morbidity (e.g., allograft atheroembolization, allograft loss [approx. 30%]) and mortality (5% cases) [125, 128, 158]. There are currently no randomized controlled trials comparing between EVI modalities.

Non-Adherence

Adherence is generally defined as the extent to which patients take medications prescribed by their health care provider. Although this definition is imperfect, it is generally used dichotomously in clinical trials, i.e.: "the patient is either taking or not taking medications." In reality, the range of adherence goes from 0 to more than 100% if one includes patients who take more than that prescribed [159]. A detailed analysis of the reasons for adherence failure is beyond the scope of this chapter. However, in a recent comprehensive review of the literature, Vella and Cohen described that approximately 22% of significant medication non-adherence occurred in the kidney transplant recipient population, which in turn could be responsible for at least 36% of allograft loss cases [160]. Morrissey et al. provided further insight into the complex nature of this huge problem. They incorporated patient's failure to follow through with medical appointments and scheduled laboratory visits and clarified the difference between the terms compliance and adherence. Of note, most data regarding adherence has been focused on immunosuppressive compliance and its association with allograft loss [161].

Recently, a small but thorough prospective cohort from Czyzewski et al. examined medication adherence including antihypertensive drugs using the Morisky–Green questionnaire [162], and found that 38% of medication non-adherence was because of forgetfulness. Despite the well-known negative association between non-adherence and adverse medical outcomes, in this study, there was no significant relationship among these variables [45].

Correcting non-adherence is complex and requires a multidisciplinary patient-centered approach. McGillicuddy et al. recently published results of a proof-of-concept 3-month small prospective randomized controlled trial that included first kidney transplant recipients with proven pre-intervention non-adherence and

HTN. By using home devices wirelessly connected to the transplant clinic: a Bluetooth BP monitor, an electronic medication tray, and a personal smartphone; they demonstrated that this protocol is feasible, safe, acceptable (>75 % of participants), enhanced adherence to medications and translated into improvement of office-based systolic BP [163].

Management

Therapeutic lifestyle modification (e.g., weight loss, exercise, low salt diet) is generally recommended as first-line therapy for patients in the general population. In truth, there are remarkably few data in the transplant population that have carefully examined the efficacy of such interventions. Guida et al. studied the effects of a 12-month dietary regimen on nutritional status and metabolic outcomes, on 46 deceased-donor kidney transplant recipients, followed prospectively during their first year post-transplantation. Adherence to dietary recommendations was related to gender (male better than female) and associated with weight loss primarily due to a decrease in fat mass, with decreases in total cholesterol and plasma glucose levels, and a concomitant increase in serum albumin level. No change in hypertension control was reported [164].

Evidence supporting the importance of blood pressure control in long-term outcomes has accrued from several sources. Mourad et al. were among the first to show evidence suggesting that by maintaining normotension, there was concomitant allograft function preservation in their cohort of cyclosporine (CsA)-treated kidney recipients, during a follow-up period of 2.5 years; limitations of this study were its small size ($n=25$) and short follow-up [165]. In 2005, Opelz and Döhler performed a larger retrospective study of 24,404 first deceased donor kidney transplant recipients (age 20 or more; mainly on CsA-based immunosuppression) between 1987 and 2000. They examined the association between BP control and kidney allograft and patient survival, and found that the best 10-year allograft and patient survival rates were obtained when systolic BP was maintained at less than or equal to 140 mmHg between 1 and 3 years post-transplantation (see Fig. 8.4) [22]. Furthermore, they showed that patients with elevated systolic BPs at 1 year post-transplantation that was subsequently controlled to less than or equal to 140 mmHg by 3 years showed significantly better 10-year allograft survival compared to those without good control [22].

Pharmacotherapy

Given the known impact of immunosuppressive therapy on blood pressure, one option to consider for patients with suboptimal hypertension control is to consider converting immunotherapy. The risks and benefits of such conversion should be

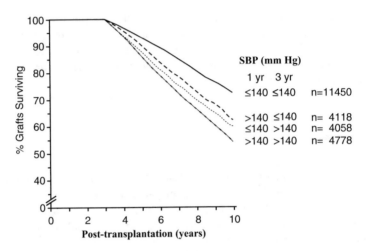

Fig. 8.4 Long-term kidney graft survival calculated from 3 to 10 years in relation to systolic BP (SBP) of <140 or ≥140 mmHg at 1 and 3 years post-transplant. The respective 1- and 3-year BPs are indicated to the right of each curve, together with number of patients studied. Adapted from: Opelz G. and Döhler B. [22]

discussed cautiously with the patient, and with input from the transplant nephrologist. Glucocorticoids (GC) may be minimized or even discontinued, although as previously mentioned, trials of steroid withdrawal have not demonstrated benefit in terms of BP control. Among the CNIs, CsA is infrequently used as first-line anti-rejection therapy currently. However, when used, its reduction or conversion to tacrolimus has been noted to promote BP control [109, 166]. The choice of immunotherapeutic drug to adjust should include consideration of individual patient's co-morbidities, allograft function, estimated rejection risk, and the transplant program's protocols. Nevertheless, these strategies alone are rarely sufficient to achieve normotension, and most kidney transplant recipients require specific antihypertensive therapy, which needs to be individualized according to rejection risk while paying attention to potential drug–drug interactions (see Table 8.6) [27, 167].

Lakkis and Weir recently published a simplified HTN management plan based on an arbitrary timeline that aligns closely to specific time-points in the first 6-months post-transplant [168]. They suggested that within the first weeks post-transplant, HTN may relate mostly to volume overload after surgery, initial high doses of CNI and glucocorticoids, thus recommending salt restriction, the use of diuretics to counteract GC- and CNI-induced salt and water retention, and calcium channel blockers (CCBs) to counteract CNI-vasoconstriction. Angiotensin-converting enzyme inhibitors (ACE-i)/angiotensin receptor blockers (ARB) are best avoided in this earlier period to allow for adequate allograft perfusion. Throughout the post-transplant timeline, β[beta]-blockers (BBs) can be generally and safely introduced.

Table 8.6 Classes of antihypertensive medications used after kidney transplantation with additional description of drug–drug immunotherapeutic interactions, benefits, and adverse effects

Class	Medication (example)	Mechanism of action	Pharmacokinetics	Drug interactions with immunotherapy	Frequency of use in transplant recipients at 1-year(*)	Beneficial effect in transplant recipients	Principal adverse effects
Dihydropyridine CCBs	Amlodipine Nifedipine	Vasodilation	Cytochrome P450 3A4 substrate	Positive May increase CNI levels through inhibition of hepatic metabolism	40 % (as a group)	Mitigates CNI-induced HTN and nephrotoxicity	Edema
Non-dihydropyridine CCBs	Diltiazem Verapamil	Vasodilation Heart rate control	Cytochrome P450 3A4 substrate and inhibitor	Strongly Positive Increases CNI levels through inhibition of hepatic metabolism		Reduced requirement for CNI/mTOR inhibitor Mitigates CNI-induced HTN and nephrotoxicity	Edema, CNI toxicity, bradycardia
ACE-i	Lisinopril Ramipril (many others)	Prevents AT-I to AT-II conversion	Lisinopril: 100 % excreted unchanged, urine 29 %, feces 69 % Ramipril: urine 60 %, feces 40 % as parent drug and metabolites	No direct PK interactions Caution with concurrent high-dose CNI due to hyperkalemia risk	24.6 % (as a group)	May reverse post-transplant erythrocytosis Mitigation of proteinuria May mitigate AMR mediated by antibodies to AT1R	Hyperkalemia, AKI, anemia

(continued)

Table 8.6 (continued)

Class	Medication (example)	Mechanism of action	Pharmacokinetics	Drug interactions with immunotherapy	Frequency of use in transplant recipients at 1-year(*)	Beneficial effect in transplant recipients	Principal adverse effects
ARB	Losartan Valsartan Candesartan Irbesartan	Selectively antagonizes AT-II; AT-I and AT-II receptor with 1000 x higher affinity for AT-I	Variable renal and fecal excretion (unchanged)	No direct PK interactions Caution with concurrent high-dose CNI due to hyperkalemia risk		Losartan may lower uric acid (ref)	Hyperkalemia, AKI, anemia
Renin inhibitors	Aliskiren	Directly inhibits renin resulting in conversion blockade of angiotensinogen to AT-I	Cytochrome P450 3A4 subtrate (minor), P-glycoprotein	CsA may increase aliskiren levels	n/a	May mitigate proteinuria Alternative to ACE-i or ARBs	Hyperkalemia (especially if used with CNIs)
Diuretics	Furosemide HCTZ	Salt and water excretion	Renal excretion	–	2.6–10% (as a group)	Useful in edema and hyperkalemia Thiazides less effective in patients with reduced GFR	Volume depletion Hypokalemia
Potassium-sparing diuretics	Amiloride	Inhibits DCT aldosterone-induced sodium resorption	Renal and fecal excretion (unchanged)	–		Useful in hypokalemia, or if there is suspected hyperaldosteronism May mitigate proteinuria	Hyperkalemia (especially if used with CNI/ACE-i)

Class	Medication (example)	Mechanism of action	Pharmacokinetics	Drug interactions with immunotherapy	Frequency of use in transplant recipients at 1-year(*)	Beneficial effect in transplant recipients	Principal adverse effects
	Spironolactone Eplerenone	Inhibits DCT aldosterone receptor	Urine (unchanged)	–			
Beta-blockers	Metoprolol tartrate or succinate (many others)	Antagonizes Beta-1 adrenergic receptors	Cytochrome P450 2D6 substrate	–	44.5– 65.5 %	Reduce risk of perioperative MI	Bradycardia Fatigue Hyperkalemia Worsening insulin resistance
Vasodilator	Hydralazine	Dilates peripheral vessels	Liver metabolism Renal and fecal excretion	–	4.8–14.5 % (as a group)	Useful in hospital post-transplant (short half-life)	SLE, headache
	Minoxidil		Renal excretion	–		May reverse tacrolimus-induced alopecia	Edema Hirsutism May exacerbate CsA-induced hypertrichosis Pericardial effusion
Alpha-blockers	Doxazosin	Antagonizes Alpha-1 adrenergic receptors	Cytochrome P450 metabolized	–	n/a	May mitigate BPH	Orthostasis

(continued)

Table 8.6 (continued)

Class	Medication (example)	Mechanism of action	Pharmacokinetics	Drug interactions with immunotherapy	Frequency of use in transplant recipients at 1-year(*)	Beneficial effect in transplant recipients	Principal adverse effects
Alpha2-adrenergic agonists	Clonidine	Stimulate central alpha-2 adrenergic receptors resulting in reduced sympathetic tone	Liver metabolism to inactive metabolites Enterohepatic circulation	–	n/a	No proved benefit in transplant population Fast acting (useful for pre-biopsy HTN control to further lower bleeding risk) Sublingual	Rebound HTN Drowsiness Headache

ACE-I angiotensin-converting enzyme inhibitor, *AKI* acute kidney injury, *AMR* antibody-mediated rejection, *ARB* angiotensin II receptor blocker, *AT* angiotensin, *AT1R* angiotensin type 1 receptor, *BPH* benign prostatic hypertrophy, *CCB* calcium channel blocker, *CNI* calcineurin inhibitor, *CsA* cyclosporine A, *DCT* distal convoluted tubule, *GFR* glomerular filtration rate, *HCTZ* hydrochlorothiazide, *HTN* hypertension, *MI* myocardial infarction, *mTOR* mammalian target of rapamycin, *PK* pharmacokinetic, *SLE* systemic lupus erythematosus. Frequency of use column data (*), from Lentine KL et al., Am J Neph, 2013;38(5):420–9 [167]

Adapted from: Rossi AP, Vella JP. Hypertension, Living Kidney Donors, and Transplantation: Where Are We Today? Advances in chronic kidney disease. 2015;22(2):154–64

Calcium Channel Blockers

Calcium channel blockers (CCBs) reduce angio-myocytes' contractility and induce vasodilation. Allograft afferent arteriole vasodilation leads to decreased mean arterial pressure and total renal vascular resistance, promoting increased renal blood flow and GFR. Both dihydropyridines ([DHP], e.g., amlodipine, nifedipine) and non-dihydropyridines (e.g., diltiazem, verapamil) have been used in transplant recipients. The former are preferred due to their lack of significant pharmacokinetic inhibitory interactions with CNIs and mTORi [169]. In a meta-analysis of 29 trials ($n = 2262$) comparing CCBs with placebo or no therapy, Cross et al. described that at 12-months post-transplant, CCBs lowered allograft loss (RR 0.75, 95 % CI 0.57–0.99; $p = 0.04$) and improved GFR by 4.5 ml/min (95 % CI 2.2–6.7 ml/min; $p < 0.0001$), but did not reduce death risk [170].

Head-to-head trials comparing DHPs with ACE-I [171] or ARBs [172] have shown similar BP control. An exception to the overall accepted safe profile that DHPs have with CNIs has been described among kidney transplant patients not expressing the cytochrome P450 CYP3A5 enzyme (an alternative metabolic pathway for CNIs), yielding an increased risk for tacrolimus toxicity with the use of oral or intravenous nicardipine [173–175].

Diuretics

The use of diuretics varies among series, at approximately 2.6–10 % at 1-year post-transplant [167], versus 34 % in the late transplant period as described by Kurnatowska et al. [176]. In this study, there was a significant trend towards higher prevalence of diuretic use that was associated with lower eGFR ($n = 54$ with eGFR <30 ml/min, 46 %, $p = 0.03$). Loop diuretics were the most commonly used, compared to 8.4 % on thiazides and 4.2 % on aldosterone antagonists. Similar findings were described on a sub-analysis from the international kidney transplant FAVORIT study [177, 178], by Carpenter et al., where thiazide use was found in 10 % of the cohort [179].

In the general population, the ALLHAT study found that thiazides, specifically chlorthalidone, were more effective than lisinopril or amlodipine in lowering systolic BP [180]; similar comparative studies had been lacking in the kidney transplant population, until the work from Taber et al., who analyzed the safety and efficacy of thiazides in a single-center retrospective cohort of 1093 adult recipients [181]. As described before, similarly in this study only 10 % of the cohort had been exposed to thiazides. These were introduced at a mean time of 2.4 ± 2.0 years post-transplant. Overall, thiazide-exposed patients had similar long-term clinical outcomes; without significant differences between groups in terms of acute rejection, allograft and patient survival, hospital re-admission rates, hypotensive events, or electrolyte imbalances. Thiazide efficacy, measured as a 10 % systolic BP reduction upon therapy initiation was achieved in 44 % of the exposed cohort. After multivariate regression analysis, factors associated with thiazide efficacy were: higher baseline systolic

BP and diastolic BP. Baseline eGFR was not associated with thiazide efficacy (HR 1.02, 95% CI 0.98–1.06; $p=0.225$).

ACE Inhibitors/ARBs

Blockade of the renin–angiotensin–aldosterone system (RAAS) is generally known to be associated with decreases of systolic BP, glomerular capillary pressure, proteinuria, and CV events. Heinze et al. retrospectively analyzed over 2000 kidney transplant recipients and found that 10-year survival rates were 74% in patients receiving either an ACEi or an ARB, while survival was significantly lower at 53% in recipients not taking these agents; showing a hazard ratio of ACEi/ARB use for mortality at 0.57 (95% CI 0.40–0.81), compared with nonuse [182]. Paoletti et al. also reported 10-year outcomes in a small randomized trial of kidney recipients (all taking CNIs, MMF, and prednisone), 36 of them on ACE inhibition versus 34 patients not on these agents, demonstrating that the ACEi group had fewer CV events, less proteinuria, and increased survival but no significant effect on allograft survival [183].

In the kidney transplant population, RAAS blockade additionally takes care of other underlying hypertension-promoters such as: native kidney renin activity, CNI-induced increased angiotensin concentration, and CNI-induced increased expression of angiotensin receptors. Furthermore, ACEi/ARBs are also potentially beneficial by preventing CNI-related fibrosis/tubular atrophy (IF/TA) [184], and disrupting the production of angiotensin-1 receptor antibodies, hence potentially preventing vascular rejection [185]. Nevertheless, despite their potential mitigation of IF/TA, enhanced allograft survival has not been conclusively attained. In the aforementioned retrospective analysis from Heinze et al., they described a 10-year actual allograft survival of 59% in the ACEi/ARB group vs only 41% in the nonusers ($p=0.0002$). In contrast, Opelz et al. from the CTS trial group, in reviewing their large cohort of 17,209 patients up until year 2004, in 33.5% of them which were taking either ACEi or ARBs, found no beneficial relationship in terms of patient or allograft survival [186]. Furthermore, in a more recent investigation, the SECRET trial was a multi-center randomized double-blind study that compared candesartan to placebo. The candesartan dose was escalated from 4 to 16 mg daily, aiming for a diastolic BP<85 mmHg. This analysis was stopped prematurely after patient randomization, because the composite primary end-point of all-cause mortality, CV morbidity, and allograft failure was much lower than expected. The treatment group experienced better systolic BP (absolute change −6.78 vs −0.60 mmHg, $p<0.001$), improved diastolic BP (absolute change −4.81 vs −1.21 mmHg, $p=0.002$), decreased proteinuria (median relative change from baseline for urinary protein/creatinine ratio −15.0% vs 23.4%, $p<0.001$), but also exhibited higher serum creatinine (increased by 10.8 vs 4.3%, $p<0.001$) and increased serum potassium levels. However, there were no significant differences in patient or allograft survival between groups [187].

Despite the conflicting data about survival, these agents are used especially after the initial post-transplant state when GFR is felt to have reached a steady state. When these drugs are considered, surveillance for known adverse effects including AKI and hyperkalemia needs to continue [188] [23, 27]. And lastly, they can decrease the hematocrit by 5–10 %[189–192], effect that might be useful in managing post-transplantation erythrocytosis (defined as a hematocrit >51 %; condition affecting around 10–15 % kidney recipients) [193], although potentially unfavorable for anemic patients. These are several reasons for the rationale of starting these drugs, when indicated, at least after the initial 3- to 6-month post-transplantation state.

Adrenergic Blockers

In a recent pharmaco-epidemiologic evaluation of 16,157 patients on their first kidney transplant anniversary, Lentine and colleagues found that BBs were the most commonly used antihypertensive agents (45–65 %), followed by CCBs at 40 % [167]. In general, β-blockers (BBs) decrease heart rate and sympathetic nervous tone; combined α[alpha]-1-β blockade additionally induces vasodilation. Their pathophysiologic impact is to mitigate increased sympathetic nervous system tone that as described is related to either the presence of native kidneys and enhanced by CNIs (see Pathogenesis) [185]. Aftab et al. performed a retrospective analysis of 321 kidney recipients followed for 10 years and found that the use of BBs was associated with better survival (HR 0.60, 95 % CI 0.26–0.98). Less than 20 % of this cohort had a history of coronary artery disease, suggesting that even patients without a previous CVD history may benefit from this drug group [194]. The vasodilating BBs with selective α[alpha]-1 blockade (e.g., carvedilol, labetalol) may be better tolerated and associated with lesser adverse metabolic effects, compared to the traditional β1-selective blockers such as metoprolol or atenolol, which previously have been linked to weight gain and worsening of insulin resistance. Atenolol is often avoided in transplant recipients due to unpredictable pharmacokinetics given its renal elimination. Nevertheless, there is no data to support the use of one group or the other in the kidney transplant population [195]. Patients on β-blocker therapy before transplantation should continue this medication perioperatively to prevent rebound HTN and tachycardia [27]. However, starting these agents in BB-naïve recipients immediately before transplant surgery is not recommended given a significantly increased risk of 30-day all-cause mortality and stroke [196, 197].

Special Considerations

Ethnicity and Gender

At present, there is no current high-grade clinical research to support specific antihypertensive therapies in the kidney recipient population based on differences in race or gender. In a recent systematic review from Brewster et al., no definitive answer was achieved when trying to understand the well-described finding that CCBs are more effective medications to lower BP in non-CKD blacks [198, 199];

nevertheless, there is no reason to suspect that this would be different in a post-transplant black recipient. Lentine et al. also found that black race was independently associated with an increased used of all classes of antihypertensives at 1-year post-transplant (CCBs adjusted OR (aOR): 1.49, 95 % CI [1.37–1.62], $p \leq 0.0001$; BBs aOR: 1.20, 95 % CI [1.10–1.31], $p \leq 0.0001$; ACE-i/ARBs aOR: 1.11, 95 % CI [1.01–1.22], $p < 0.05$–0.002) [167].

Summary

Hypertension is common in kidney transplant recipients, and it is of critical importance due to its link towards increasing the risk for allograft failure and death. Numerous mechanisms and risk factors have been described. Its diagnosis seems to be inadequate just by office BP monitoring, thus the use of ABPM has gained significant popularity, though still unproven if chronotherapy translates into better hard clinical outcomes. Transplant renal artery stenosis induced HTN continues to be a difficult clinical scenario since re-stenosis is very frequent. Post-transplant hypertension treatment is aimed at modifying the immunosuppressive medication regimen, and by judiciously using specific blood pressure lowering medications that are pharmaco-immunologically appropriate.

Disclosures Astellas, Bristol Myers Squibb (Research Grants).

References

1. Leeson S, Desai SP. Medical and ethical challenges during the first successful human kidney transplantation in 1954 at peter bent Brigham hospital, Boston. Anesth Analg. 2015;120(1):239–45.
2. Kumnig M, Rumpold G, Hofer S, Konig P, Holzner B, Giesinger J, et al. Patient-reported outcome reference values for patients after kidney transplantation. Wien Klin Wochenschr. 2014;126(1–2):15–22.
3. Muehrer RJ, Becker BN. Life after transplantation: new transitions in quality of life and psychological distress. Semin Dial. 2005;18(2):124–31.
4. Garcia GG, Harden P, Chapman J. The global role of kidney transplantation. Nephrol Dial Transplant. 2013;28(8):e1–5.
5. Costa-Requena G, Cantarell Aixendri MC, Rodriguez Urrutia A, Seron Micas D. Health related quality of life and kidney transplantation: a comparison with population values at 6 months post-transplant. Med Clin. 2014;142(9):393–6.
6. Jensen CE, Sorensen P, Petersen KD. In Denmark kidney transplantation is more cost-effective than dialysis. Dan Med J. 2014;61(3):A4796.
7. Dominguez J, Harrison R, Atal R, Larrain L. Cost-effectiveness of policies aimed at increasing organ donation: the case of Chile. Transplant Proc. 2013;45(10):3711–5.
8. Levy AR, Briggs AH, Johnston K, MacLean JR, Yuan Y, L'Italien GJ, et al. Projecting long-term graft and patient survival after transplantation. Value Health. 2014;17(2):254–60.

9. Snyder RA, Moore DR, Moore DE. More donors or more delayed graft function? A cost-effectiveness analysis of DCD kidney transplantation. Clin Transplant. 2013;27(2):289–96.
10. Schnitzler MA, Skeans MA, Axelrod DA, Lentine KL, Tuttle-Newhall JE, Snyder JJ, et al. OPTN/SRTR 2013 annual data report: economics. Am J Transplant. 2015;15(S2):1–24.
11. Linas SL, Miller PD, McDonald KM, Stables DP, Katz F, Weil R, et al. Role of the renin-angiotensin system in post-transplantation hypertension in patients with multiple kidneys. N Engl J Med. 1978;298(26):1440–4.
12. Textor SC, Canzanello VJ, Taler SJ, Wilson DJ, Schwartz LL, Augustine JE, et al. Cyclosporine-induced hypertension after transplantation. Mayo Clin Proc. 1994;69(12):1182–93.
13. First MR, Neylan JF, Rocher LL, Tejani A. Hypertension after renal transplantation. J Am Soc Nephrol. 1994;4(8 Suppl):S30–6.
14. van der Schaaf MR, Hene RJ, Floor M, Blankestijn PJ, Koomans HA. Hypertension after renal transplantation. Calcium channel or converting enzyme blockade? Hypertension. 1995;25(1):77–81.
15. Paoletti E, Gherzi M, Amidone M, Massarino F, Cannella G. Association of arterial hypertension with renal target organ damage in kidney transplant recipients: the predictive role of ambulatory blood pressure monitoring. Transplantation. 2009;87(12):1864–9.
16. Ojo AO. Cardiovascular complications after renal transplantation and their prevention. Transplantation. 2006;82(5):603–11.
17. Aakhus S, Dahl K, Wideroe TE. Cardiovascular disease in stable renal transplant patients in Norway: morbidity and mortality during a 5-yr follow-up. Clin Transplant. 2004;18(5):596–604.
18. Sarnak MJ, Levey AS, Schoolwerth AC, Coresh J, Culleton B, Hamm LL, et al. Kidney disease as a risk factor for development of cardiovascular disease: a statement from the American Heart Association Councils on Kidney in Cardiovascular Disease, High Blood Pressure Research, Clinical Cardiology, and Epidemiology and Prevention. Circulation. 2003;108(17):2154–69.
19. Kasiske BL, Anjum S, Shah R, Skogen J, Kandaswamy C, Danielson B, et al. Hypertension after kidney transplantation. Am J Kidney Dis. 2004;43(6):1071–81.
20. Mange KC, Cizman B, Joffe M, Feldman HI. Arterial hypertension and renal allograft survival. JAMA. 2000;283(5):633–8.
21. Opelz G, Wujciak T, Ritz E. Association of chronic kidney graft failure with recipient blood pressure. Collab Trans Study Kidney Int. 1998;53(1):217–22.
22. Opelz G, Dohler B. Improved long-term outcomes after renal transplantation associated with blood pressure control. Am J Transplant. 2005;5(11):2725–31.
23. Mangray M, Vella JP. Hypertension after kidney transplant. Am J Kidney Dis. 2011;57(2):331–41.
24. Ikeda N, Sapienza D, Guerrero R, Aekplakorn W, Naghavi M, Mokdad AH, et al. Control of hypertension with medication: a comparative analysis of national surveys in 20 countries. Bull World Health Organ. 2014;92(1):10-9c.
25. World Health Organization Health Statistics - Part III Global Health Indicators. 2014. Available from: http://www.who.int/gho/publications/world_health_statistics/2014/en/.
26. Blackwell DL, Lucas JW, Clarke TC. Summary health statistics for U.S. adults: National Health Interview Survey, 2012. Vital Health Stat. 2014;10(260):1–161.
27. Rossi AP, Vella JP. Hypertension, living kidney donors, and transplantation: where are we today? Adv Chronic Kidney Dis. 2015;22(2):154–64.
28. James PA, Oparil S, Carter BL, Cushman WC, Dennison-Himmelfarb C, Handler J, et al. 2014 evidence-based guideline for the management of high blood pressure in adults: report from the panel members appointed to the Eighth Joint National Committee (JNC 8). JAMA. 2014;311(5):507–20.
29. Mancia G, Fagard R, Narkiewicz K, Redon J, Zanchetti A, Bohm M, et al. 2013 ESH/ESC practice guidelines for the management of arterial hypertension. Blood Press. 2014;23(1):3–16.

30. Kidney Disease: Improving Global Outcomes Transplant Work G. KDIGO clinical practice guideline for the care of kidney transplant recipients. Am J Transplant. 2009;9 Suppl 3:S1–155.
31. Verbeke F, Lindley E, Van Bortel L, Vanholder R, London G, Cochat P, et al. A European Renal Best Practice (ERBP) position statement on the Kidney Disease: Improving Global Outcomes (KDIGO) clinical practice guideline for the management of blood pressure in non-dialysis-dependent chronic kidney disease: an endorsement with some caveats for real-life application. Nephrol Dial Transplant. 2014;29(3):490–6.
32. Wright Jr JT, Williamson JD, Whelton PK, Snyder JK, Sink KM, Rocco MV, et al. A randomized trial of Intensive versus standard blood-pressure control. N Engl J Med. 2015;373(22):2103–16.
33. Prasad GV, Nash MM, Zaltzman JS. A prospective study of the physician effect on blood pressure in renal-transplant recipients. Nephrol Dial Transplant. 2003;18(5):996–1000.
34. Stenehjem AE, Gudmundsdottir H, Os I. Office blood pressure measurements overestimate blood pressure control in renal transplant patients. Blood Press Monit. 2006;11(3):125–33.
35. Fagard RH. Dipping pattern of nocturnal blood pressure in patients with hypertension. Expert Rev Cardiovasc Ther. 2009;7(6):599–605.
36. Ibernon M, Moreso F, Sarrias X, Sarrias M, Grinyo JM, Fernandez-Real JM, et al. Reverse dipper pattern of blood pressure at 3 months is associated with inflammation and outcome after renal transplantation. Nephrol Dial Transplant. 2012;27(5):2089–95.
37. Azancot MA, Ramos N, Moreso FJ, Ibernon M, Espinel E, Torres IB, et al. Hypertension in chronic kidney disease: the influence of renal transplantation. Transplantation. 2014;98(5):537–42.
38. Minutolo R, Agarwal R, Borrelli S, Chiodini P, Bellizzi V, Nappi F, et al. Prognostic role of ambulatory blood pressure measurement in patients with nondialysis chronic kidney disease. Arch Intern Med. 2011;171(12):1090–8.
39. Angeli F, Reboldi G, Poltronieri C, Bartolini C, D'Ambrosio C, de Filippo V, et al. Clinical utility of ambulatory blood pressure monitoring in the management of hypertension. Expert Rev Cardiovasc Ther. 2014;12(5):623–34.
40. Mozdzan M, Wierzbowska-Drabik K, Kurpesa M, Trzos E, Rechcinski T, Broncel M, et al. Echocardiographic indices of left ventricular hypertrophy and diastolic function in hypertensive patients with preserved LVEF classified as dippers and non-dippers. Arch Med Sci. 2013;9(2):268–75.
41. Levy D, Garrison RJ, Savage DD, Kannel WB, Castelli WP. Prognostic implications of echocardiographically determined left ventricular mass in the Framingham Heart Study. N Engl J Med. 1990;322(22):1561–6.
42. Wadei HM, Amer H, Taler SJ, Cosio FG, Griffin MD, Grande JP, et al. Diurnal blood pressure changes one year after kidney transplantation: relationship to allograft function, histology, and resistive index. J Am Soc Nephrol. 2007;18(5):1607–15.
43. Wadei HM, Amer H, Griffin MD, Taler SJ, Stegall MD, Textor SC. Abnormal circadian blood pressure pattern 1-year after kidney transplantation is associated with subsequent lower glomerular filtration rate in recipients without rejection. J Am Soc Hypertens. 2011;5(1):39–47.
44. Fagard RH, Cornelissen VA. Incidence of cardiovascular events in white-coat, masked and sustained hypertension versus true normotension: a meta-analysis. J Hypertens. 2007;25(11):2193–8.
45. Czyzewski L, Wyzgal J, Kolek A. Evaluation of selected risk factors of cardiovascular diseases among patients after kidney transplantation, with particular focus on the role of 24-hour automatic blood pressure measurement in the diagnosis of hypertension: an introductory report. Ann Transplant. 2014;19:188–98.
46. Kayrak M, Gul EE, Kaya C, Solak Y, Turkmen K, Yazici R, et al. Masked hypertension in renal transplant recipients. Blood Press. 2014;23(1):47–53.
47. Lipkin GW, Tucker B, Giles M, Raine AE. Ambulatory blood pressure and left ventricular mass in cyclosporin- and non-cyclosporin-treated renal transplant recipients. J Hypertens. 1993;11(4):439–42.

48. Platt JF, Ellis JH, Rubin JM, DiPietro MA, Sedman AB. Intrarenal arterial Doppler sonography in patients with nonobstructive renal disease: correlation of resistive index with biopsy findings. AJR Am J Roentgenol. 1990;154(6):1223–7.

49. Sezer S, Uyar ME, Colak T, Bal Z, Tutal E, Kalaci G, et al. Left ventricular mass index and its relationship to ambulatory blood pressure and renal resistivity index in renal transplant recipients. Transplant Proc. 2013;45(4):1575–8.

50. Chobanian AV, Bakris GL, Black HR, Cushman WC, Green LA, Izzo Jr JL, et al. The Seventh Report of the Joint National Committee on Prevention, Detection, Evaluation, and Treatment of High Blood Pressure: the JNC 7 report. JAMA. 2003;289(19):2560–72.

51. Calhoun DA, Jones D, Textor S, Goff DC, Murphy TP, Toto RD, et al. Resistant hypertension: diagnosis, evaluation, and treatment: a scientific statement from the American Heart Association Professional Education Committee of the Council for High Blood Pressure Research. Circulation. 2008;117(25):e510–26.

52. Persell SD. Prevalence of resistant hypertension in the United States, 2003–2008. Hypertension. 2011;57(6):1076–80.

53. de la Sierra A, Segura J, Banegas JR, Gorostidi M, de la Cruz JJ, Armario P, et al. Clinical features of 8295 patients with resistant hypertension classified on the basis of ambulatory blood pressure monitoring. Hypertension. 2011;57(5):898–902.

54. Gago Fraile M, Fernandez Fresnedo G, Gomez-Alamillo C, de Castro SS, Arias M. Clinical and epidemiological characteristics of refractory hypertension in renal transplant patients. Transplant Proc. 2009;41(6):2132–3.

55. Arias-Rodriguez M, Fernandez-Fresnedo G, Campistol JM, Marin R, Franco A, Gomez E, et al. Prevalence and clinical characteristics of renal transplant patients with true resistant hypertension. J Hypertens. 2015

56. Covic A, Segall L, Goldsmith DJ. Ambulatory blood pressure monitoring in renal transplantation: should ABPM be routinely performed in renal transplant patients? Transplantation. 2003;76(11):1640–2.

57. Agena F, Prado Edos S, Souza PS, da Silva GV, Lemos FB, Mion Jr D, et al. Home blood pressure (BP) monitoring in kidney transplant recipients is more adequate to monitor BP than office BP. Nephrol Dial Transplant. 2011;26(11):3745–9.

58. Wen KC, Gourishankar S. Evaluating the utility of ambulatory blood pressure monitoring in kidney transplant recipients. Clin Transplant. 2012;26(5):E465–70.

59. Foley RN, Parfrey PS, Sarnak MJ. Epidemiology of cardiovascular disease in chronic renal disease. J Am Soc Nephrol. 1998;9(12 Suppl):S16–23.

60. Kasiske BL, Chakkera HA, Roel J. Explained and unexplained ischemic heart disease risk after renal transplantation. J Am Soc Nephrol. 2000;11(9):1735–43.

61. Ducloux D, Kazory A, Chalopin JM. Predicting coronary heart disease in renal transplant recipients: a prospective study. Kidney Int. 2004;66(1):441–7.

62. Luft FC, Haller H. Hypertension-induced renal injury: is mechanically mediated interstitial inflammation involved? Nephrol Dial Transplant. 1995;10(1):9–11.

63. Luke RG. Hypertension in renal transplant recipients. Kidney Int. 1987;31(4):1024–37.

64. Luke RG. Pathophysiology and treatment of posttransplant hypertension. J Am Soc Nephrol. 1991;2(2 Suppl 1):S37–44.

65. Frei U, Schindler R, Wieters D, Grouven U, Brunkhorst R, Koch KM. Pre-transplant hypertension: a major risk factor for chronic progressive renal allograft dysfunction? Nephrol Dial Transplant. 1995;10(7):1206–11.

66. Dopson SJ, Jayakumar S, Velez JC. Page kidney as a rare cause of hypertension: case report and review of the literature. Am J Kidney Dis. 2009;54(2):334–9.

67. Smyth A, Collins CS, Thorsteinsdottir B, Madsen BE, Oliveira GH, Kane G, et al. Page kidney: etiology, renal function outcomes and risk for future hypertension. J Clin Hypertens (Greenwich). 2012;14(4):216–21.

68. Ducloux D, Motte G, Kribs M, Abdelfatah AB, Bresson-Vautrin C, Rebibou JM, et al. Hypertension in renal transplantation: donor and recipient risk factors. Clin Nephrol. 2002;57(6):409–13.

69. Ojo AO. Expanded criteria donors: process and outcomes. Semin Dial. 2005;18(6):463–8.

70. Delahousse M, Chaignon M, Mesnard L, Boutouyrie P, Safar ME, Lebret T, et al. Aortic stiffness of kidney transplant recipients correlates with donor age. J Am Soc Nephrol. 2008;19(4):798–805.
71. Barenbrock M, Kosch M, Joster E, Kisters K, Rahn KH, Hausberg M. Reduced arterial distensibility is a predictor of cardiovascular disease in patients after renal transplantation. J Hypertens. 2002;20(1):79–84.
72. Bahous SA, Stephan A, Barakat W, Blacher J, Asmar R, Safar ME. Aortic pulse wave velocity in renal transplant patients. Kidney Int. 2004;66(4):1486–92.
73. Guidi E, Menghetti D, Milani S, Montagnino G, Palazzi P, Bianchi G. Hypertension may be transplanted with the kidney in humans: a long-term historical prospective follow-up of recipients grafted with kidneys coming from donors with or without hypertension in their families. J Am Soc Nephrol. 1996;7(8):1131–8.
74. Guidi E, Cozzi MG, Minetti E, Bianchi G. Donor and recipient family histories of hypertension influence renal impairment and blood pressure during acute rejections. J Am Soc Nephrol. 1998;9(11):2102–7.
75. Matas AJ, Smith JM, Skeans MA, Thompson B, Gustafson SK, Stewart DE, et al. OPTN/SRTR 2013 Annual Data Report: Kidney. Am J Transplant. 2015;15(S2):1–34.
76. Veenstra DL, Best JH, Hornberger J, Sullivan SD, Hricik DE. Incidence and long-term cost of steroid-related side effects after renal transplantation. Am J Kidney Dis. 1999;33(5):829–39.
77. Ratcliffe PJ, Dudley CR, Higgins RM, Firth JD, Smith B, Morris PJ. Randomised controlled trial of steroid withdrawal in renal transplant recipients receiving triple immunosuppression. Lancet. 1996;348(9028):643–8.
78. Hricik DE, Lautman J, Bartucci MR, Moir EJ, Mayes JT, Schulak JA. Variable effects of steroid withdrawal on blood pressure reduction in cyclosporine-treated renal transplant recipients. Transplantation. 1992;53(6):1232–5.
79. Vincenti F, Schena FP, Paraskevas S, Hauser IA, Walker RG, Grinyo J. A randomized, multicenter study of steroid avoidance, early steroid withdrawal or standard steroid therapy in kidney transplant recipients. Am J Transplant. 2008;8(2):307–16.
80. Kramer BK, Klinger M, Vitko S, Glyda M, Midtvedt K, Stefoni S, et al. Tacrolimus-based, steroid-free regimens in renal transplantation: 3-year follow-up of the ATLAS trial. Transplantation. 2012;94(5):492–8.
81. Vitko S, Klinger M, Salmela K, Wlodarczyk Z, Tyden G, Senatorski G, et al. Two corticosteroid-free regimens-tacrolimus monotherapy after basiliximab administration and tacrolimus/mycophenolate mofetil-in comparison with a standard triple regimen in renal transplantation: results of the Atlas study. Transplantation. 2005;80(12):1734–41.
82. Kramer BK, Klinger M, Wlodarczyk Z, Ostrowski M, Midvedt K, Stefoni S, et al. Tacrolimus combined with two different corticosteroid-free regimens compared with a standard triple regimen in renal transplantation: one year observational results. Clin Transplant. 2010;24(1):E1–9.
83. Woodle ES, First MR, Pirsch J, Shihab F, Gaber AO, Van Veldhuisen P. A prospective, randomized, double-blind, placebo-controlled multicenter trial comparing early (7 day) corticosteroid cessation versus long-term, low-dose corticosteroid therapy. Ann Surg. 2008;248(4):564–77.
84. Knight SR, Morris PJ. Steroid avoidance or withdrawal after renal transplantation increases the risk of acute rejection but decreases cardiovascular risk. A meta-analysis. Transplantation. 2010;89(1):1–14.
85. Knight SR, Morris PJ. Interaction between maintenance steroid dose and the risk/benefit of steroid avoidance and withdrawal regimens following renal transplantation. Transplantation. 2011;92(11):e63–4.
86. Opelz G, Dohler B. Association between steroid dosage and death with a functioning graft after kidney transplantation. Am J Transplant. 2013;13(8):2096–105.
87. Joss DV, Barrett AJ, Kendra JR, Lucas CF, Desai S. Hypertension and convulsions in children receiving cyclosporin A. Lancet. 1982;1(8277):906.

88. Cohen DJ, Loertscher R, Rubin MF, Tilney NL, Carpenter CB, Strom TB. Cyclosporine: a new immunosuppressive agent for organ transplantation. Ann Intern Med. 1984;101(5):667–82.
89. Loughran Jr TP, Deeg HJ, Dahlberg S, Kennedy MS, Storb R, Thomas ED. Incidence of hypertension after marrow transplantation among 112 patients randomized to either cyclosporine or methotrexate as graft-versus-host disease prophylaxis. Br J Haematol. 1985;59(3):547–53.
90. Palestine AG, Nussenblatt RB, Chan CC. Side effects of systemic cyclosporine in patients not undergoing transplantation. Am J Med. 1984;77(4):652–6.
91. Morris ST, McMurray JJ, Rodger RS, Farmer R, Jardine AG. Endothelial dysfunction in renal transplant recipients maintained on cyclosporine. Kidney Int. 2000;57(3):1100–6.
92. Calo LA, Davis PA, Giacon B, Pagnin E, Sartori M, Riegler P, et al. Oxidative stress in kidney transplant patients with calcineurin inhibitor-induced hypertension: effect of ramipril. J Cardiovasc Pharmacol. 2002;40(4):625–31.
93. Calo L, Semplicini A, Davis PA, Bonvicini P, Cantaro S, Rigotti P, et al. Cyclosporin-induced endothelial dysfunction and hypertension: are nitric oxide system abnormality and oxidative stress involved? Transpl Int. 2000;13 Suppl 1:S413–8.
94. Ovuworie CA, Fox ER, Chow CM, Pascual M, Shih VE, Picard MH, et al. Vascular endothelial function in cyclosporine and tacrolimus treated renal transplant recipients. Transplantation. 2001;72(8):1385–8.
95. Oflaz H, Turkmen A, Kazancioglu R, Kayacan SM, Bunyak B, Genchallac H, et al. The effect of calcineurin inhibitors on endothelial function in renal transplant recipients. Clin Transplant. 2003;17(3):212–6.
96. Van Buren DH, Burke JF, Lewis RM. Renal function in patients receiving long-term cyclosporine therapy. J Am Soc Nephrol. 1994;4(8 Suppl):S17–22.
97. Ciresi DL, Lloyd MA, Sandberg SM, Heublein DM, Edwards BS. The sodium retaining effects of cyclosporine. Kidney Int. 1992;41(6):1599–605.
98. Koomans HA, Ligtenberg G. Mechanisms and consequences of arterial hypertension after renal transplantation. Transplantation. 2001;72(6 Suppl):S9–12.
99. Klein IH, Abrahams AC, van Ede T, Oey PL, Ligtenberg G, Blankestijn PJ. Differential effects of acute and sustained cyclosporine and tacrolimus on sympathetic nerve activity. J Hypertens. 2010;28(9):1928–34.
100. Paul LC. Chronic allograft nephropathy: an update. Kidney Int. 1999;56(3):783–93.
101. Singh L, Singh G, Sharma A, Sinha A, Bagga A, Dinda AK. A comparative study on renal biopsy before and after long-term calcineurin inhibitors therapy: an insight for pathogenesis of its toxicity. Hum Pathol. 2015;46(1):34–9.
102. Hoorn EJ, Walsh SB, McCormick JA, Furstenberg A, Yang CL, Roeschel T, et al. The calcineurin inhibitor tacrolimus activates the renal sodium chloride cotransporter to cause hypertension. Nat Med. 2011;17(10):1304–9.
103. Mohebbi N, Mihailova M, Wagner CA. The calcineurin inhibitor FK506 (tacrolimus) is associated with transient metabolic acidosis and altered expression of renal acid-base transport proteins. Am J Physiol Renal Physiol. 2009;297(2):F499–509.
104. Shiba N, Chan MC, Kwok BW, Valantine HA, Robbins RC, Hunt SA. Analysis of survivors more than 10 years after heart transplantation in the cyclosporine era: Stanford experience. J Heart Lung Transplant. 2004;23(2):155–64.
105. Jardine AG. Assessing the relative risk of cardiovascular disease among renal transplant patients receiving tacrolimus or cyclosporine. Transpl Int. 2005;18(4):379–84.
106. Chatzikyrkou C, Menne J, Gwinner W, Schmidt BM, Lehner F, Blume C, et al. Pathogenesis and management of hypertension after kidney transplantation. J Hypertens. 2011;29(12):2283–94.
107. Moore J, Middleton L, Cockwell P, Adu D, Ball S, Little MA, et al. Calcineurin inhibitor sparing with mycophenolate in kidney transplantation: a systematic review and meta-analysis. Transplantation. 2009;87(4):591–605.

108. Hohage H, Bruckner D, Arlt M, Buchholz B, Zidek W, Spieker C. Influence of cyclosporine A and FK506 on 24 h blood pressure monitoring in kidney transplant recipients. Clin Nephrol. 1996;45(5):342–4.

109. Margreiter R. Efficacy and safety of tacrolimus compared with ciclosporin microemulsion in renal transplantation: a randomised multicentre study. Lancet. 2002;359(9308):741–6.

110. Bolin Jr P, Shihab FS, Mulloy L, Henning AK, Gao J, Bartucci M, et al. Optimizing tacrolimus therapy in the maintenance of renal allografts: 12-month results. Transplantation. 2008;86(1):88–95.

111. Mourer JS, Hartigh J, van Zwet EW, Mallat MJ, Dubbeld J, de Fijter JW. Randomized trial comparing late concentration-controlled calcineurin inhibitor or mycophenolate mofetil withdrawal. Transplantation. 2012;93(9):887–94.

112. Mourer JS, Ewe SH, Mallat MJ, Ng AC, Rabelink TJ, Bax JJ, et al. Late calcineurin inhibitor withdrawal prevents progressive left ventricular diastolic dysfunction in renal transplant recipients. Transplantation. 2012;94(7):721–8.

113. Mourer JS, de Koning EJ, van Zwet EW, Mallat MJ, Rabelink TJ, de Fijter JW. Impact of late calcineurin inhibitor withdrawal on ambulatory blood pressure and carotid intima media thickness in renal transplant recipients. Transplantation. 2013;96(1):49–57.

114. Roodnat JI, Hilbrands LB, Hene RJ, de Sevaux RG, Smak Gregoor PJ, Kal-van Gestel JA, et al. 15-year follow-up of a multicenter, randomized, calcineurin inhibitor withdrawal study in kidney transplantation. Transplantation. 2014;98(1):47–53.

115. Smak Gregoor PJ, de Sevaux RG, Ligtenberg G, Hoitsma AJ, Hene RJ, Weimar W, et al. Withdrawal of cyclosporine or prednisone six months after kidney transplantation in patients on triple drug therapy: a randomized, prospective, multicenter study. J Am Soc Nephrol. 2002;13(5):1365–73.

116. Hricik DE, Formica RN, Nickerson P, Rush D, Fairchild RL, Poggio ED, et al. Adverse outcomes of tacrolimus withdrawal in immune-quiescent kidney transplant recipients. J Am Soc Nephrol. 2015

117. Larsen CP, Pearson TC, Adams AB, Tso P, Shirasugi N, Strobert E, et al. Rational development of LEA29Y (belatacept), a high-affinity variant of CTLA4-Ig with potent immunosuppressive properties. Am J Transplant. 2005;5(3):443–53.

118. Vincenti F, Blancho G, Durrbach A, Friend P, Grinyo J, Halloran PF, et al. Five-year safety and efficacy of belatacept in renal transplantation. J Am Soc Nephrol. 2010;21(9):1587–96.

119. Rostaing L, Vincenti F, Grinyo J, Rice KM, Bresnahan B, Steinberg S, et al. Long-term belatacept exposure maintains efficacy and safety at 5 years: results from the long-term extension of the BENEFIT study. Am J Transplant. 2013;13(11):2875–83.

120. Charpentier B, Medina Pestana JO, Del CRM, Rostaing L, Grinyo J, Vanrenterghem Y, et al. Long-term exposure to belatacept in recipients of extended criteria donor kidneys. Am J Transplant. 2013;13(11):2884–91.

121. Curtis JJ, Galla JH, Kotchen TA, Lucas B, McRoberts JW, Luke RG. Prevalence of hypertension in a renal transplant population on alternate-day steroid therapy. Clin Nephrol. 1976;5(3):123–7.

122. Curtis JJ, Luke RG, Diethelm AG, Whelchel JD, Jones P. Benefits of removal of native kidneys in hypertension after renal transplantation. Lancet. 1985;2(8458):739–42.

123. Hausberg M, Kosch M, Harmelink P, Barenbrock M, Hohage H, Kisters K, et al. Sympathetic nerve activity in end-stage renal disease. Circulation. 2002;106(15):1974–9.

124. Zoccali C, Mallamaci F, Parlongo S, Cutrupi S, Benedetto FA, Tripepi G, et al. Plasma norepinephrine predicts survival and incident cardiovascular events in patients with end-stage renal disease. Circulation. 2002;105(11):1354–9.

125. Bruno S, Remuzzi G, Ruggenenti P. Transplant renal artery stenosis. J Am Soc Nephrol. 2004;15(1):134–41.

126. Chen W, Kayler LK, Zand MS, Muttana R, Chernyak V, DeBoccardo GO. Transplant renal artery stenosis: clinical manifestations, diagnosis and therapy. Clin Kidney J. 2015;8(1):71–8.

127. Hurst FP, Abbott KC, Neff RT, Elster EA, Falta EM, Lentine KL, et al. Incidence, predictors and outcomes of transplant renal artery stenosis after kidney transplantation: analysis of USRDS. Am J Nephrol. 2009;30(5):459–67.

128. Fervenza FC, Lafayette RA, Alfrey EJ, Petersen J. Renal artery stenosis in kidney transplants. Am J Kidney Dis. 1998;31(1):142–8.
129. Humar A, Matas AJ. Surgical complications after kidney transplantation. Semin Dial. 2005;18(6):505–10.
130. Pouria S, State OI, Wong W, Hendry BM. CMV infection is associated with transplant renal artery stenosis. QJM. 1998;91(3):185–9.
131. Audard V, Matignon M, Hemery F, Snanoudj R, Desgranges P, Anglade MC, et al. Risk factors and long-term outcome of transplant renal artery stenosis in adult recipients after treatment by percutaneous transluminal angioplasty. Am J Transplant. 2006;6(1):95–9.
132. Patel NH, Jindal RM, Wilkin T, Rose S, Johnson MS, Shah H, et al. Renal arterial stenosis in renal allografts: retrospective study of predisposing factors and outcome after percutaneous transluminal angioplasty. Radiology. 2001;219(3):663–7.
133. Benedetti E, Troppmann C, Gillingham K, Sutherland DE, Payne WD, Dunn DL, et al. Short- and long-term outcomes of kidney transplants with multiple renal arteries. Ann Surg. 1995;221(4):406–14.
134. Sankari BR, Geisinger M, Zelch M, Brouhard B, Cunningham R, Novick AC. Post-transplant renal artery stenosis: impact of therapy on long-term kidney function and blood pressure control. J Urol. 1996;155(6):1860–4.
135. Morris PJ, Yadav RV, Kincaid-Smith P, Anderton J, Hare WS, Johnson N, et al. Renal artery stenosis in renal transplantation. Med J Aust. 1971;1(24):1255–7.
136. Lacombe M. Arterial stenosis complicating renal allotransplantation in man: a study of 38 cases. Ann Surg. 1975;181(3):283–8.
137. Greenstein SM, Verstandig A, McLean GK, Dafoe DC, Burke DR, Meranze SG, et al. Percutaneous transluminal angioplasty. The procedure of choice in the hypertensive renal allograft recipient with renal artery stenosis. Transplantation. 1987;43(1):29–32.
138. Hwang JK, Kim SD, Park SC, Choi BS, Kim JI, Yang CW, et al. The long-term outcomes of transplantation of kidneys with multiple renal arteries. Transplant Proc. 2010;42(10):4053–7.
139. Becker BN, Odorico JS, Becker YT, Leverson G, McDermott JC, Grist T, et al. Peripheral vascular disease and renal transplant artery stenosis: a reappraisal of transplant renovascular disease. Clin Transplant. 1999;13(4):349–55.
140. Porter KA, Thomson WB, Owen K, Kenyon JR, Mowbray JF, Peart WS. Obliterative vascular changes in four human kidney homotransplants. Br Med J. 1963;2(5358):639–45.
141. Willicombe M, Sandhu B, Brookes P, Gedroyc W, Hakim N, Hamady M, et al. Postanastomotic transplant renal artery stenosis: association with de novo class II donor-specific antibodies. Am J Transplant. 2014;14(1):133–43.
142. Lee L, Gunaratnam L, Sener A. Transplant renal artery stenosis secondary to mechanical compression from polycystic kidney disease: a case report. Can Urol Assoc J. 2013;7(3-4):E251–3.
143. Pickering TG, Herman L, Devereux RB, Sotelo JE, James GD, Sos TA, et al. Recurrent pulmonary oedema in hypertension due to bilateral renal artery stenosis: treatment by angioplasty or surgical revascularisation. Lancet. 1988;2(8610):551–2.
144. Messerli FH, Bangalore S, Makani H, Rimoldi SF, Allemann Y, White CJ, et al. Flash pulmonary oedema and bilateral renal artery stenosis: the pickering syndrome. Eur Heart J. 2011;32(18):2231–5.
145. Gray DWR. Graft renal artery stenosis in the transplanted kidney. Transplant Rev. 1994;8(1):15–21.
146. Ghazanfar A, Tavakoli A, Augustine T, Pararajasingam R, Riad H, Chalmers N. Management of transplant renal artery stenosis and its impact on long-term allograft survival: a single-centre experience. Nephrol Dial Transplant. 2011;26(1):336–43.
147. O'Neill WC, Baumgarten DA. Ultrasonography in renal transplantation. Am J Kidney Dis. 2002;39(4):663–78.
148. Li JC, Ji ZG, Cai S, Jiang YX, Dai Q, Zhang JX. Evaluation of severe transplant renal artery stenosis with Doppler sonography. J Clin Ultrasound. 2005;33(6):261–9.

149. Loubeyre P, Abidi H, Cahen R, Tran Minh VA. Transplanted renal artery: detection of stenosis with color Doppler US. Radiology. 1997;203(3):661–5.
150. Browne RF, Tuite DJ. Imaging of the renal transplant: comparison of MRI with duplex sonography. Abdom Imaging. 2006;31(4):461–82.
151. Johnson DB, Lerner CA, Prince MR, Kazanjian SN, Narasimham DL, Leichtman AB, et al. Gadolinium-enhanced magnetic resonance angiography of renal transplants. Magn Reson Imaging. 1997;15(1):13–20.
152. Gaddikeri S, Mitsumori L, Vaidya S, Hippe DS, Bhargava P, Dighe MK. Comparing the diagnostic accuracy of contrast-enhanced computed tomographic angiography and gadolinium-enhanced magnetic resonance angiography for the assessment of hemodynamically significant transplant renal artery stenosis. Curr Probl Diagn Radiol. 2014;43(4):162–8.
153. Gagnon AL, Desai T. Dermatological diseases in patients with chronic kidney disease. J Nephropathol. 2013;2(2):104–9.
154. Touma J, Costanzo A, Boura B, Alomran F, Combes M. Endovascular management of transplant renal artery stenosis. J Vasc Surg. 2014;59(4):1058–65.
155. Henning BF, Kuchlbauer S, Boger CA, Obed A, Farkas S, Zulke C, et al. Percutaneous transluminal angioplasty as first-line treatment of transplant renal artery stenosis. Clin Nephrol. 2009;71(5):543–9.
156. Marini M, Fernandez-Rivera C, Cao I, Gulias D, Alonso A, Lopez-Muniz A, et al. Treatment of transplant renal artery stenosis by percutaneous transluminal angioplasty and/or stenting: study in 63 patients in a single institution. Transplant Proc. 2011;43(6):2205–7.
157. Biederman DM, Fischman AM, Titano JJ, Kim E, Patel RS, Nowakowski FS, et al. Tailoring the endovascular management of transplant renal artery stenosis. Am J Transplant. 2015;15(4):1039–49.
158. Seratnahaei A, Shah A, Bodiwala K, Mukherjee D. Management of transplant renal artery stenosis. Angiology. 2011;62(3):219–24.
159. Osterberg L, Blaschke T. Adherence to medication. N Engl J Med. 2005;353(5):487–97.
160. Vella JP, Cohen DJ. Transplantation NephSAP. JASN. 2013;12(5):331–4.
161. Morrissey PE, Flynn ML, Lin S. Medication noncompliance and its implications in transplant recipients. Drugs. 2007;67(10):1463–81.
162. Morisky DE, Green LW, Levine DM. Concurrent and predictive validity of a self-reported measure of medication adherence. Med Care. 1986;24(1):67–74.
163. McGillicuddy JW, Gregoski MJ, Weiland AK, Rock RA, Brunner-Jackson BM, Patel SK, et al. Mobile health medication adherence and blood pressure control in renal transplant recipients: a proof-of-concept randomized controlled trial. JMIR Res Protoc. 2013;2(2), e32.
164. Guida B, Trio R, Laccetti R, Nastasi A, Salvi E, Perrino NR, et al. Role of dietary intervention on metabolic abnormalities and nutritional status after renal transplantation. Nephrol Dial Transplant. 2007;22(11):3304–10.
165. Mourad G, Ribstein J, Mimran A. Converting-enzyme inhibitor versus calcium antagonist in cyclosporine-treated renal transplants. Kidney Int. 1993;43(2):419–25.
166. Pascual M, Curtis J, Delmonico FL, Farrell ML, Williams Jr WW, Kalil R, et al. A prospective, randomized clinical trial of cyclosporine reduction in stable patients greater than 12 months after renal transplantation. Transplantation. 2003;75(9):1501–5.
167. Lentine KL, Anyaegbu E, Gleisner A, Schnitzler MA, Axelrod D, Brennan DC, et al. Understanding medical care of transplant recipients through integrated registry and pharmacy claims data. Am J Nephrol. 2013;38(5):420–9.
168. Lakkis JI, Weir MR. Treatment-resistant hypertension in the transplant recipient. Semin Nephrol. 2014;34(5):560–70.
169. Baroletti SA, Gabardi S, Magee CC, Milford EL. Calcium channel blockers as the treatment of choice for hypertension in renal transplant recipients: fact or fiction. Pharmacotherapy. 2003;23(6):788–801.
170. Cross NB, Webster AC, Masson P, O'Connell PJ, Craig JC. Antihypertensives for kidney transplant recipients: systematic review and meta-analysis of randomized controlled trials. Transplantation. 2009;88(1):7–18.

171. Midtvedt K, Hartmann A, Foss A, Fauchald P, Nordal KP, Rootwelt K, et al. Sustained improvement of renal graft function for two years in hypertensive renal transplant recipients treated with nifedipine as compared to lisinopril. Transplantation. 2001;72(11):1787–92.

172. Cai J, Huang Z, Yang G, Cheng K, Ye Q, Ming Y, et al. Comparing antihypertensive effect and plasma ciclosporin concentration between amlodipine and valsartan regimens in hypertensive renal transplant patients receiving ciclosporin therapy. Am J Cardiovasc Drugs. 2011;11(6):401–9.

173. Sassi MB, Gaies E, Salouage I, Trabelsi S, Lakhal M, Klouz A. Involvement of CYP 3A5 in the interaction between tacrolimus and nicardipine : a case report. Curr Drug Saf. 2015.

174. Hooper DK, Fukuda T, Gardiner R, Logan B, Roy-Chaudhury A, Kirby CL, et al. Risk of tacrolimus toxicity in CYP3A5 nonexpressors treated with intravenous nicardipine after kidney transplantation. Transplantation. 2012;93(8):806–12.

175. Hooper DK, Carle AC, Schuchter J, Goebel J. Interaction between tacrolimus and intravenous nicardipine in the treatment of post-kidney transplant hypertension at pediatric hospitals. Pediatr Transplant. 2011;15(1):88–95.

176. Kurnatowska I, Krolikowski J, Jesionowska K, Marczak A, Krajewska J, Zbrog Z, et al. Prevalence of arterial hypertension and the number and classes of antihypertensive drugs prescribed for patients late after kidney transplantation. Ann Transplant. 2012;17(1):50–7.

177. Bostom AG, Carpenter MA, Kusek JW, Hunsicker LG, Pfeffer MA, Levey AS, et al. Rationale and design of the Folic Acid for Vascular Outcome Reduction in Transplantation (FAVORIT) trial. Am Heart J. 2006;152(3):448 e1–7.

178. Bostom AG, Carpenter MA, Hunsicker L, Jacques PF, Kusek JW, Levey AS, et al. Baseline characteristics of participants in the Folic Acid for Vascular Outcome Reduction in Transplantation (FAVORIT) Trial. Am J Kidney Dis. 2009;53(1):121–8.

179. Carpenter MA, Weir MR, Adey DB, House AA, Bostom AG, Kusek JW. Inadequacy of cardiovascular risk factor management in chronic kidney transplantation - evidence from the FAVORIT study. Clin Transplant. 2012;26(4):E438–46.

180. Major outcomes in high-risk hypertensive patients randomized to angiotensin-converting enzyme inhibitor or calcium channel blocker vs diuretic: The Antihypertensive and Lipid-Lowering Treatment to Prevent Heart Attack Trial (ALLHAT). JAMA. 2002;288(23):2981–97.

181. Taber DJ, Srinivas TM, Pilch NA, Meadows HB, Fleming JN, McGillicuddy JW, et al. Are thiazide diuretics safe and effective antihypertensive therapy in kidney transplant recipients? Am J Nephrol. 2013;38(4):285–91.

182. Heinze G, Mitterbauer C, Regele H, Kramar R, Winkelmayer WC, Curhan GC, et al. Angiotensin-converting enzyme inhibitor or angiotensin II type 1 receptor antagonist therapy is associated with prolonged patient and graft survival after renal transplantation. J Am Soc Nephrol. 2006;17(3):889–99.

183. Paoletti E, Bellino D, Marsano L, Cassottana P, Rolla D, Ratto E. Effects of ACE inhibitors on long-term outcome of renal transplant recipients: a randomized controlled trial. Transplantation. 2013;95(6):889–95.

184. Burdmann EA, Andoh TF, Nast CC, Evan A, Connors BA, Coffman TM, et al. Prevention of experimental cyclosporin-induced interstitial fibrosis by losartan and enalapril. Am J Physiol. 1995;269(4 Pt 2):F491–9.

185. Thomas B, Taber DJ, Srinivas TR. Hypertension after kidney transplantation: a pathophysiologic approach. Curr Hypertens Rep. 2013;15(5):458–69.

186. Opelz G, Zeier M, Laux G, Morath C, Dohler B. No improvement of patient or graft survival in transplant recipients treated with angiotensin-converting enzyme inhibitors or angiotensin II type 1 receptor blockers: a collaborative transplant study report. J Am Soc Nephrol. 2006;17(11):3257–62.

187. Philipp T, Martinez F, Geiger H, Moulin B, Mourad G, Schmieder R, et al. Candesartan improves blood pressure control and reduces proteinuria in renal transplant recipients: results from SECRET. Nephrol Dial Transplant. 2010;25(3):967–76.

188. Curtis JJ, Laskow DA, Jones PA, Julian BA, Gaston RS, Luke RG. Captopril-induced fall in glomerular filtration rate in cyclosporine-treated hypertensive patients. J Am Soc Nephrol. 1993;3(9):1570–4.

189. Vlahakos DV, Canzanello VJ, Madaio MP, Madias NE. Enalapril-associated anemia in renal transplant recipients treated for hypertension. Am J Kidney Dis. 1991;17(2):199–205.

190. Gaston RS, Julian BA, Barker CV, Diethelm AG, Curtis JJ. Enalapril: safe and effective therapy for posttransplant erythrocytosis. Transplant Proc. 1993;25(1 Pt 2):1029–31.

191. Gaston RS, Julian BA, Curtis JJ. Posttransplant erythrocytosis: an enigma revisited. Am J Kidney Dis. 1994;24(1):1–11.

192. Julian BA, Brantley Jr RR, Barker CV, Stopka T, Gaston RS, Curtis JJ, et al. Losartan, an angiotensin II type 1 receptor antagonist, lowers hematocrit in posttransplant erythrocytosis. J Am Soc Nephrol. 1998;9(6):1104–8.

193. Nankivell BJ, Allen RD, O'Connell PJ, Chapman JR. Erythrocytosis after renal transplantation: risk factors and relationship with GFR. Clin Transplant. 1995;9(5):375–82.

194. Aftab W, Varadarajan P, Rasool S, Kore A, Pai RG. Beta and angiotensin blockades are associated with improved 10-year survival in renal transplant recipients. J Am Heart Assoc. 2013;2(1), e000091.

195. Weir MR, Salzberg DJ. Management of hypertension in the transplant patient. J Am Soc Hypertens. 2011;5(5):425–32.

196. Lentine KL, Costa SP, Weir MR, Robb JF, Fleisher LA, Kasiske BL, et al. Cardiac disease evaluation and management among kidney and liver transplantation candidates: a scientific statement from the American Heart Association and the American College of Cardiology Foundation: endorsed by the American Society of Transplant Surgeons, American Society of Transplantation, and National Kidney Foundation. Circulation. 2012;126(5):617–63.

197. Devereaux PJ, Yang H, Yusuf S, Guyatt G, Leslie K, Villar JC, et al. Effects of extended-release metoprolol succinate in patients undergoing non-cardiac surgery (POISE trial): a randomised controlled trial. Lancet. 2008;371(9627):1839–47.

198. Brewster LM, van Montfrans GA, Kleijnen J. Systematic review: antihypertensive drug therapy in black patients. Ann Intern Med. 2004;141(8):614–27.

199. Brewster LM, Seedat YK. Why do hypertensive patients of African ancestry respond better to calcium blockers and diuretics than to ACE inhibitors and beta-adrenergic blockers? A systematic review. BMC Med. 2013;11:141.

Chapter 9
Hypertensive Urgencies and Emergencies

Hina K. Trivedi, Dipti Patel, and Matthew R. Weir

Epidemiology

Hypertension is a common medical condition affecting nearly a billion people worldwide [1]. Of those, one to two percent of patients will present with acute hypertensive crises requiring medical treatment [2]. The true prevalence of hypertensive crisis may be underestimated as few prospective studies have been done. Many, if not most, of these patients have previously diagnosed hypertension. Risk factors for hypertensive crisis include lack of a primary care physician, pain, emotional stress, female race, obesity, coronary artery disease (CAD), underlying hypertension requiring multiple medications and more often, non-adherence to medications [3].

Similarly, chronic kidney disease (CKD) is a highly prevalent disease affecting 13.1% of the US population, corresponding to just over 26 million people. Individuals with CKD are at increased risk for morbidity and mortality from cardiovascular disease (CVD) [4]. The goal of CKD management is to stabilize kidney function and prevent further progression to end stage renal disease (ESRD). One of the most important risk factors contributing to CKD is hypertension. Blood pressure management in CKD patients can be challenging, and may frequently require multiple antihypertensive agents to achieve recommended blood pressure goals.

The frequency of hypertensive emergencies and urgencies in the CKD population, including those with ESRD on dialysis, has not been well described. This may be in part due to an under recognition and/or under-reporting of hypertensive crises in this patient population.

H.K. Trivedi, DO • D. Patel, MD • M.R. Weir, MD (✉)
Department of Nephrology, University of Maryland Medical Center, Baltimore, MD, USA
e-mail: mweir@medicine.umaryland.edu

© Springer Science+Business Media New York 2016
A.K. Singh, R. Agarwal (eds.), *Core Concepts in Hypertension in Kidney Disease*, DOI 10.1007/978-1-4939-6436-9_9

Hypertensive crises are separated into hypertensive urgencies and hypertensive emergencies. There is no universally defined blood pressure threshold for hypertensive urgencies or emergencies. Classically, a hypertensive urgency is defined as severely elevated blood pressure, typically >180/120 mmHg. This blood pressure elevation occurs in the absence of acute end organ damage. Examples of urgencies include hypertensive patients with CAD or chronic kidney disease (CKD), patients with a kidney transplant, preoperative and postoperative hypertension, and hypertension associated with burns. Hypertensive emergency refers to blood pressure elevation that is associated with target organ damage. Examples of emergencies include accelerated/ malignant hypertension, hypertensive encephalopathy, acute left ventricular failure/ pulmonary edema, acute aortic dissection, intracranial hemorrhage, pheochromocy- toma/adrenergic crisis, eclampsia, substance/drug-induced hypertension, retinal hem- orrhage, papilledema, acute myocardial infarction, stroke, acute renal dysfunction, epistaxis, and hypertension after coronary bypass or vascular surgery [5–7].

Indeed, it is likely that while hypertension is an important etiologic factor for kid- ney disease, intrinsic kidney disease likely predisposes patients to hypertensive crises as it is a risk factor for the development of hypertension. Both non-dialysis dependent and dialysis-dependent CKD patients often have elevated blood pressure either before or, and more often, after the diagnosis of CKD. Physicians should be mindful of the relationship between blood pressure elevation and chronic kidney disease.

Pathophysiology

If one considers the equation of cardiac output $(CO) = $ heart rate $(HR) \times$ stroke vol- ume (SV), and blood pressure $ = CO \times$ total peripheral resistance (TPR), then one can better understand the pathophysiological processes that lead to accelerated increases in blood pressure.

The pathophysiology of hypertensive crises is poorly understood. A sudden rise in PVR causes an acute elevation in blood pressure leading to vasoconstriction via activation of hormonal systems such as the renin–angiotensin system (RAS), cate- cholamines, endothelin, and vasopressin [8]. This subsequently increases mechani- cal stress on the vessel wall leading to endothelial injury.

The endothelium plays a central role in the regulation of blood pressure. Through the secretion of various molecules, vascular tone is adjusted for any given blood pressure. Nitric oxide is secreted by the endothelium in response to sheer stress and is under the influence of stress hormones. This causes vasodilation, which is the initial compensatory mechanism in response to rapid blood pressure elevation. When this response is overwhelmed, subsequent endothelial injury may occur [8]. Additionally, upregulation of proinflammatory markers, cytokines, and endothelial adhesion molecules endorse local inflammation further contributing to the loss of endothelial function. This stress and sympathetic activation causes activation of the coagulation cascade, platelets, and promotes fibrin deposition leading to a cycle of vascular injury, increased endothelial permeability, and higher blood pressures [3].

In a prospective, cross-sectional study by Derhaschnig et al., patients with hypertensive emergency were found to have elevated markers of thrombogenesis, fibrinolysis, and markers of inflammation as compared to patients with hypertensive urgency. While the study does not suggest a cause–effect relationship, endothelial dysfunction plays a role in altering biomarkers, specifically in hypertensive emergencies [9]. Furthermore, a pressure diuresis can occur, leading to volume contraction, diminished effective arterial blood volume, and activation of the renin–angiotensin system.

Multiple mechanisms exist which affect the hemodynamic environment of the renal vasculature. Intrinsic vasoactive mechanisms within the kidney can alter intrarenal vascular resistance to maintain renal blood flow. Renal autoregulation allows the kidneys to maintain adequate, yet stable glomerular filtration across a wide range of perfusion pressures. This is thought to be mediated by two mechanisms: the myogenic response of the glomerular vasculature and the tubuloglomerular feedback system (TGF) of the macula densa [10, 11]. The TGF mechanism senses and responds to the volume and composition of the glomerular filtrate. When distal delivery of filtrate is increased, the afferent arteriole is stimulated to constrict and limit filtration [11]. The second mechanism, the myogenic system, responds directly to changes in local pressure. For example, with decreased effective arterial blood pressure, afferent glomerular vascular resistance decreases to maintain renal blood flow, and angiotensin II-mediated efferent glomerular arteriolar vasoconstriction results in a restoration of glomerular pressure necessary for filtration. Conversely, intrarenal vascular resistance increases in response to increased arterial pressures. This is associated with a myogenic response of the afferent glomerular arteriole to vasoconstrict and reduce potentially damaging levels of systemic arterial pressure from entering the glomerular capillaries which usually see pressures approximately one half to two thirds of systemic pressure [11]. These changes occur rapidly, to protect the glomerulus from sudden changes in arterial pressures. However, when these autoregulatory systems are overwhelmed, for example in the setting of rapid changes in blood pressure, the glomeruli are susceptible to hypertensive injury hydraulic injury [12]. Furthermore, in the setting of CKD, the autoregulatory mechanisms are impaired and even modest increases in blood pressure may lead to glomerular capillary damage [11, 13].

A number of factors appear to contribute to the challenges with blood pressure control in CKD patients. These factors center primarily around increased sodium and fluid retention. This is due to ineffective pressure-natriuresis that often occurs with chronic renal impairment. With progressive kidney disease, there is an inability to suppress tubular sodium reabsorption due to increased RAAS and sympathetic nervous system activity. This dysregulation of these systems are often targets of blood pressure control in the CKD population [14].

In ESRD patients, increased salt and fluid intake and excessive interdialytic weight gain are major contributing factors to resistant hypertension. Additionally, inadequate ultrafiltration with dialysis sessions may also lead to interdialytic hypertension. Increased renin secretion occurs in the setting of an ultrafiltration rate that exceeds the plasma refill rate during hemodialysis [15]. This topic is further discussed in another chapter.

Sympathetic nervous activity from increased catecholamine release has also been noted in dialysis patients, leading to increased vasoconstriction. Another factor leading to difficult blood pressure control involves alterations in endothelin and nitric oxide (NO). Specifically, asymmetric dimethylarginine (ADMA), a chemical which accumulates in patients on dialysis, inhibits NO thereby leading to vasoconstriction. Another cause of vasoconstriction is erythropoietin therapy. Erythropoietin therapy has been known to cause a hypercoagulable state which can lead to hemoconcentration induced vasoconstriction. Lastly, increased intracellular calcium from hyperparathyroidism can lead to vasoconstriction and elevated blood pressure as well [16].

Approaching the Patient

As previously mentioned, the clinical feature distinguishing hypertensive urgency from hypertensive emergency is evidence of end organ injury or dysfunction. The recognition of these signs and symptoms should prompt the individualization of treatment as will be discussed below.

A patient's presenting complaints can vary, but are often related to the acute elevation in blood pressure. Common symptoms include chest pain, shortness of breath, headache, confusion, and focal neurologic complaints. A focused history including comorbid conditions, prescribed medications, use of over-the-counter medications, medication adherence, and use of recreational drugs should be taken. Confirmation of the blood pressure should be made with manual blood pressure measurements of both arms. The physical exam should focus on identifying evidence of target organ damage. A fundoscopic exam may reveal retinopathy with hemorrhage, exudates, or papilledema. Neurologic exam to identify focal neurologic deficits may point towards intracranial pathology.

Initial laboratory tests should include a basic metabolic panel to evaluate for electrolyte abnormalities and renal dysfunction. A complete blood count with differential with low platelets suggests microangiopathic hemolysis and a peripheral blood smear should be examined if thrombocytopenia is present. A urinalysis with blood and protein points towards underlying renal disease and possible hemolysis. An electrocardiogram should be performed in all patients to look for signs of ischemia. A chest X-ray is useful to quickly evaluate for aortic dissection. If clinical suspicion for aortic dissection is high, a CT angiogram of the chest should be pursued. A chest X-ray can also evaluate for pulmonary edema or other pulmonary processes. A renal ultrasound is warranted in patients with renal dysfunction. A CT or MRI of the brain is needed to determine if the patient is having a hemorrhagic or ischemic stroke.

The clinical presentation of CKD and ESRD patients can be similar to the general population with hypertensive crisis, presenting with end organ damage in a variety of forms including congestive heart failure, papilledema, hemorrhagic strokes, left ventricular hypertrophy, and acute coronary syndromes. This patient population though can have volume overload as a more prominent feature of their presentation. For example, CKD and ESRD patients often present with acute pulmonary symptoms and evaluation should be focused on determining the volume status of the patient [16].

Treatment

Treatment should be tailored to the clinical scenario, the degree of blood pressure elevation, and the presence or absence of end organ injury. Typically, therapies are first instituted in the emergency department.

Hypertensive Emergency

If the patient is having a hypertensive emergency, they should be hospitalized, preferably in an intensive care unit (ICU). The goal is to prevent and reverse end organ damage by lowering blood pressure in a monitored setting. Moreover, the duration of action of a medication should be considered so as to not cause significant hypotension and subsequent ischemic brain injury. Treating the blood pressure takes priority over determining the cause of the hypertensive crisis.

The choice of parenteral or oral medications for treatment depends on the patient's comorbidities and clinical scenario. Generally, if the patient has a hypertensive emergency and is admitted to the ICU, parenteral medications are the treatment of choice. This allows for careful and controlled changes in blood pressure which are largely predictable to minimize the risk for worsening target organ injury.

How much should one lower the blood pressure? As will be discussed later, there are different targets depending on the target organ injury. The rule of thumb is lowering the mean arterial pressure (MAP) no more than 15–25 % [17] within the first few hours of a hypertensive emergency or no lower than 100 mmHg diastolic blood pressure (DBP). Aim to lower systolic blood pressure (SBP) by 20–40 mmHg within the first half hour using parenteral medications. Another general recommendation is to lower blood pressure cautiously to 140/90 mmHg [6].

Generally, IV medications used to treat a patient over 12–24 h will allow for cerebrovascular autoregulation to re-establish. After this time, the provider should transition from parenteral to oral medications and monitor for postural hypotension. When treating this patient population, one must consider that often a pressure-natriuresis occurs due to substantial vasoconstriction. For this reason, diuretics should not be used initially unless there is clinical evidence of volume overload, and at times, fluids are given to prevent too rapid a drop in blood pressure [6].

Additional Considerations in the CKD/Dialysis Population

The rules of managing hypertensive emergencies and urgencies in the general population are applicable to the CKD population as well. Here, we illustrate using various clinical scenarios:

CASE #1: A 52-year-old man with a history of systolic heart failure, hypertension, diabetes mellitus type 2, coronary artery disease presents to the emergency room with hypertensive emergency. He has a history of tobacco abuse, without drug or alcohol use. Home medications include metformin, carvedilol, amlodipine, furosemide, and aspirin. He denies shortness of breath but complains of increased leg edema bilaterally. Vital signs are significant for a blood pressure of 200/110 mmHg, heart rate of 89 bpm, and oxygen saturation of 86 % on room air, which improved to 94 % on 6 l oxygen via nasal cannula. On physical exam, he is dyspneic, with crackles to the mid-lung, and 2+ lower extremity edema. CXR shows bilateral pleural effusions and vascular congestion. Upon lab review, serum creatinine is increased from his baseline creatinine 1.6 to creatinine 2.3, with an eGFR of 28 ml/min. How would you manage this patient?

Answer #1: Particular attention should be paid to the volume status of CKD patients and treatment of hypertensive crises should incorporate management of volume overload in this patient population. This includes not only the standard treatments as listed, but also the aggressive use of diuretic agents and renal replacement therapy in certain clinical scenarios. While diuretics generally should not be used as single agents in the treatment of hypertensive crises, they can be used in combination with other drug classes for blood pressure control.

If this patient's CKD was more advanced, one could consider renal replacement therapy with ultrafiltration as a possible therapy.

In this clinical scenario, we would recommend starting nicardipine or labetalol IV infusion to lower blood pressure by 20 % within the first few hours of treatment. Concurrently, given his presentation of volume overload, diuretic therapy with IV furosemide infusion should also be considered. If his CKD were more advanced in the setting of volume overload, dialysis with ultrafiltration would likely need to be initiated for blood pressure management.

CASE #2: A 67-year-old African American female with a history of diabetes mellitus type 2, hypertension, and ESRD on dialysis for 1 year presents to the emergency room with fatigue, dyspnea with exertion, and nausea. Her last dialysis session was 5 days ago. She is anuric. On admission, her vitals are significant for blood pressure 240/114 mmHg, heart rate of 92 bpm, and oxygen saturation of 88 % on room air improved to 96 % on BiPAP. Physical exam is significant for elevated jugular venous pressure, bibasilar crackles, and 1+ lower extremity edema. CXR shows increased interstitial markings consistent with pulmonary edema. What is the best management for this patient?

Answer #2: Again, this patient shows signs of volume overload. However, this patient is a chronic dialysis patient who has been non-adherent to her outpatient dialysis regimen. Interdialytic fluid intake, physical exam, and interdialytic weight gain are important markers that help determine the patient's dry weight. In the setting of volume overload, antihypertensive medications are of limited utility. In the acute setting, dialysis is best for volume removal and blood pressure control. The patient should have blood pressure lowered safely by 20 % to prevent cerebral hypoperfusion. If blood pressure is not adequately controlled with dialysis alone, she may require a labetalol or nicardipine drip for adequate blood pressure control.

Undoubtedly, in ESRD patients, dialysis with ultrafiltration is central to blood pressure management. Careful evaluation of volume status should first be performed, as volume depletion can also sometimes present as severe hypertension. Target dry weight requires frequent evaluation and adjustment dependent on the physician's clinical assessment of the patient. Adherence to scheduled dialysis treatments must be emphasized to the patient to avoid hypertensive crises as presented here.

Parenteral Medications for Hypertensive Emergencies

See Table 9.1 for a listing of parenteral medications for hypertensive emergencies, including doses and onset of action.

Vasodilators

Diazoxide—benzothiadiazine drug, a pure arterial vasodilator [18, 19]. Usually begin 1 mg/kg and administer every 5–15 min to prevent sudden dangerous drops in blood pressure. Dosage reduction is required in the presence of renal disease because of prolonged half-life. An increase in cardiac output and heart rate occur, which could provoke cardiac ischemia in some patients. Concurrent beta blocker and diuretic administration is needed due to reflex vasodilatory responses and salt and water retention. This medication is removed by hemodialysis and peritoneal dialysis but with low clearance due to high protein binding [5, 6].

Hydralazine hydrochloride—a direct acting vasodilator which relaxes vascular smooth muscle. Given IV or IM, it causes hypotension, but in an unpredictable manner. The onset of action is 10–30 min and the effect lasts up to 6 h [18, 19]. Hydralazine is considered a safe choice for patients with eclampsia. Side effects include reflex tachycardia as well as salt and water retention.

Sodium nitroprusside—a potent vasodilator. It acts on the excitation contraction coupling of vascular smooth muscle, dilating both arterioles and venous vessels. It has the benefit of rapid onset and offset. This drug should be avoided in patients with high intracranial pressure and those with renal impairment. Cyanide accumulation may occur in patients with CKD.
Nitroglycerin.

Nitroglycerin—weak systemic arteriolar vasodilation with a dose-related response.

Its rapid onset of action, within 2–5 min, allows it to be a good choice to dilate coronary vessels increasing blood supply to ischemic regions in cases of unstable angina or acute myocardial infarction. Nitroglycerin reduces preload and cardiac output at lower dosages, and reduces afterload at higher doses. Side effects include headache, nausea, and vomiting. Prolonged use may lead to tolerance.

Table 9.1 Parenteral drugs used to treat hypertensive emergencies

Drug	Starting dose	Titration/Usual dose	Maximum dose	Onset of action	Peak effect	Duration of action
Nitroprusside	0.3 μg/kg/min	2–4 μg/kg/min	8 μg/kg/min × 10 min	Immediate	1–2 min	2–5 min
Nicardipine	5 mg/h	Titrate by 2.5 mg/h at 5–15 min intervals	max 15 mg/h	5–10 min	45 min	50 h
Labetalol	2 mg/min or 0.25 mg/kg	20 mg over 2 min, then 4–80 mg at 10 min intervals	Up to 300 mg total or 2 mg/kg	5 min	10 min	3–6 h
Enalaprilat	0.625 mg–5.0 mg over 5 min	0.625–1.25 mg every 6 h	5 mg/dose	5–15 min	1–4 h	6 h
Esmolol	80–500 μg/kg over 1 min	50–100 μg/kg/min for maintenance	300 μg/kg/min	1–2 min	5 min	0–30 min
Phentolamine	0.5–1.0 mg/min infusion or 2.5–5.0 mg bolus	–	–	Immediate	3–5 min	10–15 min
Nitroglycerin	5 μg/min	Titrate by 5 μg/min at 3–5 min intervals, can go up by 10–20 μg/min if no response seen at 20 μg/min	100 μg/min	1–2 min	2–5 min	3–5 min
Hydralazine	0.5–1.0 mg/min infusion or 10–50 mg IM	Can give q 30 min intervals	–	1–5 min	10–80 min	3–6 h
Clevidipine	16 mg/h	–	–	1–2 min	5–6 min	15 min
Fenoldopam	0.01–1.6 μg/min	Constant infusion	–	5–15 min	30 min	5–10 min
Diazoxide	7.5–30 mg/min infusion or 1 mg/kg	May bolus q5–15 min	300 mg max	1–5 min	30 min	4–12 h
Methyldopa	250–500 mg bolus	Bolus q6 h	2 g max	2–3 h	3–5 h	6–12 h
Trimethaphan	0.5–10 mg/min infusion bolus over 2 min	–	300 mg max	Immediate	1–2 min	5–10 min

Calcium Channel Blockers

Nicardipine hydrochloride—a dihydropyridine calcium channel blocker (CCB) with fast onset of action, with a final steady state after 50 h. Begin the infusion 5.0 mg/h and titrate up. There is a dose dependent decrease in blood pressure. Nicardipine is effective in treating pediatric hypertensive emergencies [20, 21].

   Clevidipine butyrate—a short-acting, third generation dihydropyridine calcium channel blocker. It is metabolized by blood esterases and therefore can be used in cases of renal and liver impairment. It is also highly protein bound. Blood levels drop rapidly after terminating the infusion. The elimination half-life is 15 min. Adverse effects include sinus tachycardia, headache, nausea, and chest discomfort [22]. In the ECLIPSE trial, in patients with preoperative HTN, clevidipine treatment resulted in lower mortality rates than compared to those treated with nitroprusside.

Adrenergic Agents

Labetalol—a combined alpha 1 and beta 2 adrenergic receptor antagonist with rapid onset of action. The drug can be given parenterally or orally [18, 23]. If given IV, the dose administered is 0.5–2.0 mg/min which will cause a rapid but not abrupt decrease in blood pressure. Avoid in patients experiencing acute heart failure, asthma, and AV block. Its main indications include aortic dissection, acute coronary syndrome, hypertensive encephalopathy, adrenergic crisis, and particularly useful and safe in pregnancy induced hypertensive crisis.

   Esmolol hydrochloride—a beta 1 selective blocker which acts immediately and has a short duration of action, with negligible concentrations at 30 min after discontinuation. It also produces negative chronotropic and inotropic activity. It must be diluted to a concentration of 10 mg/ml. Extravasation can cause local irritation or skin necrosis. A loading dose and then infusion of a maintenance dose of the drug allows for steady state blood concentration to be achieved (see Table 9.1). It is used in patients with hypertensive crisis that are also tachycardic with increased cardiac output, such as in post-surgical patients. Esmolol is also used in patients with post-operative hypertension. Use cautiously in patients with renal insufficiency [18, 23].

   Methyldopa—a central alpha 2 adrenergic agent that is administered IV as a bolus. It has an unpredictable effect on blood pressure with delayed onset of action and peak effect.

   Phentolamine—an alpha receptor antagonist with a short lived effect that is used more often in cases of increased circulating catecholamines (i.e., pheochromocytoma crisis, monoamine oxidase inhibitor and drug food interaction, clonidine withdrawal syndrome). The duration of action is 10–15 min with a short half-life (19 min) [18, 23]. Phentolamine may cause angina/cardiac arrhythmias.

Other Parenteral Medications

Trimethaphan camsylate—a ganglionic blocking agent with immediate onset of action. It decreases peripheral vascular resistance and usually decreases cardiac output due to venous dilation and peripheral pooling of blood [18, 23]. Intra-arterial blood pressure monitoring is required. The patient must be supine to receive trimethaphan. Start the infusion at 1 mg/min and titrate up as needed. Trimethaphan is effective in the setting of acute aortic dissection. Watch for tachyphylaxis from volume expansion if infused for 48 h or more as well as histamine release.

Enalaprilat—the active metabolite of enalapril, is administered IV slowly over 5 min that is 1/4th the oral dose [24]. Onset of action is within 15 min and maximal effect is seen within 1–4 h. Initial dose in patients with renal insufficiency should be no more than 0.625 mg [6]. Enalaprilat is contraindicated in patients with renal artery stenosis and those who are pregnant.

Fenoldopam mesylate—a dopamine(D1)-like receptor agonist which causes arteriolar vasodilation with a half-life of 5 min. Steady state concentrations are reached within 20 min. It increases blood flow in hypertensive and normotensive individuals [25, 26]. Fenoldopam is helpful in those with renal impairment as its target receptors are located in the renal and splanchnic arteries. Adverse effects include increased intraocular pressures, reflex tachycardia, headache, flushing, hypotension, and nausea.

Diuretics[1]

Furosemide, torsemide, bumetanide—loop diuretics, blocks NaK2Cl channel in the thick ascending limb of the Loop of Henle, preventing sodium and chloride reabsorption. Can be given as an IV bolus, IV continuous infusion [27].

Renal Replacement Therapy

Hemodialysis/isolated ultrafiltration—intermittent hemodialysis is more predictable than peritoneal dialysis for acute fluid removal as the ultrafiltration rate is set by the provider.

Hypertensive Urgency

Patients with chronically elevated blood pressure and those with hypertensive urgencies should have slower reduction of their blood pressure, preferably over 24–48 h and may not need hospitalization. Generally, blood pressure in a

---

[1]Not used in hypertensive emergencies in the general population, but may be considered in the CKD population if eveidence of volume overload.

hypertensive urgency is >200/130 mmHg but lacks target organ damage. Gradual lowering of blood pressure is necessary due to changes in autoregulation of cerebral blood flow. Normally, cerebral blood flow is regulated so perfusion is maintained at lower blood pressures. Perfusion is diminished in states of chronic hypertension to prevent cerebral edema. Rapid lowering could lead to cerebral ischemia or infarction. Sudden drops in blood pressure can even lead to myocardial ischemia, infarction, or arrhythmia. Patients with hypertensive urgency should be treated with oral medications rather than parenteral medications.

In patients with hypertensive urgency, a quiet dark room can decrease BP by 20/10 mmHg. Treatment of pain is also important in order to prevent hypotension after the administration of antihypertensive medications. Preferably, one should start with oral medications such as clonidine or captopril, which have a quick onset of action and shorter half-life to allow for gradual blood pressure drop in the setting of a higher autoregulatory threshold [28, 29]. Then, longer acting medications can be added. Avoid IV hydralazine and sublingual nifedipine as these medications have been shown to cause severe and uncontrolled hypotension [2]. Sublingual nifedipine capsules have been linked to stroke and heart attack in hypertensive subjects due to the overshooting of the blood pressure target [2].

The goal of antihypertensive treatment is to reduce or reverse end organ damage while at the same time preventing hypoperfusion and ischemic injury. There is a higher risk of ischemia, coma, and death when diastolic pressure is lowered below 90 mmHg or when initial blood pressure is dropped by 35% [19].

Patients with asymptomatic severe hypertension, as frequently seen in chronically hypertensive patients who either do not have a primary care physician or are non-adherent with their medication regimen, do not need emergent treatment. If non-adherent, their medication should be restarted, and efforts should be made to encourage compliance.

Oral Medications for Hypertensive Urgency

See Table 9.2 for a list of oral medications for use during hypertensive urgent treatment.

Nifedipine—rapid onset of action, can cause reflex tachycardia, useful for hypertensive crisis. Can cause symptomatic hypotension. For this reason, one should only use long-acting preparations.

Clonidine—a central alpha 2 agonist that allows for an immediate antihypertensive effect but requires repetitive dosing which can lead to drowsiness.

Captopril or enalapril—maximum effect in 2 h. Does not cause tachycardia.

Minoxidil—direct vasodilator, 2.5–10 mg given every 4–6 h initially for hypertensive emergency. Use with an adrenergic blocker or diuretic.

Labetalol—an alpha 1 and beta antagonist, effective within 1–3 h but has an unpredictable dose response.

Table 9.2 Rapid acting oral drugs for treating hypertensive emergencies

Drug	Dose	Onset of action	Peak effect	Duration of action
Labetalol	100–400 mg q12h, max 2400 mg	1–2 h	2–4 h	8–12 h
Clonidine	0.2 mg initially, then 0.1 mg/h (0.8 mg max)	30–60 min	2–4 h	6–8 h
Diltiazem	30–120 mg q8h (480 mg max)	<15 min	2–3 h	8 h
Verapamil	80–120 mg q8h (480 mg max)	<60 min	2–3 h	8 h
Captopril	12.5–25 mg q6h (150 mg max)	<15 min	1 h	6–12 h
Enalapril	2.5–10 mg q6h (40 mg max)	<60 min	4–8 h	12–24 h
Prazosin	1–5 mg q2h (20 mg max)	<60 min	2–4 h	6–12 h

Clinical Scenarios

Malignant and Accelerated HTN

From a historical perspective, there is no blood pressure which defines either malignant or accelerated hypertension. Accelerated hypertension involves marked elevation of blood pressure which may be associated with headache, weight loss from pressure-natriuresis, retinopathy, and renal failure. The signs and symptoms of accelerated hypertension relate to the vascular injury due to uncontrolled hypertension. If papilledema is also found, this indicates malignant hypertension. In patients with malignant hypertension, patients may also have occipital headache, blurry vision, and confusion. Preferably, patients should be treated in the ICU in order to monitor and stabilize them. Again, treatment goal is to prevent and reverse end organ damage. Parenteral or any of the oral medications listed in Table 9.2 may be used. Malignant or accelerated hypertension is older terminology which has been removed from the National and International Blood Pressure Control guidelines and is referred to as hypertensive emergency [2, 6, 17].

Hypertensive Encephalopathy

Hypertensive encephalopathy can occur from severe hypertension or in cases of malignant hypertension and is associated with a poor prognosis if not quickly recognized and treated. More often than not, patients with hypertensive encephalopathy also have renal impairment. The full syndrome can take 12–48 h to develop [6]. Symptoms include marked hypertension, headache, nausea, vomiting, papilledema (but can also be absent and should not exclude the diagnosis), visual issues, transient focal neurologic deficits. Progressive worsening of symptoms can result without treatment leading to coma and death. One must rule out ischemic or hemorrhagic stroke as well as uremic encephalopathy in the setting of renal failure. If symptoms improve rapidly with treatment, the diagnosis is likely hypertensive encephalopathy.

Blood pressure should be lowered within 3–4 h but the DBP should remain >100 mmHg to avoid risk of cerebral ischemia. Parenteral therapy is preferred over oral medications, especially in light of these patients having nausea and vomiting. Parenteral therapy should be continued for 8–12 h. If nausea has resolved, then the patient could be transitioned to oral medications such as minoxidil or nifedipine. Avoid medications that will cause cerebral vasodilation in the setting of hypertensive encephalopathy or central nervous system hemorrhage.

Cerebral Infarction/CNS Bleeding

The approach to managing blood pressure in patients who are status post a cerebral thrombotic or hemorrhagic event is as follows: (1) Begin antihypertensive therapy if SBP>220 mmHg or SBP>130 mmHg. (2) Avoid thrombolytics unless the SBP<180 mmHg or DBP<110 mmHg. (3) In the case of a hemorrhagic stroke, SBP>180 mmHg or SBP>30 mmHg should be targeted. (4) Sodium nitroprusside should be avoided as initial therapy as it increases intracranial pressure. In the case of an ischemic or hemorrhagic infarction, autoregulation may not be normal. For this reason, managing such patients is problematic, without any clear guidelines. (5) Avoid lowering the blood pressure by more than 20 % and not lowering SBP below 100 mmHg, at least initially [6].

Acute Aortic Dissection

Patients with acute aortic dissection present with severe chest, back, neck, or intrascapular pain, syncope, headache, blindness, hemoptysis, dyspnea, nausea, vomiting, and even melena or hematemesis [6]. Abrupt pain is often the most characteristic sign. As patients may be unstable, stat CT angiography is most often used to diagnose an acute dissection. Direct vasodilators are contraindicated as they could reflexively stimulate the heart. Sodium nitroprusside along with labetalol or esmolol are considerations to bring blood pressure down in a smooth and controlled way. Trimethaphan can also be used as it has a negative inotropic effect, slowing down the pulsatile wave generated by the heart.

Acute Left Ventricular Failure/Pulmonary Edema (Refractory to Conventional Medical Therapy)

The left ventricle must work harder when blood pressure is higher. In settings of severe hypertension, the left ventricle could fail leading to pulmonary edema. Sodium nitroprusside, diuretics, and other intravenous drugs should be used in this situation. Sodium nitroprusside lowers both afterload and preload allowing for increased cardiac output [5, 6].

Pheochromocytoma/Adrenergic Crisis

Patients with pheochromocytoma present with sustained or episodic hypertension associated with sweating, tachycardia, numbness and tingling of the feet and hands [5, 6]. The frequency of blood pressure elevation varies as the episodes can occur multiple times a day or only once a month. Plasma free metanephrines can be falsely positive in patients with chronic kidney disease (CKD) [30]. For this reason, plasma catecholamines may be a more useful screening tool in patients with advancing CKD. Phentolamine is preferable as it helps reduce blood pressure in the setting of alpha adrenergic-mediated hypertension [18]. A beta blocker like labetalol can be used after phentolamine or phenoxybenzamine is administered.

An adrenergic crisis can occur in any state of catecholamine excess. This condition may be seen in cases of abrupt clonidine or methyldopa withdrawal, acute spinal cord injuries which lead to automatic hyperreflexia, sympathomimetic drug use (i.e., cocaine, amphetamines), and interaction of tyramine containing compounds with monoamine oxidase inhibitors. These scenarios respond well to phentolamine or nitroprusside. However, it is important to avoid beta blockers as they can worsen a hypertensive crisis.

Conclusion

Hypertensive urgencies and emergencies are clinical syndromes caused by various clinical scenarios. The goal is to prevent end organ damage, or reverse it, if possible. It is important to distinguish between these two clinical syndromes as this helps direct treatment strategies, need for hospitalization, and level of care. Careful individualization is always necessary. Progressive control of blood pressure in a prompt and controlled manner is essential to prevent hypoperfusion to vital organs. One must always consider why the crisis occurred, i.e. due to non-adherence or progression of the underlying secondary cause of hypertension, as this will assist in management and prevention.

In patients with CKD and those on dialysis, hypertensive crises are frequently seen. Management of those patients often involves targeting volume overload either with parenteral medications and/or renal replacement therapy with ultrafiltration.

References

1. Kearney PM, Whelton M, Reynolds K, Muntner P, Whelton PK, He J. Global burden of hypertension: analysis of worldwide data. Lancet. 2005;365:217–23.
2. Marik PE, Rivera R. Hypertensive emergencies: an update. Curr Opin Crit Care. 2011;17:569–80.
3. Marik PE, Varon J. Hypertensive crises: challenges and management. Chest. 2007;131:1949–62.
4. Coresh J, Selvin E, Stevens LA, et al. Prevalence of chronic kidney disease in the United States. JAMA. 2007;298:2038–47.
5. Sarafidis PA, Bakris GL. Evaluation and treatment of hypertensive urgencies and emergencies. In: Johnson R, Feehally J, Floege J, editors. Comprehensive clinical nephrology. 5th ed. Philadelphia: Elsevier Saunders; 2014. p. 439–46.
6. Ram C, Venkata S. Hypertensive urgencies and emergencies: considersations for treatment. In: Weir MR, editor. Hypertension. Philadelphia: American College of Physicians; 2005. p. 203–20.
7. Muiesan ML, Salvetti M, Amadoro V, et al. An update on hypertensive emergencies and urgencies. J Cardiovasc Med (Hagerstown). 2015;16:372–82.
8. Vaughan CJ, Delanty N. Hypertensive emergencies. Lancet. 2000;356:411–7.
9. Derhaschnig U, Testori C, Riedmueller E, Aschauer S, Wolzt M, Jilma B. Hypertensive emergencies are associated with elevated markers of inflammation, coagulation, platelet activation and fibrinolysis. J Hum Hypertens. 2013;27:368–73.
10. Carlstrom M, Wilcox CS, Arendshorst WJ. Renal autoregulation in health and disease. Physiol Rev. 2015;95:405–511.
11. Loutzenhiser R, Griffin KA, Bidani AK. Systolic blood pressure as the trigger for the renal myogenic response: protective or autoregulatory? Curr Opin Nephrol Hypertens. 2006;15:41–9.
12. Bidani AK, Griffin KA, Williamson G, Wang X, Loutzenhiser R. Protective importance of the myogenic response in the renal circulation. Hypertension. 2009;54:393–8.
13. Loutzenhiser R, Griffin K, Williamson G, Bidani A. Renal autoregulation: new perspectives regarding the protective and regulatory roles of the underlying mechanisms. Am J Physiol Regul Integr Comp Physiol. 2006;290:R1153–67.
14. Khawaja Z, Wilcox CS. Role of the kidneys in resistant hypertension. Int J Hypertens. 2011;2011:143471.
15. Inrig JK. Intradialytic hypertension: a less-recognized cardiovascular complication of hemodialysis. Am J Kidney Dis. 2010;55:580–9.
16. Singapuri MS, Lea JP. Management of hypertension in the end-stage renal disease patient. J Clin Outcomes Manage. 2010;17:87–95.
17. Pak KJ, Hu T, Fee C, Wang R, Smith M, Bazzano LA. Acute hypertension: a systematic review and appraisal of guidelines. Ochsner J. 2014;14:655–63.
18. Elliott WJ. Hypertensive emergencies. Crit Care Clin. 2001;17:435–51.
19. Grossman E, Messerli FH, Grodzicki T, Kowey P. Should a moratorium be placed on sublingual nifedipine capsules given for hypertensive emergencies and pseudoemergencies? JAMA. 1996;276:1328–31.
20. Michael J, Groshong T, Tobias JD. Nicardipine for hypertensive emergencies in children with renal disease. Pediatr Nephrol. 1998;12:40–2.

21. Neutel JM, Smith DH, Wallin D, et al. A comparison of intravenous nicardipine and sodium nitroprusside in the immediate treatment of severe hypertension. Am J Hypertens. 1994;7:623–8.
22. Deeks ED, Keating GM, Keam SJ. Clevidipine: a review of its use in the management of acute hypertension. Am J Cardiovasc Drugs. 2009;9:117–34.
23. Grossman E, Ironi AN, Messerli FH. Comparative tolerability profile of hypertensive crisis treatments. Drug Saf. 1998;19:99–122.
24. Hirschl MM, Binder M, Bur A, et al. Clinical evaluation of different doses of intravenous enalaprilat in patients with hypertensive crises. Arch Intern Med. 1995;155:2217–23.
25. Murphy MB, Murray C, Shorten GD. Fenoldopam: a selective peripheral dopamine-receptor agonist for the treatment of severe hypertension. N Engl J Med. 2001;345:1548–57.
26. Oparil S, Aronson S, Deeb GM, et al. Fenoldopam: a new parenteral antihypertensive: consensus roundtable on the management of perioperative hypertension and hypertensive crises. Am J Hypertens. 1999;12:653–64.
27. Prisant LM. Pharmacology of antihypertensive drugs. In: Weir MR, editor. Hypertension. Philadelphia: American College of Physicians; 2005. p. 89.
28. Daugirdas JT, Blake PG, Ing TS. Handbook of dialysis. 5th ed. Lippincott Williams & Wilkins; 2014.
29. Gales MA. Oral antihypertensives for hypertensive urgencies. Ann Pharmacother. 1994;28:352–8.
30. Judd E, Calhoun DA. Management of hypertension in CKD: beyond the guidelines. Adv Chronic Kidney Dis. 2015;22:116–22.

Chapter 10
Management of Hypertension in Chronic Kidney Disease

Jordana B. Cohen and Raymond R. Townsend

Blood Pressure Goals in Chronic Kidney Disease

Chronic kidney disease (CKD) and hypertension have an undeniably complex relationship. Hypertension is both a product of underlying kidney disease and a risk factor for the development and progression of CKD [1]. The complexity of this relationship likely contributes to disagreement in the literature, and thus among experts, regarding optimal blood pressure goals in patients with CKD. Sufficient blood pressure control can significantly reduce the rate of worsening renal function in patients with CKD [2]. Although there have been no blood pressure target trials specifically focused on cardiovascular events, patients with concomitant hypertension and CKD are at increased risk of adverse cardiovascular and cerebrovascular outcomes. Thus, careful attention to the management of blood pressure in these patients is critical [3].

In the 2014 Evidence-Based Management of Hypertension in Adults report, those empanelled as the Eighth Joint National Committee (JNC8) performed an intensive, systematic review of the existing literature; the 2014 report used data from Fair- to Good-quality randomized controlled trials (RCTs), and resorted to expert opinion in areas where RCTs were either not available, conflicting in their conclusions, or failed to address a particular question [4]. The report recommended that individuals <70 years of age with reduced kidney function (defined as an estimated glomerular filtration rate [eGFR] of <60 mL/min/1.73 m^2) and patients with albuminuria (defined as >30 mg/g) at any level of eGFR, with or without diabetes, should be initiated on antihypertensive therapy for a systolic blood pressure of ≥140 mmHg or a diastolic blood pressure of ≥90 mmHg. Treatment should be titrated to achieve a goal systolic blood pressure of <140 mmHg and a goal diastolic

J.B. Cohen, MD (✉) • R.R. Townsend, MD
Renal, Electrolyte, Hypertension Division, Department of Medicine,
University of Pennsylvania, 3400 Spruce St, 1 Founders, Philadelphia, PA, USA
e-mail: jco@mail.med.upenn.edu

© Springer Science+Business Media New York 2016
A.K. Singh, R. Agarwal (eds.), *Core Concepts in Hypertension in Kidney Disease*, DOI 10.1007/978-1-4939-6436-9_10

blood pressure of <90 mmHg [4–7]. RCTs demonstrate no added benefit from stricter blood pressure control in patients with CKD with regard to progression of renal disease and adverse cardiovascular outcomes [8–10].

The Kidney Disease Improving Global Outcomes (KDIGO) Clinical Practice Guideline for the Management of Blood Pressure in CKD published in December 2012 provided comprehensive guidance regarding an extensive range of topics in the management of hypertension in patients with CKD (Table 10.1) [11]. The KDIGO guidelines systematically and transparently drew from a broader body of evidence, scrutinizing and denoting the quality of the available data for each subject addressed. The KDIGO guidelines have similar recommendations to those empanelled as JNC8 with regard to non-proteinuric patients with CKD. KDIGO recommends that non-diabetic and diabetic adults with CKD and no albuminuria (defined as <30 mg per 24 h) should be treated with antihypertensive medications to maintain a goal blood pressure of ≤140 mmHg systolic and ≤90 mmHg diastolic [11].

Blood Pressure Goals with Albuminuria

The increased risk of adverse cardiovascular and cerebrovascular outcomes in patients with concomitant hypertension and CKD is further exacerbated by the presence of proteinuria [3]. Post-hoc analysis of the MDRD study indicated that patients with >3 g per 24 h of proteinuria had greater renal benefit, defined as the slope of GFR change over time, from a blood pressure goal of <130/80 [8]. However, this finding was not consistent with primary analyses of other RCTs [9, 10]. As a result of the mixed available evidence, the recommendations regarding patients with albuminuria differ across treatment guidelines. Those empanelled as JNC8 recommend a goal systolic blood pressure of <140 mmHg and a goal diastolic blood pressure of <90 mmHg in these patients [4]. Acknowledging the limitations of the MDRD post-hoc analyses, the KDIGO report suggests that non-diabetic and diabetic adult CKD patients with any amount of albuminuria ≥ 30 mg per 24 h should be treated with antihypertensive medications to maintain a blood pressure of ≤130 mmHg systolic and ≤80 mmHg diastolic [8, 11].

Blood Pressure Goals in the Elderly

Those empanelled as JNC8 recommend that patients who are ≥60 years of age without CKD should be treated with antihypertensive therapy to achieve a goal systolic blood pressure of <150 mmHg and a goal diastolic blood pressure of <90 mmHg [4–7]. The group noted that there is no clear evidence regarding optimal blood pressure treatment goals in individuals with CKD who are ≥70 years of age. They recommend that elderly patients be evaluated and treated on an individualized

Table 10.1 Summary of the KDIGO 2012 guidelines for blood pressure management in CKD patients [11]

General guidelines
Individualize blood pressure targets and agents based on age, comorbidities, and side effects
Monitor for orthostatic hypotension, particularly in the elderly
Recommend lifestyle modification
Achieve or maintain a body mass index of 20–25 kg/m²
Lower sodium intake to <2 g per day
Exercise at least 30 min 5 times per week
Limit alcohol intake to 2 drinks per day in men, 1 drink per day in women
Blood pressure management in diabetic and non-diabetic CKD patients
Urine Albumin Excretion <30 mg per 24 h
Initiate therapy for blood pressure >140 mmHg systolic or >90 mmHg diastolic
Maintain blood pressure consistently ≤140 mmHg systolic and ≤90 mmHg diastolic
Urine Albumin Excretion ≥30 mg per 24 h
Initiate therapy for blood pressure >130 mmHg systolic or >80 mmHg diastolic
Maintain blood pressure consistently ≤130 mmHg systolic and ≤80 mmHg diastolic
ARB or ACE-I is recommended
Blood pressure management in the elderly
Tailor blood pressure regimen based on age, comorbidities, and risk of medication interactions
Gradual escalation of therapy
Close monitoring for adverse effects
Orthostatic hypotension, acutely worsening azotemia, and electrolyte abnormalities

basis, taking into account other associated comorbidities and risk of adverse effects from treatment [4].

The KDIGO guidelines recommend a similar individualized approach to blood pressure targets according to age and coexisting comorbidities [11]. The authors noted that multiple studies in non-CKD elderly populations demonstrate a J-shaped relationship between both systolic and diastolic blood pressure and survival [12–14], but that it appears to be safe to treat elevated blood pressures in elderly patients without CKD to a target level of <150/80 mmHg [5]. Much like JNC8, the KDIGO report states that the available data cannot be appropriately extrapolated to patients with CKD, and that it is not possible to provide a specific blood pressure target in elderly patients with CKD. The KDIGO report suggests an approach using the same goals as in younger patients with CKD, but emphasizes that treatment of hypertension in the elderly with CKD must be undertaken with greater caution and that treatment goals should be achieved gradually. The KDIGO guidelines also promote asking about dizziness and assessing for postural hypotension, noting that elderly patients with CKD undergoing treatment for hypertension are particularly prone to orthostatic hypotension, which can be exacerbated by volume depletion from diuretic therapy [11, 15].

Target Versus Achieved Blood Pressure

The disparity in recommendations regarding blood pressure goals in patients with CKD across different guidelines may be attributable in part to perceived differences in target versus achieved blood pressures. Achieved blood pressures in clinical practice may not consistently correlate with target blood pressures [16], raising concern that target blood pressures should be made lower in order to reach optimum blood pressure control in a greater number of patients and avoid treatment inertia. Critics of more lenient target blood pressures argue that observational data supporting lower blood pressure goals are evidence of the discrepancy between target and actually achieved blood pressures in "real world" settings. These critics also argue that RCT populations are not always generalizable to "real world" settings, where patients tend to have decreased motivation and adherence and increased heterogeneity compared to trial participants [11, 16].

Historically, some guidelines addressed the issue of achieved versus target blood pressure by recommending titration of treatment to a blood pressure that is lower than the recommended target blood pressure. The potential pitfalls of this approach include increased risk of adverse effects from medications, hypotension, and potential decreased survival in certain populations [12–14]. The KDIGO authors address the issue of achieved versus target blood pressure by recommending repeated office blood pressure measurements, and by wording their guidelines to recommend that patients *consistently* meet their target blood pressure [11]. Additionally, ambulatory blood pressure monitoring and home blood pressure monitoring are superior options to office-based measurements for prognostication of renal and cardiovascular outcomes in patients with chronic kidney disease, and allow for more reliable assessment of achieved blood pressure [17, 18].

Management of Hypertension in CKD

Non-Pharmacologic Therapy

RCT and observational data support lifestyle modifications such as decreased sodium intake [19], increased exercise [20], weight loss [21], and reduction in alcohol intake [22] for the management of blood pressure in the general population [23]. Existing evidence indicates that blood pressure reduction through lifestyle modifications can significantly improve cardiovascular and renal outcomes. Although mainly observational data are available in the CKD population, non-pharmacologic management with lifestyle modifications has become a key factor in the treatment of hypertension in patients with CKD. That said, most patients will require a combination of non-pharmacologic and pharmacologic treatment in order to achieve blood pressure targets (Table 10.2).

Reduced Sodium Intake

Excess sodium and water retention is a major contributing factor to elevated blood pressure in patients with CKD [24, 25]. Patients with reduced GFR have impaired filtering of sodium and water, resulting in expansion of the extracellular volume and thus an increase in systemic blood pressure. High amounts of sodium intake in patients with CKD contribute to volume expansion (which can occur in the absence of peripheral edema) [26], increased filtration fraction resulting in increased proteinuria [27], and hypo-responsiveness to pharmacologic antihypertensive therapies [28]. Since their elevated blood pressure is in part driven by this impairment in sodium excretion, patients with CKD tend to be sensitive to reductions in sodium intake. Although no RCTs have been performed evaluating the long-term effect of dietary sodium reduction in CKD patients, short duration RCTs have demonstrated that reduced sodium intake improves responsiveness to pharmacologic antihypertensive therapy in these patients [29–31].

There is no high-quality data on the ideal level of sodium intake in patients with CKD, however recent guidelines recommend a reduction in sodium intake to less than 2–2.3 g daily; more stringent sodium restriction does not appear to be beneficial [11, 32]. Patient education on interpreting food labels and provider-initiated feedback on sodium reduction using 24 h urine sodium collection are valuable tools in effectively implementing sodium reduction in hypertensive patients [33].

Potassium Supplementation

A number of studies in non-CKD patients demonstrate that low dietary potassium intake increases sodium sensitivity in patients with normal renal function, and that dietary potassium intake is inversely proportional to blood pressure [34, 35].

Table 10.2 Summary of non-pharmacologic and pharmacologic management options in CKD

Non-pharmacologic	Summary of the literature
Reduced sodium intake	Reduce sodium intake to less than 2–2.3 g per day
Potassium supplementation	Benefit in hypertension in inconclusive
	Not recommended in CKD due to risk of hyperkalemia
Exercise	Aerobic exercise 30 to 40 min, five to seven times weekly
Weight loss	Reduce or maintain body mass index <25 kg/m^2
Reduced alcohol intake	No studies in CKD
	Recommendations per KDIGO; limit to 2 drinks per day in men, 1 drink per day in women
Smoking cessation	No studies in CKD; strong evidence in diverse populations to support cessation
Pharmacologic	
ACE-I/ARB	Recommended as first-line therapy in most patients; best evidence is in the setting of proteinuria
	No benefit from dual ACE-I and ARB therapy, with increased risk of hyperkalemia and azotemia
Direct renin inhibition	Increased risk of nonfatal stroke, azotemia, hyperkalemia, and hypotension when given with ARB
	Not currently recommended in CKD in combination with ACE-I or ARB
Diuretics	Thiazides have long-term benefit in CKD, but are less effective than loop diuretics in advanced CKD
	Chlorthalidone is more potent than hydrochlorothiazide; electrolyte abnormalities persist in CKD
	Metolazone is useful for short-term adjunctive therapy along with loop diuretics
K-sparing diuretics and	Triamterene and amiloride not recommended due to risk of hyperkalemia
Mineralocorticoid antagonists	Spironolactone and eplerenone may be helpful as adjunct to ACE-I/ARB, however increase risk of hyperkalemia
Calcium channel blockers	Dihydropyridines may exacerbate extravascular volume expansion and albuminuria
	Non-dihydropyridines may reduce albuminuria; however, increase risk of bradycardia
Beta blockers	Avoid giving with non-dihydropyridines due to risk of atrioventricular block and bradycardia
	Atenolol and bisoprolol are renally eliminated
	Atenolol may have greater mortality benefit than metoprolol in older patients
Centrally acting alpha agonists	No interaction with other antihypertensives; useful as adjunctive therapy
	Moxonide accumulates in kidney disease, and has increased risk of mortality in heart failure
	Guanfacine has higher risk of sedation, postural hypotension, and sexual dysfunction

(continued)

Table 10.2 (continued)

Non-pharmacologic	Summary of the literature
Alpha blockers	Increased risk of heart failure in high-risk hypertensive patients
	High risk of postural hypotension, tachycardia, and falls, particularly in the elderly
Direct vasodilators	Hydralazine not generally recommended for long-term therapy due to need for frequent dosing
	Minoxidil is useful in very resistant hypertension; however, high risk of side effects
	Minoxidil should be administered with a beta blocker and diuretic due to risk of myocardial ischemia and volume expansion

Although some studies demonstrate that potassium supplementation can attenuate the effect of sodium on blood pressure, data on the effectiveness of potassium supplementation in the treatment of hypertension is inconclusive [36]. One proposed explanation for the inconsistent evidence is that both reduction in dietary sodium and increase in dietary potassium intake work synergistically to reduce sodium retention [37]. Regardless, potassium excretion is significantly impaired in the setting of reduced GFR, increasing the risk for hyperkalemia in patients with CKD. Given the limited evidence and potentially grave risk, there is no indication for potassium supplementation in the management of hypertension in patients with CKD.

Exercise

Multiple RCTs demonstrate that aerobic exercise lasting 30–40 min four to seven times weekly contributes to a significant reduction in blood pressure in the general population [20]. Resistance training at least 3 days per week, including three to four sets of eight to twelve repetitions, also significantly reduces blood pressure in non-CKD patients, but to a lesser degree than aerobic exercise [20]. Multiple RCTs exist evaluating the role of aerobic exercise in CKD populations. These studies demonstrated a significant though modest reduction in systolic blood pressure and no overall reduction in diastolic blood pressure in CKD patients who undergo at least 8 weeks of aerobic exercise intervention compared to controls [38]. No studies exist evaluating the role of resistance training in blood pressure reduction in patients with CKD.

Weight Loss

Excess adipose tissue contributes to increased sympathetic nervous activity and increased renin, angiotensin, and aldosterone activity [39–41]. Modest weight loss significantly decreases muscle sympathetic nerve activity [42] and renin-angiotensin activity [43] in non-CKD obese patients. Based on multiple RCTs, remission of hypertension is observed in 75 % of non-CKD patients who lose weight after undergoing bariatric surgery [21]. Observational studies demonstrate a significant reduction in blood pressure with both surgical and non-surgical weight loss in patients with CKD (with 9 mmHg reduction and 22.6 mmHg reduction observed, respectively) [44]. Although elevated body mass index may be protective in dialysis populations [45], evidence suggests that increased adipose tissue increases the rate of progression of CKD in pre-dialysis patients [46]. Due to the role of excess adipose tissue in increased blood pressure and deterioration of renal function, current guidelines recommend normalization of body weight to a body mass index of less than 25 kg/m^2 in hypertensive patients with CKD [11].

Reduced Alcohol Intake

In non-CKD patients, reduction of alcohol intake results in a significant decrease in both systolic and diastolic blood pressure [22]. No studies have specifically evaluated the effect of reduction in alcohol intake on blood pressure in CKD patients, although there is also no evidence to suggest that the effect would vary significantly from non-CKD patients. The KDIGO guidelines recommend a maximum of two alcoholic drinks per day for men and one drink per day for women with CKD, consistent with current guidelines for the general population [11].

Smoking Cessation

Multiple observational studies demonstrate a significant improvement in systolic and diastolic blood pressure following smoking cessation in diverse non-CKD populations [47–49]. No studies specifically evaluate the effect of smoking cessation on blood pressure in patients with CKD. However, given the clear cardiovascular benefits of smoking cessation across all populations of patients, smoking cessation is strongly recommended in CKD patients to aid in the reduction of overall cardiovascular risk [11].

Pharmacologic Management

Patients with elevated blood pressure in CKD will likely benefit most from a step-wise approach to the management of their hypertension using a combination of lifestyle modifications and antihypertensive agents. Although adequate blood pressure control has clear renal, cardiac, and cerebrovascular benefits, selection of specific antihypertensive medications should be made on an individual patient basis, particularly taking into account the potential for adverse effects [11].

General Principles

Angiotensin converting enzyme inhibitors (ACE-Is) and angiotensin receptor blockers (ARBs) are strongly recommended as first-line therapy in patients with proteinuric CKD [4, 11, 50]; in patients with non-proteinuric CKD, there is no compelling evidence to support the use of ACE-Is or ARBs as first-line therapy, however these agents are still generally used for initial treatment of hypertension in most CKD patients [4]. The vast majority of patients with CKD will require a minimum of two to three antihypertensive medications in order to achieve target blood pressures [51]. No RCTs exist comparing different approaches to adjusting antihypertensive regimens in these patients. Based on expert opinion, if patients fail to meet the appropriate treatment goal within 1 month of initiation of an intervention, either the dose of the initial therapy should be increased as tolerated or an additional therapy may be introduced [4]. When selecting second and third-line therapies, patient-specific comorbidities and patient tolerance of the respective treatment should be taken strongly into consideration. Given the particularly high incidence of cardiac disease in patients with CKD, close attention should be paid to the coexistence of cardiovascular disease or congestive heart failure [52]. Treatment regimens should be tailored accordingly in order to optimize cardiac remodeling, afterload reduction, and other end organ effects of these frequently associated comorbidities.

Taking into account the often complex treatment regimens required to achieve adequate blood pressure control in these patients, certain combinations of medications should be addressed with caution or altogether avoided due to increased risks of adverse outcomes. Combination of ACE-I and ARB therapy is not currently recommended in patients with diabetic and non-diabetic CKD due to the amplified risk of hyperkalemia and azotemia, with no clear added benefit based on RCTs [53, 54]. Although there is anti-proteinuric benefit, the addition of an aldosterone antagonist to ACE-I or ARB therapy remains a point of controversy as well due to the potential increased risk of hyperkalemia [55]. The combination of non-dihydropyridine calcium channel blockers and beta blockers should be avoided due to the possibility of developing atrioventricular block or symptomatic bradycardia [56]. On the other hand, minoxidil should only be used in combination with both a beta blocker and high-dose loop diuretic due to the increased risk of tachycardia, myocardial ischemia, and tubular sodium retention when it is used as monotherapy [57].

ACE-Is, ARBs, and Renin Inhibitors

Reduction of proteinuria can be achieved both with adequate blood pressure control and blockade of the renin-angiotensin system, and plays a critical role in decreasing the rate of progression of CKD [2]. ACE-Is or ARBs significantly decrease the degree of proteinuria and delay the progression to end stage renal disease in diabetic and non-diabetic nephropathies when compared to both placebo and other antihypertensive therapies [58–61]. Additionally, ACE-Is and ARBs have greater renoprotective effect at higher degrees of baseline proteinuria [59, 60]. Consequently, patients with proteinuria should receive an ACE-I or ARB as first-line therapy [4, 11, 50]. There is no strong evidence to support first-line treatment with ACE-Is or ARBs in non-proteinuric patients with CKD, however experts do generally recommend initial therapy with ACE-Is or ARBs in non-black patients with CKD. Black patients with non-proteinuric kidney disease may be initiated on treatment with a thiazide-type diuretic, calcium channel blocker, ACE-I, or ARB, with second-line addition of an ACE-I or ARB if not used as initial therapy [4, 62].

Aliskiren is a direct renin inhibitor that prevents the conversion of angiotensinogen to angiotensin I. There are limited data on the use of aliskiren in patients with CKD. One small RCT in patients with diabetic nephropathy demonstrated a slight improvement in proteinuria and no improvement in blood pressure when aliskiren was used as an adjunct to ARB therapy [63]. Another, larger scale RCT of combination aliskiren and ARB therapy in patients with diabetic nephropathy was terminated early due to an increased risk of adverse events (including nonfatal stroke, azotemia, hyperkalemia, and hypotension) in the absence of any clear benefit [64]. Accordingly, direct renin inhibition in combination with an ACE-I or ARB is not currently recommended in the management of hypertension in patients with chronic kidney disease [11].

Diuretics

Given the high sensitivity of CKD patients to sodium and water retention, diuretic therapy is a critical component of blood pressure management in these patients [24, 25]. Diuretic therapy augments the antihypertensive and renoprotective effects of ACE-I or ARB therapy [29–31]. Additionally, diuretics can help to attenuate the increased risk of hyperkalemia that occurs as a result of treatment with ACE-Is or ARBs. Patients with CKD require relatively high doses of diuretics due to decreased secretion of diuretics by the renal tubules in the setting of impaired renal function [25]. Although loop diuretics are the mainstay of treatment in patients with advanced CKD (i.e., GFR <30 mL/min/1.73 m^2), multiple small RCTs support the use of thiazide diuretics as monotherapy or in conjunction with loop diuretics in patients with CKD [65, 66]. Thiazides may also decrease peripheral vascular resistance, contributing to greater long-term benefit on blood pressure in addition to the acute improvement in volume expansion [25]. However, thiazide diuretics are overall less effective than loop diuretics in patients with more advanced CKD, likely due to decreased filtered sodium load reaching the distal tubule [67]. Additionally, thiazide diuretics may induce or exacerbate diabetes and hyperlipidemia [68].

Unlike traditional thiazide diuretics, metolazone remains effective in the setting of renal dysfunction [69]. However, the bioavailability of metolazone is unpredictable, and the medication should only be used for short durations of treatment, in combination with loop diuretics, and under close monitoring of serum electrolytes [67]. Observational data in patients with normal renal function demonstrates improved long-term cardiovascular outcomes with thiazide-like diuretics (chlorthalidone) compared to thiazide diuretics (hydrochlorothiazide) [70], though the results are not upheld across all studies [71], and chlorthalidone is more highly associated with hypokalemia and hyponatremia in these patients. No evidence is available comparing the effectiveness of these medications in CKD patients; nonetheless, the increased potency of chlorthalidone is advantageous in the setting of reduced GFR, but the risk of hypokalemia persists [72, 73].

Potassium-Sparing Diuretics and Mineralocorticoid Antagonists

Potassium-sparing diuretics, including triamterene and amiloride, are not typically recommended in patients with CKD due to the added risk of hyperkalemia. Strong evidence supports the use of spironolactone, an aldosterone antagonist, and eplerenone, a mineralocorticoid receptor blocker, as adjunctive therapy in the treatment of resistant hypertension and congestive heart failure in the absence of CKD [25, 74, 75]. Eplerenone is favorable due to the absence of estrogen-like effects, though both medications are thought to be similarly effective. In patients with CKD, several RCTs demonstrate enhanced anti-proteinuric effects of ACE-Is or ARBs when given in combination with mineralocorticoid antagonists [55, 76], though the long-term efficacy of this combination of medications remains unclear. The added benefit of aldosterone antagonism in the treatment of CKD patients is thought to be due to a phenomenon identified as aldosterone escape, which occurs via non-ACE activation of angiotensin II [77]. Additionally, aldosterone is thought to play a role in renal fibrosis, which is attenuated by treatment with an aldosterone antagonist in animal studies [78]. Although many studies demonstrate no increased risk of adverse effects (specifically azotemia or hyperkalemia) from the use of aldosterone antagonists along with ACE-Is or ARBs [76], a meta-analysis suggests greater than twofold increase in relative risk of hyperkalemia with combination therapy [55]. If utilized, combination of aldosterone antagonism and renin-angiotensin system blockade should be handled with caution, including close monitoring of renal function and potassium.

Calcium Channel Blockers

Dihydropyridine calcium channel blockers, including amlodipine and nifedipine, are primarily selective for vascular smooth muscle, resulting in vasodilation. These medications are often associated with the development of peripheral edema. Dihydropyridine calcium channel blockers also primarily act on the afferent glomerular arteriole, resulting in increased albuminuria when used as monotherapy [79]. On the other hand, non-dihydropyridine calcium channel blockers, including diltiazem and verapamil, have a greater effect on the myocardium; these medications confer an increased risk of atrioventricular block or bradycardia, particularly when prescribed in combination with beta blockers [56]. Non-dihydropyridine calcium channel blockers have a vasodilatory effect on both the efferent and afferent glomerular arterioles, resulting in decreased albuminuria. While both subclasses of medications have a similar capacity to lower blood pressure, non-dihydropyridines are preferred in patients with existing albuminuria, particularly if there is a contraindication to concomitant treatment with an ACE-I or ARB [79]. Due to the differential mechanisms of the calcium channel blocker subclasses, potential benefit of combination dihydropyridine and non-dihydropyridine therapy in hypertensive patients has been proposed [80]; however, this has not been studied in CKD patients.

Beta Blockers

Beta blockers are particularly useful in targeting specific cardiac comorbidities in patients with CKD, including cardiovascular disease, congestive heart failure, and tachyarrhythmias. Of note, elimination of atenolol and bisoprolol is highly dependent on renal function, extending their duration of action in patients with renal dysfunction [81]. Metoprolol and carvedilol have the greatest mortality benefit in non-CKD patients with congestive heart failure [81, 82]. Nonetheless, a recent large-scale observational study demonstrated that atenolol was associated with lower 90-day mortality than metoprolol in older patients, including patients with CKD; there was a similar risk of hospitalization for bradycardia or hypotension with both beta blockers, regardless of renal function [83].

Centrally Acting Alpha Agonists

Clonidine, methyldopa, guanfacine, and moxonidine are centrally acting alpha$_2$ agonists that act by decreasing central sympathetic outflow, resulting in vasodilation. While extensive data are not available in CKD patients, alpha$_2$ agonists do not tend to interact with other antihypertensive medications; they can therefore be used as relatively safe adjunctive therapy in CKD patients with resistant hypertension who are already being treated with multiple other medications [50]. Of note, moxonidine is associated with increased mortality in non-CKD patients with advanced heart failure [84]. Significant renal excretion of moxonidine requires dose-reduction in the setting of CKD [85]. Guanfacine, an alpha$_2$ agonist also utilized in the treatment of attention deficit hyperactivity disorder and anxiety, is associated with a higher frequency of sedation, orthostatic hypotension, and sexual dysfunction than the other alpha$_2$ agonists [86].

Alpha Blockers

Alpha$_1$ blockers cause peripheral vasodilation resulting in reduction in blood pressure. Alpha$_1$ blockers may be useful in men who also have symptoms of benign prostatic hyperplasia. However, alpha$_1$ blockers are highly associated with postural hypotension, tachycardia, and increased risk of falls, particularly in the elderly [87].

Additionally, the alpha$_1$ blocker arm of the Antihypertensive and Lipid-Lowering Treatment to Prevent Heart Attack Trial (ALLHAT) was terminated early based on an increased risk of combined cardiovascular events, particularly congestive heart failure, in high-risk hypertensive patients who received an alpha$_1$ blocker as opposed to chlorthalidone [88]. Consequently, alpha$_1$ blockers are not recommended as first-line therapy in CKD patients due to an increased risk of adverse events compared to other antihypertensive agents.

Direct Vasodilators

Hydralazine and minoxidil have a direct vasodilatory effect on vascular smooth muscle, resulting in a reduction in blood pressure. Given its short duration of action and need for frequent dosing, hydralazine is not generally recommended in the treatment of chronic hypertension in patients with CKD [50]. Minoxidil may have a role in the treatment of CKD patients with highly resistant hypertension, however it is often poorly tolerated due to a considerable range of side effects, including hirsutism, pericardial effusion, severe volume expansion, and potentially myocardial ischemia. Minoxidil should only be administered along with a high dose diuretic and beta blocker, in order to limit adverse events [50, 57].

Pseudo-Resistant Hypertension in CKD

CKD patients frequently require complex antihypertensive regimens, resulting in a high pill-burden. Poor adherence is a common issue in these patients, and may result in misperceived resistance to medication. As a result, patients may be prescribed a greater number of medications, at higher doses than indicated by their degree of hypertension, increasing the risk of hypotension and other adverse effects when they do take their medications. Pill counting and monitoring of prescription renewals may provide clues into the occurrence of this phenomenon, but are suboptimal options in the usual treatment setting. Ambulatory blood pressure monitoring can be particularly helpful in the identification of these patients [89]. Additionally, providing empathy and carefully interviewing patients can shed light on specific barriers to appropriate use of medications, such as financial restraints, insufficient motivation, poor understanding of the benefits of medications, adverse effects, and high pill-burden [23]. Prescribers are encouraged to educate patients accordingly, and to employ strategies to try to help minimize pill-burden and maximize patient adherence. Examples of potential approaches include the use of less expensive or generic medications, as well as carefully coordinated and decreased frequency of dosing when possible, including the use of combination pills [11, 23, 89, 90].

References

1. Rao MV, Qiu Y, Wang C, Bakris G. Hypertension and CKD: Kidney Early Evaluation Program (KEEP) and National Health and Nutrition Examination Survey (NHANES), 1999-2004. Am J Kidney Dis. 2008;51(4 Suppl 2):S30–7.
2. Pohl MA, Blumenthal S, Cordonnier DJ, De Alvaro F, Deferrari G, Eisner G, et al. Independent and additive impact of blood pressure control and angiotensin II receptor blockade on renal outcomes in the irbesartan diabetic nephropathy trial: clinical implications and limitations. J Am Soc Nephrol. 2005;16(10):3027–37.
3. Chronic Kidney Disease Prognosis Consortium, Matsushita K, van der Velde M, Astor BC, Woodward M, Levey AS, et al. Association of estimated glomerular filtration rate and albuminuria with all-cause and cardiovascular mortality in general population cohorts: a collaborative meta-analysis. Lancet. 2010;375(9731):2073–81.
4. James PA, Oparil S, Carter BL, Cushman WC, Dennison-Himmelfarb C, Handler J, et al. 2014 evidence-based guideline for the management of high blood pressure in adults: report from the panel members appointed to the Eighth Joint National Committee (JNC 8). JAMA. 2014;311(5):507–20.
5. Beckett NS, Peters R, Fletcher AE, Staessen JA, Liu L, Dumitrascu D, et al. Treatment of hypertension in patients 80 years of age or older. N Engl J Med. 2008;358(18):1887–98.
6. JATOS Study Group. Principal results of the Japanese trial to assess optimal systolic blood pressure in elderly hypertensive patients (JATOS). Hypertens Res. 2008;31(12):2115–27.
7. SHEP Cooperative Study Group. Prevention of stroke by antihypertensive drug treatment in older persons with isolated systolic hypertension. Final results of the Systolic Hypertension in the Elderly Program (SHEP). SHEP Cooperative Research Group. JAMA. 1991;265(24):3255–64.
8. Klahr S, Levey AS, Beck GJ, Caggiula AW, Hunsicker L, Kusek JW, et al. The effects of dietary protein restriction and blood-pressure control on the progression of chronic renal disease. Modification of Diet in Renal Disease Study Group. N Engl J Med. 1994;330(13):877–84.
9. Ruggenenti P, Perna A, Loriga G, Ganeva M, Ene-Iordache B, Turturro M, et al. Blood-pressure control for renoprotection in patients with non-diabetic chronic renal disease (REIN-2): multicentre, randomised controlled trial. Lancet. 2005;365(9463):939–46.
10. Wright Jr JT, Bakris G, Greene T, Agodoa LY, Appel LJ, Charleston J, et al. Effect of blood pressure lowering and antihypertensive drug class on progression of hypertensive kidney disease: results from the AASK trial. JAMA. 2002;288(19):2421–31.
11. KDIGO Clinical practice guideline for the management of blood pressure in chronic kidney disease. Kidney Int Suppl. 2012;2(5):337–414.
12. Somes GW, Pahor M, Shorr RI, Cushman WC, Applegate WB. The role of diastolic blood pressure when treating isolated systolic hypertension. Arch Intern Med. 1999;159(17):2004–9.
13. Oates DJ, Berlowitz DR, Glickman ME, Silliman RA, Borzecki AM. Blood pressure and survival in the oldest old. J Am Geriatr Soc. 2007;55(3):383–8.
14. Protogerou AD, Safar ME, Iaria P, Safar H, Le Dudal K, Filipovsky J, et al. Diastolic blood pressure and mortality in the elderly with cardiovascular disease. Hypertension. 2007;50(1):172–80.
15. Acelajado MC, Oparil S. Hypertension in the elderly. Clin Geriatr Med. 2009;25(3):391–412.
16. Lewis JB. Blood pressure control in chronic kidney disease: is less really more? J Am Soc Nephrol. 2010;21(7):1086–92.
17. Agarwal R, Andersen MJ. Prognostic importance of ambulatory blood pressure recordings in patients with chronic kidney disease. Kidney Int. 2006;69(7):1175–80.
18. Agarwal R, Andersen MJ. Blood pressure recordings within and outside the clinic and cardiovascular events in chronic kidney disease. Am J Nephrol. 2006;26(5):503–10.
19. Graudal N, Jurgens G, Baslund B, Alderman MH. Compared with usual sodium intake, low- and excessive-sodium diets are associated with increased mortality: a meta-analysis. Am J Hypertens. 2014.

20. Pal S, Radavelli-Bagatini S, Ho S. Potential benefits of exercise on blood pressure and vascular function. J Am Soc Hypertens. 2013;7(6):494–506.
21. Chang SH, Stoll CR, Song J, Varela JE, Eagon CJ, Colditz GA. The effectiveness and risks of bariatric surgery: an updated systematic review and meta-analysis, 2003–2012. JAMA Surg. 2014;149(3):275–87.
22. Dickinson HO, Mason JM, Nicolson DJ, Campbell F, Beyer FR, Cook JV, et al. Lifestyle interventions to reduce raised blood pressure: a systematic review of randomized controlled trials. J Hypertens. 2006;24(2):215–33.
23. Chobanian AV, Bakris GL, Black HR, Cushman WC, Green LA, Izzo Jr JL, et al. The Seventh Report of the Joint National Committee on Prevention, Detection, Evaluation, and Treatment of High Blood Pressure: the JNC 7 report. JAMA. 2003;289(19):2560–72.
24. Borst JG, Borst-De Geus A. Hypertension explained by starling's theory of circulatory homoeostasis. Lancet. 1963;1(7283):677–82.
25. Sinnakirouchenan R, Kotchen TA. Role of sodium restriction and diuretic therapy for "resistant" hypertension in chronic kidney disease. Semin Nephrol. 2014;34(5):514–9.
26. De Nicola L, Minutolo R, Bellizzi V, Zoccali C, Cianciaruso B, Andreucci VE, et al. Achievement of target blood pressure levels in chronic kidney disease: a salty question? Am J Kidney Dis. 2004;43(5):782–95.
27. Weir MR, Dengel DR, Behrens MT, Goldberg AP. Salt-induced increases in systolic blood pressure affect renal hemodynamics and proteinuria. Hypertension. 1995;25(6):1339–44.
28. Krikken JA, Laverman GD, Navis G. Benefits of dietary sodium restriction in the management of chronic kidney disease. Curr Opin Nephrol Hypertens. 2009;18(6):531–8.
29. Slagman MC, Waanders F, Hemmelder MH, Woittiez AJ, Janssen WM, Lambers Heerspink HJ, et al. Moderate dietary sodium restriction added to angiotensin converting enzyme inhibition compared with dual blockade in lowering proteinuria and blood pressure: randomised controlled trial. BMJ. 2011;343:d4366.
30. Esnault VL, Ekhlas A, Delcroix C, Moutel MG, Nguyen JM. Diuretic and enhanced sodium restriction results in improved antiproteinuric response to RAS blocking agents. J Am Soc Nephrol. 2005;16(2):474–81.
31. Vogt L, Waanders F, Boomsma F, de Zeeuw D, Navis G. Effects of dietary sodium and hydrochlorothiazide on the antiproteinuric efficacy of losartan. J Am Soc Nephrol. 2008;19(5):999–1007.
32. Strom BL, Yaktine AL, Oria M. Sodium intake in populations: assessment of evidence. Washington: National Academic Press; 2013.
33. Agarwal R. Resistant hypertension and the neglected antihypertensive: sodium restriction. Nephrol Dial Transplant. 2012;27(11):4041–5.
34. Intersalt: an international study of electrolyte excretion and blood pressure. Results for 24 hour urinary sodium and potassium excretion. Intersalt Cooperative Research Group. BMJ. 1988;297(6644):319–28.
35. Mente A, O'Donnell MJ, Rangarajan S, McQueen MJ, Poirier P, Wielgosz A, et al. Association of urinary sodium and potassium excretion with blood pressure. N Engl J Med. 2014;371(7):601–11.
36. Dickinson HO, Nicolson DJ, Campbell F, Beyer FR, Mason J. Potassium supplementation for the management of primary hypertension in adults. Cochrane Database Syst Rev. 2006;3, CD004641.
37. Kotchen TA, McCarron DA. Dietary electrolytes and blood pressure: a statement for healthcare professionals from the American Heart Association Nutrition Committee. Circulation. 1998;98(6):613–7.
38. Heiwe S, Jacobson SH. Exercise training in adults with CKD: a systematic review and meta-analysis. Am J Kidney Dis. 2014;64(3):383–93.
39. Thethi T, Kamiyama M, Kobori H. The link between the renin-angiotensin-aldosterone system and renal injury in obesity and the metabolic syndrome. Curr Hypertens Rep. 2012;14(2):160–9.
40. DeMarco VG, Aroor AR, Sowers JR. The pathophysiology of hypertension in patients with obesity. Nat Rev Endocrinol. 2014;10(6):364–76.

41. Amann K, Benz K. Structural renal changes in obesity and diabetes. Semin Nephrol. 2013;33(1):23–33.
42. Straznicky NE, Grima MT, Lambert EA, Eikelis N, Dawood T, Lambert GW, et al. Exercise augments weight loss induced improvement in renal function in obese metabolic syndrome individuals. J Hypertens. 2011;29(3):553–64.
43. Chagnac A, Weinstein T, Herman M, Hirsh J, Gafter U, Ori Y. The effects of weight loss on renal function in patients with severe obesity. J Am Soc Nephrol. 2003;14(6):1480–6.
44. Navaneethan SD, Yehnert H, Moustarah F, Schreiber MJ, Schauer PR, Beddhu S. Weight loss interventions in chronic kidney disease: a systematic review and meta-analysis. Clin J Am Soc Nephrol. 2009;4(10):1565–74.
45. Jialin W, Yi Z, Weijie Y. Relationship between body mass index and mortality in hemodialysis patients: a meta-analysis. Nephron Clin Pract. 2012;121:102–11.
46. Bonnet F, Deprele C, Sassolas A, Moulin P, Alamartine E, Berthezene F, et al. Excessive body weight as a new independent risk factor for clinical and pathological progression in primary IgA nephritis. Am J Kidney Dis. 2001;37(4):720–7.
47. Takami T, Saito Y. Effects of smoking cessation on central blood pressure and arterial stiffness. Vasc Health Risk Manag. 2011;7:633–8.
48. Minami J, Ishimitsu T, Matsuoka H. Effects of smoking cessation on blood pressure and heart rate variability in habitual smokers. Hypertension. 1999;33(1 Pt 2):586–90.
49. Oncken CA, White WB, Cooney JL, Van Kirk JR, Ahluwalia JS, Giacco S. Impact of smoking cessation on ambulatory blood pressure and heart rate in postmenopausal women. Am J Hypertens. 2001;14(9 Pt 1):942–9.
50. Kidney Disease Outcomes Quality Initiative. K/DOQI clinical practice guidelines on hypertension and antihypertensive agents in chronic kidney disease. Am J Kidney Dis. 2004;43(5 Suppl 1):S1–290.
51. Muntner P, Anderson A, Charleston J, Chen Z, Ford V, Makos G, et al. Hypertension awareness, treatment, and control in adults with CKD: results from the Chronic Renal Insufficiency Cohort (CRIC) Study. Am J Kidney Dis. 2010;55(3):441–51.
52. Foster MC, Rawlings AM, Marrett E, Neff D, Willis K, Inker LA, et al. Cardiovascular risk factor burden, treatment, and control among adults with chronic kidney disease in the United States. Am Heart J. 2013;166(1):150–6.
53. Yusuf S, Teo KK, Pogue J, Dyal L, Copland I, Schumacher H, et al. ONTARGET Investigators. Telmisartan, ramipril, or both in patients at high risk for vascular events. N Engl J Med. 2008;358(15):1547–59.
54. Fried LF, Emanuele N, Zhang JH, Brophy M, Conner TA, Duckworth W, et al. Combined angiotensin inhibition for the treatment of diabetic nephropathy. N Engl J Med. 2013;369(20):1892–903.
55. Navaneethan SD, Nigwekar SU, Sehgal AR, Strippoli GFM. Aldosterone antagonists for preventing the progression of chronic kidney disease: a systematic review and meta-analysis. Clin J Am Soc Nephrol. 2009;4:542–51.
56. DeWitt CR, Waksman JC. Pharmacology, pathophysiology and management of calcium channel blocker and beta-blocker toxicity. Toxicol Rev. 2004;23(4):223–38.
57. Slim HB, Black HR, Thompson PD. Older blood pressure medications-do they still have a place? Am J Cardiol. 2011;108(2):308–16.
58. Kshirsagar AV, Joy MS, Hogan SL, Falk RJ, Colindres RE. Effect of ACE inhibitors in diabetic and nondiabetic chronic renal disease: a systematic overview of randomized placebo-controlled trials. Am J Kidney Dis. 2000;35(4):695–707.
59. Chiurchiu C, Remuzzi G, Ruggenenti P. Angiotensin-converting enzyme inhibition and renal protection in nondiabetic patients: the data of the meta-analyses. J Am Soc Nephrol. 2005;16 Suppl 1:S58–63.
60. Kunz R, Friedrich C, Wolbers M, Mann JF. Meta-analysis: effect of monotherapy and combination therapy with inhibitors of the renin angiotensin system on proteinuria in renal disease. Ann Intern Med. 2008;148(1):30–48.

61. Randomised placebo-controlled trial of effect of ramipril on decline in glomerular filtration rate and risk of terminal renal failure in proteinuric, non-diabetic nephropathy. The GISEN Group (Gruppo Italiano di Studi Epidemiologici in Nefrologia). Lancet. 1997;349(9069): 1857–63.
62. ALLHAT Officers. Major outcomes in high-risk hypertensive patients randomized to angiotensin-converting enzyme inhibitor or calcium channel blocker vs diuretic: The Antihypertensive and Lipid-Lowering Treatment to Prevent Heart Attack Trial (ALLHAT). JAMA. 2002;288(23):2981–97.
63. Parving HH, Persson F, Lewis JB, Lewis EJ, Hollenberg NK, Investigators AS. Aliskiren combined with losartan in type 2 diabetes and nephropathy. N Engl J Med. 2008;358(23):2433–46.
64. McMurray JJ, Abraham WT, Dickstein K, Kober L, Massie BM, Krum H. Aliskiren, ALTITUDE, and the implications for ATMOSPHERE. Eur J Heart Fail. 2012;14(4):341–3.
65. Knauf H, Mutschler E. Diuretic effectiveness of hydrochlorothiazide and furosemide alone and in combination in chronic renal failure. J Cardiovasc Pharmacol. 1995;26(3):394–400.
66. Dussol B, Moussi-Frances J, Morange S, Somma-Delpero C, Mundler O, Berland Y. A randomized trial of furosemide vs hydrochlorothiazide in patients with chronic renal failure and hypertension. Nephrol Dial Transplant. 2005;20(2):349–53.
67. Ernst ME, Moser M. Use of diuretics in patients with hypertension. N Engl J Med. 2009;361(22):2153–64.
68. Salvetti A, Ghiadoni L. Thiazide diuretics in the treatment of hypertension: an update. J Am Soc Nephrol. 2006;17(4 Suppl 2):S25–9.
69. Paton RR, Kane RE. Long-term diuretic therapy with metolazone of renal failure and the nephrotic syndrome. J Clin Pharmacol. 1977;17(4):243–51.
70. Roush GC, Holford TR, Guddati AK. Chlorthalidone compared with hydrochlorothiazide in reducing cardiovascular events: systematic review and network meta-analyses. Hypertension. 2012;59(6):1110–7.
71. Dhalla IA, Gomes T, Yao Z, Nagge J, Persaud N, Hellings C, et al. Chlorthalidone versus hydrochlorothiazide for the treatment of hypertension in older adults: a population-based cohort study. Ann Intern Med. 2013;158(6):447–55.
72. Cirillo M, Marcarelli F, Mele AA, Romano M, Lombardi C, Bilancio G. Parallel-group 8-week study on chlorthalidone effects in hypertensives with low kidney function. Hypertension. 2014;63(4):692–7.
73. Agarwal R, Sinha AD, Pappas MK, Ammous F. Chlorthalidone for poorly controlled hypertension in chronic kidney disease: an interventional pilot study. Am J Nephrol. 2014;39(2):171–82.
74. Gaddam KK, Nishizaka MK, Pratt-Ubunama MN, Pimenta E, Aban I, Oparil S, et al. Characterization of resistant hypertension: association between resistant hypertension, aldosterone, and persistent intravascular volume expansion. Arch Intern Med. 2008;168(11):1159–64.
75. Vaclavik J, Sedlak R, Plachy M, Navratil K, Plasek J, Jarkovsky J, et al. Addition of spironolactone in patients with resistant arterial hypertension (ASPIRANT): a randomized, double-blind, placebo-controlled trial. Hypertension. 2011;57(6):1069–75.
76. Bomback AS, Kshirsagar AV, Amamoo MA, Klemmer PJ. Change in proteinuria after adding aldosterone blockers to ACE inhibitors or angiotensin receptor blockers in CKD: a systematic review. Am J Kidney Dis. 2008;51(2):199–211.
77. Sato A, Saruta T. Aldosterone breakthrough during angiotensin-converting enzyme inhibitor therapy. Am J Hypertens. 2003;16(9 Pt 1):781–8.
78. Fujisawa G, Okada K, Muto S, Fujita N, Itabashi N, Kusano E, et al. Spironolactone prevents early renal injury in streptozotocin-induced diabetic rats. Kidney Int. 2004;66(4):1493–502.
79. Bakris GL, Weir MR, Secic M, Campbell B, Weis-McNulty A. Differential effects of calcium antagonist subclasses on markers of nephropathy progression. Kidney Int. 2004;65(6): 1991–2002.
80. Sica DA. Current concepts of pharmacotherapy in hypertension: combination calcium channel blocker therapy in the treatment of hypertension. J Clin Hypertens (Greenwich). 2001;3(5): 322–7.

81. Frishman WH, Alwarshetty M. Beta-adrenergic blockers in systemic hypertension: pharmacokinetic considerations related to the current guidelines. Clin Pharmacokinet. 2002;41(7):505–16.
82. Badve SV, Roberts MA, Hawley CM, Cass A, Garg AX, Krum H, et al. Effects of beta-adrenergic antagonists in patients with chronic kidney disease: a systematic review and meta-analysis. J Am Coll Cardiol. 2011;58(11):1152–61.
83. Fleet JL, Weir MA, McArthur E, Ozair S, Devereaux PJ, Roberts MA, et al. Kidney function and population-based outcomes of initiating oral atenolol versus metoprolol tartrate in older adults. Am J Kidney Dis. 2014;64(6):883–91.
84. Cohn JN, Pfeffer MA, Rouleau J, Sharpe N, Swedberg K, Straub M, et al. Adverse mortality effect of central sympathetic inhibition with sustained-release moxonidine in patients with heart failure (MOXCON). Eur J Heart Fail. 2003;5(5):659–67.
85. Fenton C, Keating GM, Lyseng-Williamson KA. Moxonidine: a review of its use in essential hypertension. Drugs. 2006;66(4):477–96.
86. Sorkin EM, Heel RC. Guanfacine. A review of its pharmacodynamic and pharmacokinetic properties, and therapeutic efficacy in the treatment of hypertension. Drugs. 1986;31(4):301–36.
87. Hajjar I. Postural blood pressure changes and orthostatic hypotension in the elderly patient: impact of antihypertensive medications. Drugs Aging. 2005;22(1):55–68.
88. Major cardiovascular events in hypertensive patients randomized to doxazosin vs chlorthalidone: the antihypertensive and lipid-lowering treatment to prevent heart attack trial (ALLHAT). ALLHAT Collaborative Research Group. JAMA. 2000;283(15):1967–75.
89. Burnier M, Wuerzner G. Ambulatory blood pressure and adherence monitoring: diagnosing pseudoresistant hypertension. Semin Nephrol. 2014;34(5):498–505.
90. Gupta AK, Arshad S, Poulter NR. Compliance, safety, and effectiveness of fixed-dose combinations of antihypertensive agents: a meta-analysis. Hypertension. 2010;55(2):399–407.

Chapter 11
Genetic Syndromes of Renal Hypertension

Hakan R. Toka

Introduction

As outlined in the other chapters in this book, hypertension is a substantial public health problem affecting at least 25 % of the adult population in industrialized societies and over one billion people worldwide [1]. Hypertension is the major risk factor for cardiovascular morbidity [2] and as an independent risk factor may affect up to ~13 % of all deaths worldwide [3].

Despite the important role of hypertension as a common cause of cardiovascular disease and death, its pathogenesis still remains largely unknown. Extensive investigations over the last century led to the conclusion that hypertension has a multifactorial etiology, including both polygenic and environmental factors. The first physician to address the inheritance of hypertension was Wilhelm Weitz (1881–1969) from the Tubingen University in Germany. Weitz routinely measured blood pressure in all of his clinic patients, noticing that individuals with hypertension (at the time defined as blood pressure >160/110 mmHg) suffered strokes and heart attacks at a higher frequency than his normotensive patients. Weitz also observed that first degree relatives of hypertensives were twice as likely to have elevated blood pressure themselves. He therefore checked blood pressure in entire families including twins, and based on his observations proposed that hypertension is a genetic disorder, inherited in autosomal dominant fashion [4]. More than two decades later, the British physician Robert (Baron) Platt proposed a similar model [5], suggesting bimodal distribution of blood pressure with hypertensive individuals as a distinct subpopulation. In contrast to the theories of Weitz and Platt, Sir George Pickering, another British physician, believed that blood pressure variation follows a Gaussian distribution and that the etiology of hypertension is multifactorial, caused by multiple genes [6].

H.R. Toka, MD, PhD (✉)
Graduate Medical Education, Manatee Memorial Hospital, Bradenton, FL, USA
e-mail: hrtoka@gmail.com

© Springer Science+Business Media New York 2016
A.K. Singh, R. Agarwal (eds.), *Core Concepts in Hypertension in Kidney Disease*, DOI 10.1007/978-1-4939-6436-9_11

Sir Pickering's viewpoint was that blood pressure levels vary continuously, with hypertensives representing the upper end of the Bell curve. Although Platt's model was favored during the 1940s and 1950s, Sir Pickering's view ultimately dominated and has become the basis of today's understanding of hypertension as a cardiovascular disease risk factor, determined by many components, including demographic, dietary, and numerous genetic factors.

The demographic components for hypertension are many, including age, gender, and body mass [7]. Various dietary factors have been implicated, mainly sodium, potassium, and calcium intake [8]. The role of genetic factors on blood pressure was demonstrated by extensive twin studies involving biological versus adopted siblings. Twin studies have made a remarkable contribution, not only to the study of the genetics of hypertension, but also to the inheritance of complex diseases in general, addressing nature (inheritance) versus nurture (environmental) contributions. They clearly demonstrated an inheritable component of blood pressure. Monozygotic twins have by far greater concordance of blood pressure variation than dizygotic twins or biological siblings [9], whose blood pressure values might not differ significantly from adopted siblings [10]. A more recent twin study compared the contribution of genetic influences on blood pressure variation over time, studying $n = 1577$ individuals over nearly three decades (~1/3 identical twins and ~2/3 nonidentical siblings) [11]. The analysis allowed for comparison of the relative contribution of genetic and environmental factors across the first half of the participant's life span, comparing blood pressure levels of twins or siblings at four age ranges (averaging ages ~17, ~32, ~37, and ~44 years). The study analyses demonstrated heritability of blood pressure variation for all age groups (~48–60 % for systolic blood pressure and ~34–67 % for diastolic blood pressure) and that blood pressure levels can be explained by the same genetic factors across time.

In addition to twin studies, demonstrating heritability of hypertension, investigating molecular mechanisms of blood pressure variation has been of great value. The identification of genes with large effects on blood pressure variation helped tremendously to define primary physiologic mechanisms and revealed previously unknown disease mechanisms, leading to development of novel drug therapies. Different approaches have been made to study the molecular basis of blood pressure variation including in vitro and in vivo studies, animal models, and population genetics (genome-wide association studies). The most successful approach, however, has been the investigation of Mendelian (monogenic) forms of arterial hypertension and low blood pressure phenotypes, where single genes have large effects on blood pressure [12]. Many disease-causing mutations and their mechanisms have been identified [13]. In the early 1990s, this was mainly accomplished by studying large pedigrees of individuals with noticeable blood pressure variation in conjunction with advances in genotyping technology and computational (linkage) analysis. Advances in studying polymorphic "microsatellite" markers on a genome-wide level were followed by single nucleotide polymorphism (SNP) technology in the 2000s. An additional approach was candidate gene analysis in conditions that had been previously studied in great detail. In the last decade, new advances in sequencing so-called next generation sequencing technology and computational tools have made it possible to identify additional disease genes in small pedigrees and even in single individuals with "extreme" phenotypes of blood pressure variation [14, 15]. The relevance of recognizing rare disease genes has been substantiated in genetic studies in the general population by showing that rare allelic variation of Mendelian disease genes can have implications for the genetic structure of blood pressure variation in the general population [16].

In the following paragraphs, rare genetic syndromes of hypertension and also renal salt wasting (lower blood pressure) are reviewed, comparing distinct molecular pathways of blood pressure control.

Genetic Syndromes of Renal Hypertension

Enhanced Sodium Reabsorption in the Collecting Duct

Glucocorticoid-Remediable Aldosteronism (Familial Hyperaldosteronism Type 1)

The blood pressure in patients with glucocorticoid-remediable aldosteronism (GRA) is salt-sensitive, increasing with dietary salt intake. Laboratory tests reveal mild hypokalemia and metabolic alkalosis (see Table 11.1). Renin levels are typically low while aldosterone values can be normal or elevated. Patients with this condition are often suspected of having primary hyperaldosteronism. Computerized tomography scanning of the adrenal glands will be negative for (unilateral) adrenal adenomas. Family history of high blood pressure is often positive, suggesting autosomal dominant inheritance. The blood pressure in GRA improves typically with diuretics, including blockers of the epithelial sodium channel (ENaC) in the distal nephron. A distinguishing biochemical feature of GRA is the presence of steroid metabolites, which normally are not present in the urine. Urine testing in affected individuals will be positive for 18-hydroxycortisol and 18-oxocortisol. Recognition of these abnormal steroid products helped recognize the etiology of this condition. Computational analysis of a large kindred with GRA localized the responsible gene to chromosome 8q21. The enzyme 11-β-hydroxylase (encoded by the Cytochrome P450, Family 11, Subfamily B, Polypeptide 1 gene *CYP11B1*), expressed in the zona fasciculata of the adrenal gland, resides within this locus. 11-β-hydroxylase is adrenocorticotropic hormone (ACTH)-responsive and part of the terminal steps of glucocorticoid biosynthesis. "Neighboring" *CYP11B1* on chromosome 8q21 resides the gene for aldosterone synthase (*CYP11B2*), which has a highly similar nucleotide sequence (~95 % identical to *CYB11B1*). Aldosterone synthase plays an important role in the final steps of mineralocorticoid synthesis. In individuals with GRA, a chimeric gene is formed by the unequal crossing over at the chromosomal location 8q21, consisting of the regulatory region of the 11-β-hydroxylase gene and the main structural portion of aldosterone synthase (see Fig. 11.1). The protein of this *CYP11B1/CYP11B2*-chimeric gene performs all of the same actions as aldosterone,

Table 11.1 Inherited forms of hypertension due to enhanced sodium reabsorption in the distal nephron

Syndrome	Mode of inheritance	K^+	Serum pH	Renin	Aldo	Treatment	Gene locus	Disease gene(s)
Glucocorticoid-remediable aldosteronism (GRA)	AD	→	↑	→	N (↑)	Corticosteroid therapy	8q24	Chimeric gene: 11β-hydroxylase/aldosterone synthase
Apparent mineralocorticoid excess (AME)	AR	→	↑	→	→	Spironolactone (ENaC inhibitors)	16q22	11β-hydroxysteroid dehydrogenase
Liddle's	AD	→	↑	→	→	ENaC inhibitors	16p12	ENaC (Epithelial sodium channel)
Mineralocorticoid receptor (MR) activating mutation	AD	→	↑	→	→	ENaC inhibitors	4q31	NR3C2
Aldosterone-producing adrenal adenomas (APA)	de novo[a] de novo de novo de novo	→	↑	→	↑	Spironolactone (adrenal adenomectomy)	11q24 3p21 1p13 Xq28	KCNJ5 CACNA1D ATP1A1 ATP2B3
Congenital Adrenal Hyperplasia (CAH)	AR	→	↑	→	→	Corticosteroid therapy	10q24 8q24	17α-hydroxylase 11β-hydroxylase
Pseudohypoaldosteronism type 2 (PAH II)	AD AR/de novo	↑	→	→	N (↑)	Thiazide diuretics	12p13 17q21 5q31 2q36	WNK1 WNK4 Kelch-like3 Cullin3

AD autosomal dominant; *AR* autosomal recessive; *N* normal; *KCNJ5* K+ inwardly rectifying channel, subfamily J, member 5; *CACNA1D* calcium channel, voltage-dependent, L type, α-1D subunit; *ATP1A1* Na+/K+ ATPase α-1 subunit; *ATP2B3* ATPase, Ca++ transporting, plasma membrane3.

[a]Rarely, can be inherited in Mendelian (autosomal dominant) fashion

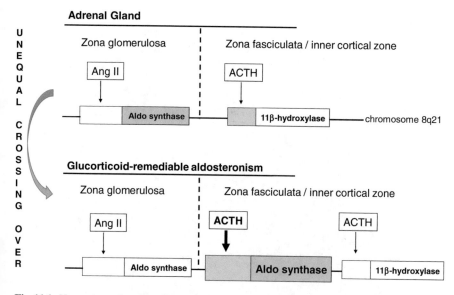

Fig. 11.1 Unequal crossing over of two neighboring genes, encoding for 11β-hydroxylase (*CYP11B1*) and aldosterone synthase (*CYP11B2*), leads to gene fusion/duplication. The resulting chimeric gene consists of the regulatory 5' region of the 11-β-hydroxylase gene and the structural portion of aldosterone synthase gene. The protein of the *CYP11B1/CYP11B2*-chimeric gene performs all of the same actions as aldosterone, however is regulated by ACTH (adrenocorticotropic hormone)

however protein expression is regulated by ACTH and not angiotensin 2. Metabolism of the *CYP11B1/CYP11B2* protein results in unusual urine metabolites mentioned above. Steroid treatment with prednisone ameliorates hypertension in GRA patients by suppressing the adrenal zona fasciculata, giving this condition its name [17, 18].

Apparent Mineralocorticoid Excess

The biochemical presentation of apparent mineralocorticoid excess (AME) is similar to GRA (see Table 11.1). However, in contrary to GRA, urine analysis is negative for abnormal steroid metabolites. Instead, the urinary free cortisol-to-cortisone ratio is abnormally increased (ratio >0.5) in the presence of normal serum cortisol levels. This finding was useful in identifying the disease gene for AME, a condition inherited in autosomal recessive fashion. While the affinity of mineralocorticoid receptors (MR) for aldosterone is higher than that for cortisol, circulating concentrations of cortisol are several orders of magnitude higher than aldosterone. A mechanism that serves to prevent MR activation by cortisol is the activity of 11β-hydroxysteroid dehydrogenase (11-β-HSD), which rapidly oxidizes cortisol to its "inactive" metabolite cortisone. This mechanism facilitates mineralocorticoid pathway regulation of the MR by aldosterone (angiotensin 2). Candidate gene analysis demonstrated that individuals with AME have bi-allelic loss-of-function mutations in the kidney

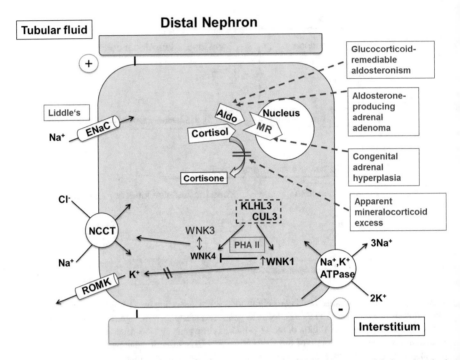

Fig. 11.2 Schematic illustration of one distal tubular epithelial cell, showing several defects (marked in *red*) leading to increased salt reabsorption and hypertension in the distal nephron (distal convoluted tubule or collecting duct). The main mechanism is increased activation of the MR (mineralocorticoid receptor), including a gain-of-function mutation increasing constitutive activity of the receptor. *WNK1* gain-of-function mutations lead to increased suppression of WNK4, which have dual functions, NCCT activation, and ROMK (renal outer medullary potassium channel) suppression. Mutations in *CUL3* (cullin 3) and *KLHL3* (Kelch-like 3), which form an E3 ligase ubiquitination system that regulates substrates WNK1 and WNK4, can also lead to dysregulation of NCCT and ROMK in the distal nephron. *Red double lines* indicate loss-of-function effect on downstream targets. *PHA* pseudohypoaldosteronism, ENaC epithelial sodium channel, NCCT Na/Cl cotransporter

isoform of 11β-hydroxysteroid dehydrogenase (11-β-HSD2), rendering this enzyme incapable of converting cortisol to cortisone (see Fig. 11.2). The hypertension in this condition responds to both spironolactone and ENaC blockers. Individuals ingesting large amounts of licorice or other glycyrrhetinic acid-containing substances (certain liquors, chewing tobaccos, carbenoxolone, etc.) can develop features of AME, because glycyrrhetinic acid inhibits 11-β-HSD2 [19, 20].

Liddle's Syndrome

In 1963, Grant W. Liddle was the first to describe patients with an autosomal dominant form of hypertension associated with hypokalemia, metabolic alkalosis, and low aldosterone level [21]. He speculated that his patients had a genetic defect,

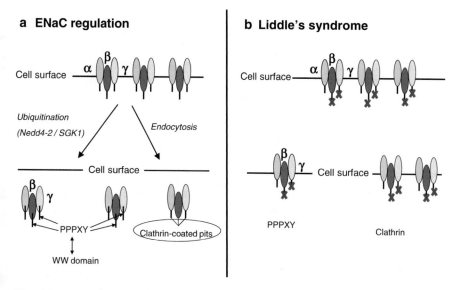

Fig. 11.3 (**a**) ENaC is a heteromeric membrane channel protein consisting of three subunits (α, β, and γ), whose surface expression is regulated by ubiquitination and endocytosis. Proline-rich PY motif (peptide sequence PPPXY) in the cytoplasmic tails of the ENaC subunits interact with tryptophan-rich WW-domains of proteins, such as NEDD4-2, known to ubiquitinate and degrade cell surface proteins. NEDD4-2 is regulated by the aldosterone-induced kinase SKG1 (Serum/Glucocorticoid Regulated Kinase 1). The clathrin-based endocytic machinery plays also a role in internalization of ENaC. (**b**) Missense mutations or deletions in the PY motif of either the β- or the γ-subunit lead to impaired deactivation of ENaC from the cell surface in the distal nephron and increased sodium reabsorption

enhancing sodium reabsorption in the distal tubule segment. Renal transplantation in "Liddle's patients," who developed renal failure, "cured" hypertension, suggesting that the etiology of this condition resided within the kidney. Hypertension in this syndrome was not responsive to spironolactone treatment, suggesting that the molecular defect was downstream of the mineralocorticoid receptor. This hypothesis was supported by significant improvement of hypertension with ENaC blockers [22]. Candidate gene analysis of ENaC identified gain-of-function mutations in two out of three subunits as cause for Liddle's syndrome (see Fig. 11.3). Missense mutations or deletions in the cytoplasmic tails of the β- or the γ-subunit of ENaC, which share ~35 % identity in their amino acid sequences, led to impaired deactivation of the channel from the cell surface in distal nephron epithelial cells [23, 24]. Disease-causing mutations typically occur in a proline-rich PY motif (PPPXY) of the cytoplasmic tails of these subunits, which interact with WW-domains of proteins that are known for ubiquitination and degradation of cell surface proteins, e.g. NEDD4-2 (neural precursor cell-expressed developmentally downregulated gene 4-2). The PY motif of the cytoplasmic tails is also believed to have an important role for endocytosis via clathrin-coated pits [25]. As a consequence, internalization of the ENaC channels is impaired and they remain active on the apical cell surface, leading to increased sodium reabsorption (see Fig. 11.3). This mechanism explains the superb efficacy of ENaC blockers (amiloride, triamterene) in the treatment of this disease (see Table 11.1). Amiloride is the preferred drug due to longer half-life and decreased risk of crystallizing in urine, which can occur transiently with triamterene in acidic urine and in some cases lead to irreversible renal tubular injury [26].

Activating Mutation of the Mineralocorticoid Receptor

Candidate screening of the mineralocorticoid receptor (MR) gene (NR3C2) in patients with features resembling Liddle's syndrome, who were tested negative for ENaC mutations, led to the identification of individuals with NR3C2-activating mutations [27]. The index case had a heterozygous mutation at codon 810 of the MR, resulting in a leucine (L) amino acid substitution for serine (S). All four affected family members carried the same S810L mutation, whereas unaffected members were all negative. The mode of transmission was autosomal dominant (see Table 11.1). Interestingly, affected women in this family exhibited a significant worsening of their hypertension in pregnancy, suggesting that other steroids could act as an agonist of the mutated MR-S810L. Structural protein analysis revealed that mutated MR allowed for activation by steroids lacking the 21-hydroxyl group (e.g., progesterone), which under normal conditions is not possible. Leucine at position 810 within helix 5 of the ligand-binding domain of the MR creates a novel interaction with alanine of MR helix 3. This modification explains why in in vitro studies compounds that are normally antagonists, such as spironolactone, can act as agonists of MR-S810L [27].

Aldosterone-Producing Adrenal Adenomas (Familial Hyperaldosteronism Type III)

Approximately 5–10 % of patients referred for evaluation of secondary hypertension have aldosterone-producing adrenal adenomas (APA) or adrenal hyperplasia [28]. As in GRA and AME, these patients show findings consistent with excessive aldosterone secretion (see Table 11.1). Family history is typically negative. Patients are identified due to hypokalemia and frequently feature a characteristic adrenal mass on computerized tomography. Adrenal vein sampling demonstrates predominant aldosterone secretion from the gland harboring the tumor and is crucial for the diagnosis, allowing to distinguish APA from idiopathic hyperaldosteronism. Surgical removal of the affected adrenal gland ameliorates hypertension in most patients [28]. Exome sequencing performed in 22 adrenal adenoma tissues showed that ~1/3 of all adenomas harbored novel somatic mutations at highly conserved residues (G151R and L168R) of the inwardly rectifying potassium channel KCNJ5

(Kir3.4) [29]. Boulkroun and colleagues screened 380 adrenal tissue from individuals with APA and confirmed that ~1/3 carried the same somatic *KCNJ5* mutations previously identified [30]. *KCNJ5* was further implicated as a rare cause of a Mendelian form of primary aldosteronism in one family (father and both daughters) with familial adrenal adenomas associated with severe hypertension [31]. Mutational analysis revealed a novel germline mutation within a highly conserved residue of *KCNJ5* (T158A). Structural proteomics and in vitro experiments suggest that these rare *KCNJ5* mutations alter Kir3.4 channel function, leading to chronic depolarization of adrenal zona glomerulosa cells and causing constitutive aldosterone production as well as adrenal cell proliferation [32]. Since the discovery of *KCNJ5* as cause for APA, somatic mutations in other genes, all expressed in adrenal glands, have also been recognized. These include somatic gain-of-function mutations in *CACNA1D* [33], encoding a voltage-gated calcium channel [33], loss-of-function mutation in *ATP1A1* [34], encoding the Na/K ATPase α1-subunit, and loss of function in *ATP2B3* [35], encoding a Ca (2+) ATPase. Interestingly, there is a gender discrepancy in the frequency of APA gene mutations; at least twice as many more females than males carry somatic mutations in *KCNJ5* [30], whereas mostly males will have somatic mutations in *ATP1A1* and *ATP2B3* [35].

Congenital Adrenal Hyperplasia

Congenital adrenal hyperplasia (CAH) refers to conditions inherited in autosomal recessive fashion that result from mutations of genes encoding for enzymes mediating biochemical steroidogenesis in the adrenal gland (see Fig. 11.4). In CAH, the adrenal glands secrete excessive or deficient amounts of sex hormones and mineralocorticoids during prenatal development [36]. Poor cortisol production is a hallmark of all CAH types, which are classified into the common, classical (so-called salt-wasting or simple virilizing) CAH, mostly due to 21α-hydroxylase deficiency, and the rare, non-classical forms (<5–10 %), which are associated with hypertension, caused by increased ACTH levels, leading to increased production of mineralocorticoid precursors (11-deoxy corticosterone and corticosterone). Loss-of-function mutations in *CYP11B1* (11β-hydroxylase) and *CYP17A1* (cytochrome P450 17A1; 17α-hydroxylase) are both causes of these rare forms of CAH associated with hypertension [36]. Both cortisol and sex steroids are decreased. Patients typically develop hypertension in childhood due to volume expansion and feature hypokalemia and metabolic alkalosis (see Table 11.1). Treatment with glucocorticoids suppresses ACTH, thereby decreasing mineralocorticoid precursor production and lowering blood pressure [37]. Female virilization (in 11β-hydroxylase deficiency) and ambiguous genitalia in genetic males or failure of the ovaries to function at puberty in genetic females (in 17-α-hydroxylase deficiency) are co-features of CAH.

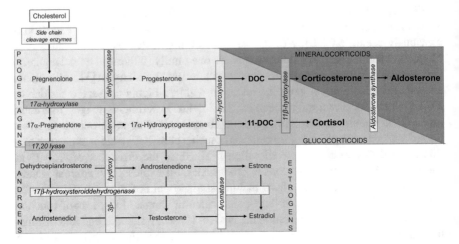

Fig. 11.4 Steroidogenesis. The enzymes affected in congenital adrenal hyperplasia (CAH) are represented by *yellow* (salt-wasting, ~95 % of CAH) or *green bars* (salt-retaining, ~5 % of CAH) in the diagram. Depending upon which enzyme is unavailable, there is increased (21-hydroxylase, 11β-hydroxylase) or decreased production of androgens (3β-HSD, 17α-hydroxylase), shown in the left low corner. Increased production of mainly mineralocorticoid precursors (*upper right*) occurs with bi-allelic loss-of-function mutations in *CYP11B1* (encoding for 11β-hydroxylase) and in *CYP17A1* (encoding for both 17α-hydroxylase and 17,20 lyase)

Pathway of Enhanced Salt Reabsorption in the Distal Convoluted Tubule

Pseudohypoaldosteronism Type 2

Pseudohypoaldosteronism type 2 (PHA II) also known as Gordon's syndrome is a unique form of hypertension syndrome associated with hyperkalemia and metabolic acidosis with mostly autosomal dominant inheritance [38] (see Table 11.1). Hypercalciuria has been reported in some cases, making this syndrome a near mirror image of Gitelman's syndrome [39]. In PHA II, renin activity is typically suppressed and aldosterone levels can be normal or slightly elevated due to hyperkalemia. The hypertension is chloride-dependent because the exchange of bicarbonate or citrate infusions instead of chloride can ameliorate BP elevation [40]. In recent years, several genes have been identified for the etiology of PHA II. Intronic deletions in the With-No-Lysine(K) kinase *WNK1* and missense mutations in *WNK4* have been identified in large pedigrees by computational analysis [41]. Both kinases are expressed in the distal nephron and have been implicated in the regulation of several transporters and channels since their discovery (see Fig. 11.2). The mutation in *WNK1* or *WNK4* leads to increased salt reabsorption in the distal nephron via activation of the Na⁺-Cl⁻ cotransporter (NCCT) regardless of volume status; this results in salt-sensitive hypertension and inhibition of K⁺ excretion despite marked hyperkalemia. The role of NCCT activation in the pathophysiology of PHA II explains why this condition is so susceptible to treatment with thiazide diuretics. Thiazide diuretics are very effective in this syndrome, normalizing all features of this rare condition.

The exact functions of the WNKs are still under investigation; at baseline, WNK1 appears to function as a suppressor of WNK4 by associating with WNK4 in a protein complex involving the kinase domains. In addition to NCCT, WNK4 was also found to regulate the renal outer medullary K$^+$ channel (ROMK) in the DCT [42], explaining why loss of function leads to decreased ROMK activation and hyperkalemia. WNK kinase regulation of NCCT and probably also ENaC contributes to aldosterone's ability to increase sodium reabsorption in the DCT and CCD in response to hypovolemia, and increase potassium excretion in response to hyperkalemia. A WNK kinase cascade (including SPAK-OSR1) is believed to regulate the SGK1/Nedd4-2/ENaC pathway in the cortical collecting duct by still unclear mechanisms, which are being elucidated [43]. Since their discovery, extra-renal WNK kinases have been identified in numerous other tissues, making them a potential drug target not only for blood pressure regulation and potassium handling, but also potential targets for treatment of cystic fibrosis and central nervous system disorders, including autism, epilepsy, and stroke [44].

Recently, two more gene defects for PHA II have been identified by exome sequencing [45]; the study was motivated by the fact that the majority of patients with PHA II were negative for WNK mutations and did not display the usual autosomal dominant inheritance, but suggested a recessive model or de novo occurrence. Novel, protein-altering allelic variants were identified primarily in 2 genes; 24 PHA II index cases revealed novel mutations in the gene *KLHL3* (Kelch-like 3) that were predominantly at positions conserved among orthologs. Amid the remaining index cases of PHA II without mutations in *WNK1*, *WNK4* or *KLHL3*, 17 were identified with novel allelic variants in the gene *CUL3* (Cullin 3). Eight of these mutations were *de novo* and not present in parents. The molecular mechanism of KLHL3 and CUL3 in causing PHA II is not entirely unclear, however both proteins are expressed in the DCT and co-localize with WNK1, WNK4, and NCCT. Cullin3 and KLHL3 form an E3 ligase ubiquitination system and probably regulate WNK1 and WNK4 as substrates. Impaired ubiquitination of NCCT from the luminal cell surface in the DCT has been speculated as mechanism for PHA II in patients with KLHL3 and CUL3 mutations [45].

All PHA II genes lead to increased stability and/or function of NCCT at the cell surface, ultimately resulting in hyperkalemic hypertension associated with metabolic acidosis. However, the phenotype of patients with PHA II varies greatly. Whereas patients with CUL3 defects appear more severely affected as they develop PHA II at younger age, present with more severe hyperkalemia and acidosis, and also failure to thrive, patients with WNK1 mutations often feature only mild hyperkalemia and hypertension occurring at later age. Nevertheless, thiazide diuretics are a very effective treatment for all forms of PHA II, regardless of which gene is defective and the severity of presenting features [39].

Pathways Affecting Autonomic (Sympathetic) Regulation of Blood Pressure

Hereditary Familial Pheochromocytoma

Pheochromocytoma (PCC) is caused by catecholamine-producing adrenal tumors and is associated with various symptoms depending on the type and secretory pattern of the produced catecholamine(s). Hypertension can present as paroxysmal, labile hypertension, complicated by orthostatic hypotension, as well as persistent hypertension. Hypokalemia can often be found, and renin and aldosterone levels can be elevated due to decreased intravascular volume and regulation of renin secretion by the sympathetic nervous system [46]. The frequency of hereditary, familial forms of PCC was reported to be ~25 %. The majority of these are associated with the type II multiple endocrine neoplasia syndrome (MEN II) and caused by gain-of-function mutations in the *RET* proto-oncogene [47]. Besides PCC, MEN II features medullary thyroid cancer (type IIA and IIB), hyperparathyroidism (type IIA), and mucosal neuromas (type IIB). Including *RET*, more than 10 gene defects were associated with PCC. Other examples are neurofibromatosis type 1 (*NF1*), Von Hippel-Lindau disease (*VHL*), and familial extra-adrenal paragangliomas (*SDHB*, *SDHC*, *SDHD*) [47]. The genes encoding for the succinate dehydrogenase subunits B (*SDHB*), C (*SDHB*), and D (*SDHD*) are three of four proteins forming the succinate dehydrogenase protein complex, which participates in the Krebs cycle and the mitochondrial electron chain transport. More recently, a study utilizing exome sequencing from PCC tissues discovered novel, non-silent (amino acid-changing) somatic mutations in genes associated with apoptosis-related pathways. Mutations in one "cancer" gene, lysine (K)-specific methyltransferase 2D (*KMT2D*), were discovered more frequently (~14 %, 14 out of 99 PCC tissues). KMT2D expression was upregulated in PCC tissues compared to normal adrenal gland tissue and KMT2D overexpression positively affected cell migration in vitro. Similar to somatic mutations in *KCJN5*, responsible for ~1/3 of all aldosterone-producing adrenal adenomas, *KMT2D* represents a recurrently mutated gene with potential implication for the development of PCC [48].

The treatment of choice for PCCs is surgical resection of the affected adrenal gland(s) or paraganglioma, respectively. Treatment with irreversible alpha-blockade prior to surgery is mandatory to prevent hypertensive complications [46].

Autosomal Dominant Hypertension Associated with Brachydactyly Type E

The autosomal dominant hypertension syndrome associated with brachydactyly (HBS) was first described in 1973 [49]. Affected family members were short in stature, developed hypertension in childhood, and died often before the age of 50. Short metacarpal bones (brachydactyly type E), cone-shaped epiphysis, and short end-phalanx of the thumb (brachydactyly type B) are found in all affected family members with hypertension [50]. Contrary to previously described syndromes, HBS does typically not feature any associated biochemical abnormalities; blood pressure appears not salt-sensitive. Evaluation of the renin–angiotensin–aldosterone axis, as well as catecholamines, revealed no abnormalities [51]. Diuretics were not found to play a particular role in the treatment of this condition and patients typically require multiple anti-hypertensive medications [52]. Autonomic nervous system testing revealed an abnormal baroreceptor reflex response, resulting in an excessive increase of blood pressure with sympathetic stimuli [53]. Affected individuals have increased sensitivity to the alpha-agonist phenylephrine at baseline compared to controls. This difference is diminished when the baroreceptor reflex is blocked with trimethaphan. All tested affected patients feature neurovascular anomalies at the left ventrolateral medulla oblongata in MRI studies [54]. The gene locus was mapped to chromosome 12p [50], containing a complex chromosomal rearrangement in all affected individuals across all identified families. The significance of this rearrangement is poorly understood [55]. A recent study showed that affected individuals from six different families displayed novel gain-of-function mutations in highly conserved residues of the Phosphodiesterase 3A gene *PDE3A* [56]. In vitro analyses of mesenchymal stem cell-derived vascular smooth muscle cells (VSMCs) and chondrocytes from affected individuals suggest that these mutations increase protein kinase A-mediated PDE3A phosphorylation, increasing cAMP-hydrolytic activity and thereby enhance cell proliferation. The level of phosphorylated VASP (vasodilator-stimulated phosphoprotein) was diminished in VSMCs, suggesting altered vascular smooth muscle cell biology. In addition, PTHrP levels were found to be dysregulated in chondrocytes. Cell-based studies demonstrated that available PDE3A inhibitors suppress these mutant isoforms [57]. Increasing cGMP levels to indirectly inhibit the PDE3A enzyme seemed to be effective in in vitro studies. Although the exact molecular mechanism of PDE3A mutations regulating blood pressure is still being investigated, VSMC-expressed PDE3A could be an interesting new therapeutic target for the treatment of hypertension.

Pathway with Unclear Mechanism: Mitochondrial Gene Mutation Resembling Metabolic Syndrome

Lifton and coworkers described a familial form of hypertension, hypomagnesemia, and hyperlipidemia along the maternal lineage of a large family, indicating mitochondrial inheritance of this novel syndrome [58]. Sequencing of the mitochondrial genome of the maternal lineage identified a homoplasmic mutation substituting cytidine for uridine immediately 5-prime to the mitochondrial tRNA anti-codon for Isoleucin (Ile). In silico analysis showed that uridine at this position is nearly invariant among tRNAs stabilizing the tRNA anti-codon loop. Hypertension, hypomagnesemia, and hypercholesterolemia each showed 50 % penetrance among adults on the maternal lineage. The prevalence of hypertension showed marked age dependence, increasing from 5 % in subjects under age of 30 years to 95 % in those over the age of 50 years. The mechanism of blood pressure elevation in this syndrome is unexplained. In vivo nuclear magnetic resonance (NMR) spectroscopy of skeletal muscle in one affected individual showed decreased ATP production (in the setting of normal Krebs cycle function) [58]. Given the known loss of mitochondrial function with aging due to increased mitochondrial mutations, increased blood pressure could be due to loss of ATP production which has been associated with hypertension in the animal models [58]. Another possibility is the increased presence of reactive oxygen species (ROS) secondary to mitochondrial dysfunction that has also been associated with hypertension [59]. Epidemiological studies have shown that children of hypertensive mothers are more likely to develop hypertension, also suggesting that the mitochondrial genome could be associated with inheriting hypertension [60, 61].

Genetic Syndromes of Decreased Blood Pressure

Pathways of Renal Salt Wasting in the TAL: Bartter's Syndrome

The apical membrane of the thick ascending limb (TAL) of Henle's loop reabsorbs ~25 % to ~35 % of the sodium load filtered in the glomeruli. The main driving force is the luminal Na-K-2Cl co-transporter NKCC2. The chloride imported by NKCC2 exits the basolateral side of TAL epithelial cells via the chloride channel CLCNKB, which has an adjacent β-subunit called Barttin, co-localizing with CLCNKB at the basolateral membrane and regulating its intracellular trafficking and function (see Fig. 11.5). Barttin also serves as β-subunit for a related chloride channel, CLCNKA, in potassium-secreting epithelial cells of the inner ear. The sodium imported from the TAL lumen via NKCC2 leaves the basolateral side of the cell via the Na/K--ATPase. Because chloride carries a negative charge, exit of unaccompanied chloride through basolateral CLCNKB depolarizes the TAL cell. The stoichiometry of the Na/K ATPase, three sodium outward per two potassium inward, partly counters this depolarization, however additional repolarization of the cell is accomplished by the apical potassium channel ROMK (renal outer medullary K channel), which recycles the potassium imported into the cell via NKCC2 back into the lumen. The coordinated operation of these apical and basolateral transporters and channels generates a lumen-positive electrical potential across the TAL (see Fig. 11.4). Reduced function of any one of these transporters or channels, secondary either to pharmacological inhibition (loop diuretics) or genetic mutation, is associated with renal salt-wasting [62]. Patients with loss-of-function mutations in the above transporters or channels feature varying degrees of hypokalemic metabolic alkalosis, hypokalemia, and low(er) BP with elevated renin levels (known as Bartter's syndrome). In addition, hypercalciuria can be seen, mainly in Bartter's types 1, 2, and 5. Five different disease genes were identified for this syndrome, four genes encoding for the proteins mentioned above, and a fifth gene, the Calcium-Sensing Receptor (CASR), in which gain-of-function mutations can lead to a phenocopy of Bartter's syndrome (see Table 11.2).

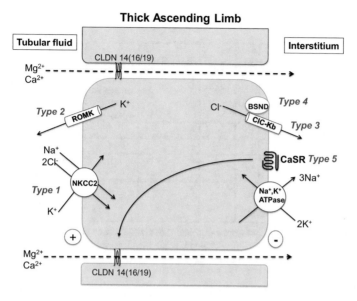

Fig. 11.5 Mutations in five genes expressed in TAL epithelia lead to Bartter's syndrome. NKCC1 and ROMK mutations cause neonatal Bartter's associated with nephrocalcinosis. CLCNKB defects lead to clinically milder type 3 or "classic" Bartter's. BSND mutations (type 4) has similar clinical features, but is associated with sensorineural deafness. Type 5 is caused by CASR gain-of-function mutations, decreasing paracellular transport of calcium and magnesium, thereby altering the electrochemical driving force in the TAL. CASR is believed to increase Claudin 14 activity, which is a negative regulator of the paracellular claudin 16/19 cation channel complex. All defects can lead to renal salt wasting in TAL epithelia associated with low(er) blood pressure. *NKCC2* Na-K-2Cl cotransporter, *ROMK* renal outer medullary K+ channel, *CLCNKB* Chloride Channel, Voltage-Sensitive Kb, *BSND* Barttin, *CASR* calcium-sensing receptor, *CLDN* Claudin

The various types of Bartter's syndrome can differ in disease severity. Neonatal Bartter's syndrome is the most common form (~90 % of all patients) and is typically noticed during pregnancy due to polyhydramnios (excess amniotic fluid). Neonatal infants feature severe polyuria and polydipsia. Life-threatening volume contraction may result if the infant does not receive adequate fluids after birth. The majority of infants are hypercalciuric and will develop nephrocalcinosis, which often progresses to renal failure. Failure to thrive is a typical occurrence in children with neonatal Bartter's, caused either by loss-of-function mutations in *NKCC2* (type 1) or *ROMK* (type 2) [63, 64]. In comparison, type 3 or "classic" Bartter's is caused by loss-of-function mutations in CLCNKB and is usually diagnosed at school age or later, although symptoms of renal salt wasting may occur earlier in life [65]. In classic Bartter's syndrome, increased urinary calcium excretion is significantly milder and kidney stones can develop later in life if at all. Renal function is typically normal, however, progression to end-stage renal disease has been described [66]. Type 4 Bartter's is caused by mutations in Barttin (*BSND*), the accessory β-subunit of the CLCNKB [67]. Since Barttin is also expressed in the inner ear, affected individuals also suffer from sensorineural deafness. Gain-of-function mutations in the *CASR* can feature renal salt wasting and hypercalciuria [68]. Although PTH levels are

Table 11.2 *Bartter's syndrome*: Renal salt-wasting in the thick ascending limb (TAL) associated with hypercalciuria

Syndrome	Inheritance	K$^+$	pH	Renin	Aldosterone	Treatment	Gene Locus	Gene
1	AR	↓	↑	↑	↑	Increase salt intake (for all types)	15q21	*SLC12A1* (NKCC2)
2	AR	↓	↑	↑	↑		11q24	*KCNJ1* (ROMK)
3	AR	↓	↑	↑	↑		1p36	*CLCNKB*
4	AR	↓	↑	↑	↑		1p32	*BSND* (associated with deafness)
5	AD	↓	↑	↑	↑		3q21	*CASR* (also known as Autosomal Dominant Hypocalcemia)

AR autosomal recessive; *AD* autosomal dominant; *SLC12A1* solute carrier family 12, member 1; *KCNJ1* potassium inwardly rectifying channel, subfamily J, member 1; *CLCNKB* chloride channel, voltage-sensitive Kb; *BSND* Barttin; *CASR* calcium-sensing receptor

severely suppressed in this syndrome, which is also known as autosomal dominant hypocalcemia, this condition is classified by some as Bartter's type 5 due to the expression of CASR on the basolateral membrane of TAL epithelia.

Pathways of Renal Salt Wasting in the Distal Nephron

Gitelman's Syndrome

Patients with Gitelman's syndrome present with symptoms identical to those who are on thiazide diuretics. Richard Lifton and colleagues performed linkage analysis in several unrelated families with Gitelman's syndrome and identified the locus for the thiazide-sensitive NCCT gene (*SLC12A3*). Several homozygous or compound heterozygous loss-of-function mutations in *SLC12A3* were identified [69], which inactivate NCCT expressed in the apical membrane of DCT epithelia. The clinical symptoms include hypochloremic metabolic alkalosis, hypokalemia, hypomagnesemia, and hypocalciuria (see Table 11.3). Affected individuals are typically asymptomatic, however muscular cramps, weakness/fatigue, and irritability have been described. More severe symptoms such as tetany and paralysis are rare. Individuals with heterozygous loss-of-function mutations in NCCT may have a survival benefit due to lower BP and increased bone mineral density [16, 70].

Pseudohypoladosteronism Type 1 (PHA I)

PHA I is characterized by salt wasting resulting from renal unresponsiveness to mineralocorticoids [71, 72]. Patients may present with neonatal renal salt wasting with hyperkalemic acidosis despite high aldosterone levels (see Table 11.3). Two genetic subtypes can be distinguished, type I A, which is inherited in an autosomal dominant fashion, and type I B, which is transmitted in an autosomal recessive pattern. PHA I A is caused by mutations in the MR gene and is typically milder than PHA I B [71]. Patients improve with age and usually become asymptomatic without treatment when they reach adulthood. Some adult patients are found to have elevated aldosterone levels, however, they lack a history of the disease. This observation suggested that only those infants whose salt homeostasis is "stressed" by intercurrent illness and volume depletion develop clinically recognized PHA I. The recessive form, PHA 1B, is caused by loss-of-function mutations in any one of the three genes encoding for the α-, β-, or γ-subunits of ENaC leading to decreased channel activity and renal salt wasting (see Fig. 11.3) [72]. Patients with this form can feature a severe systemic disorder starting in infancy and persisting into adulthood.

Epilepsy, Ataxia, Sensorineural Deafness, and (Salt-Wasting) Tubulopathy (EAST Syndrome)

EAST also known as SeSAME (Seizures, Sensorineural deafness, Ataxia, Mental retardation, and Electrolyte imbalance) syndrome features renal salt wasting and electrolyte imbalance, and added considerable new insight into renal electrolyte handling in the distal nephron [73, 74]. The mode of inheritance is autosomal recessive and consanguinity has been described in some families. The responsible gene *KCNJ10*, identified by linkage analysis, encodes for the potassium channel Kir4.1, expressed in the basolateral membranes of distal convoluted tubule (DCT), connecting tubule (CNT), and collecting duct epithelia. The identified electrolyte and acid base abnormalities are similar to the one seen in Gitelman's syndrome, including hypokalemia, hypomagnesemia, and metabolic alkalosis (see Table 11.3). Renin and aldosterone levels are elevated. Patients typically have normal blood pressure values but still crave salt, suggesting that they compensate for renal salt losses with increased consumption of salt, thereby maintaining normal blood pressure values [73]. In vitro studies suggest that loss-of-function mutations in *KCNJ10* impair the activity of the Na/K-ATPase, which is also located at the basolateral membrane of epithelia of the same nephron segments. Loss of Kir4.1 function probably impairs potassium cycling at the basolateral membrane and thereby inhibits the Na/K-ATPase function and sodium reabsorption [74]. The additional features seen in this syndrome are due to expression of Kir4.1 in neuronal tissue and in cells of the inner ear. *KCNJ10*-deficient mice exhibit striking pathology of the entire central nervous system and display renal salt wasting and volume contraction [75].

Severe Hypotension Due to Renal Tubular Dysgenesis (RTD)

Autosomal recessive RTD is a severe developmental disorder of abnormal renal tubular formation associated with persistent fetal oligoanuria and frequently in utero or perinatal death [76]. Parental consanguinity is present in ~1/3 of all reported

Table 11.3 Renal salt-wasting syndromes associated with lower blood pressure caused by defects in the distal nephron

Syndrome	Inheritance	K⁺	pH	Renin	Aldosterone	Treatment	Gene Locus	Gene
Gitelman	AR	↓	↑	↑	↑	Increase salt intake	16q13	SLC12A3 (NCCT)
EAST (SeSAME)	AR	↓	↑	↑	↑	Increase salt intake	1q23	KCNJ10 (Kir4.1)
Pseudohypoaldosteronism type 1 (PHA I)	AD AR AR AR	↑	↓	↑	↑	Increase salt intake	4q31 12p13 16p13 16p13	NR3C2 (type 1A) SCNN1A (type 1B) SCNN1B (type 1B) SCNN1G (type 1B)
Renal Tubular Dysgenesis (RTD)	AR	↑	↓	↑ or ↓	↓	Vasopressors	1q32 1q42 3q24 17q23	REN AGT ACE AGT1R

AR autosomal recessive; *AD* autosomal dominant; *EAST* Epilepsy, Ataxia, Sensorineural deafness, Tubulopathy; *SeSAME* Seizures, Sensorineural deafness, Ataxia, Mental retardation, and Electrolyte imbalance; *Kir 4.1* inward rectifier-type K⁺-channel, member 4.1; *NR3C2* nuclear receptor subfamily 3, group C, member 2; *SCNN1A, 1B or 1C* sodium channel, non-voltage-gated 1, α-subunit, β-subunit or γ-subunit (genes encoding for ENaC subunits); *REN* renin; *AGT* angiotensinogen; *ACE* angiotensin-converting-enzyme; *AGT* angiotensin 2 type 1 receptor families [77]. Surviving newborn infants display severe and refractory hypotension requiring vasopressors, and typically need in addition respiratory assistance and dialysis after birth. Death likely occurs due to pulmonary hypoplasia and respiratory failure from early-onset oligohydramnios (Potter sequence). Only few individuals with RTD survived after days or weeks of intensive care [77]. Absence or paucity of differentiated proximal tubules is the histopathologic hallmark of this disorder, which is often associated with postnatal skull ossification defects (hypocalvaria). In RTD, all tubules appear abnormally developed, primitive and reminiscent of collecting tubules. RTD can also be found in children of women using angiotensin-converting-enzyme inhibitors (ACEi) during pregnancy. Hypocalvaria is also present in this acquired (secondary) form of RTD, also known as ACEi fetopathy [78]. The genetic forms of RTD are caused by loss-of-function mutations in four genes encoding for proteins of the renin–angiotensin system (RAS). The genes shown in Table 11.2 include REN (renin), AGT (angiotensinogen), ACE, and AGT1R (angiotensin II receptor type 1). No correlation could be established between clinical course of disease and the type of mutations in 160 RTD cases [77].

Conclusion

The lessons learned from rare, inherited syndromes of blood pressure variation have been profound. They have led us to understand the primary physiology of blood pressure regulation and taught us disease mechanisms, which can lead to arterial hypertension, lower blood pressure, and associated disturbances of electrolyte and acid base homeostasis. Some of the genes discussed in this chapter (NCCT, NKCC2, and ROMK) were screened in participants of the Framingham Heart Study (FHS) population; rare, functional allelic variations were identified and associated with decreased blood pressure, based on comparative genomics, genetics, and biochemistry [16]. It is likely that the combined effects of rare independent mutations may account for a substantial fraction of blood pressure variation in the general population. The study of these rare conditions continues to be of great importance, helping us to improve our understanding of hypertension, its treatment and prevention.

References

1. Kearney PM, Whelton M, Reynolds K, Muntner P, Whelton PK, He J. Global burden of hypertension: analysis of worldwide data. Lancet. 2005;365(9455):217–23. Epub 2005/01/18.
2. Mosterd A, D'Agostino RB, Silbershatz H, Sytkowski PA, Kannel WB, Grobbee DE, et al. Trends in the prevalence of hypertension, antihypertensive therapy, and left ventricular hypertrophy from 1950 to 1989. N Engl J Med. 1999;340(16):1221–7. Epub 1999/04/22.
3. WHO. Global health risks: mortality and burden of disease attributable to selected major risks. WHO Library Cataloguing-in-Publication Data. 2009.
4. Weitz W. Zur Ätiologie der genuinen Hypertonie. Klin Med. 1923;96:151.

5. Platt R. Heredity in hypertension. Q J Med. 1947;16(3):111–33. Epub 1947/07/01.
6. Pickering GW. The genetic factor in essential hypertension. Ann Intern Med. 1955;43(3): 457–64. Epub 1955/09/01.
7. Stanton JL, Braitman LE, Riley Jr AM, Khoo CS, Smith JL. Demographic, dietary, life style, and anthropometric correlates of blood pressure. Hypertension. 1982;4(5 Pt 2):III135–42. Epub 1982/09/01.
8. Appel LJ, Moore TJ, Obarzanek E, Vollmer WM, Svetkey LP, Sacks FM, et al. A clinical trial of the effects of dietary patterns on blood pressure. DASH Collaborative Research Group. N Engl J Med. 1997;336(16):1117–24. Epub 1997/04/17.
9. Feinleib M, Garrison RJ, Fabsitz R, Christian JC, Hrubec Z, Borhani NO, et al. The NHLBI twin study of cardiovascular disease risk factors: methodology and summary of results. Am J Epidemiol. 1977;106(4):284–5. Epub 1977/10/01.
10. Rice T, Vogler GP, Perusse L, Bouchard C, Rao DC. Cardiovascular risk factors in a French Canadian population: resolution of genetic and familial environmental effects on blood pressure using twins, adoptees, and extensive information on environmental correlates. Genet Epidemiol. 1989;6(5):571–88. Epub 1989/01/01.
11. Hottenga JJ, Boomsma DI, Kupper N, Posthuma D, Snieder H, Willemsen G, et al. Heritability and stability of resting blood pressure. Twin Res Hum Genet. 2005;8(5):499–508. Epub 2005/10/11.
12. Lifton RP, Gharavi AG, Geller DS. Molecular mechanisms of human hypertension. Cell. 2001;104(4):545–56. Epub 2001/03/10.
13. Toka HR, Luft FC. Monogenic forms of human hypertension. Semin Nephrol. 2002;22(2):81–8. Epub 2002/03/14.
14. Bockenhauer D, Medlar AJ, Ashton E, Kleta R, Lench N. Genetic testing in renal disease. Pediatr Nephrol. Epub 2011/05/28.
15. Bailey-Wilson JE, Wilson AF. Linkage analysis in the next-generation sequencing era. Hum Hered. 72(4):228–36. Epub 2011/12/23.
16. Ji W, Foo JN, O'Roak BJ, Zhao H, Larson MG, Simon DB, et al. Rare independent mutations in renal salt handling genes contribute to blood pressure variation. Nat Genet. 2008;40(5):592–9. Epub 2008/04/09.
17. Lifton RP, Dluhy RG, Powers M, Rich GM, Cook S, Ulick S, et al. A chimaeric 11 beta-hydroxylase/aldosterone synthase gene causes glucocorticoid-remediable aldosteronism and human hypertension. Nature. 1992;355(6357):262–5. Epub 1992/01/16.
18. Lifton RP, Dluhy RG, Powers M, Rich GM, Gutkin M, Fallo F, et al. Hereditary hypertension caused by chimaeric gene duplications and ectopic expression of aldosterone synthase. Nat Genet. 1992;2(1):66–74. Epub 1992/09/11.
19. Mune T, Rogerson FM, Nikkila H, Agarwal AK, White PC. Human hypertension caused by mutations in the kidney isozyme of 11 beta-hydroxysteroid dehydrogenase. Nat Genet. 1995;10(4):394–9. Epub 1995/08/01.
20. White PC, Mune T, Agarwal AK. 11 beta-Hydroxysteroid dehydrogenase and the syndrome of apparent mineralocorticoid excess. Endocr Rev. 1997;18(1):135–56. Epub 1997/02/01.
21. Liddle GW, Bledsoe T, Coppage Jr WS. A familial renal disorder stimulating primary aldosteronism but with negligible aldosterone secretion. Trans Assoc Am Phys. 1963;76:199–213.
22. Botero-Velez M, Curtis JJ, Warnock DG. Brief report: Liddle's syndrome revisited–a disorder of sodium reabsorption in the distal tubule. N Engl J Med. 1994;330(3):178–81. Epub 1994/01/20.
23. Shimkets RA, Warnock DG, Bositis CM, Nelson-Williams C, Hansson JH, Schambelan M, et al. Liddle's syndrome: heritable human hypertension caused by mutations in the beta subunit of the epithelial sodium channel. Cell. 1994;79(3):407–14. Epub 1994/11/04.
24. Hansson JH, Nelson-Williams C, Suzuki H, Schild L, Shimkets R, Lu Y, et al. Hypertension caused by a truncated epithelial sodium channel gamma subunit: genetic heterogeneity of Liddle syndrome. Nat Genet. 1995;11(1):76–82. Epub 1995/09/01.
25. Rotin D, Kanelis V, Schild L. Trafficking and cell surface stability of ENaC. Am J Physiol Renal Physiol. 2001;281(3):F391–9. Epub 2001/08/15.

26. Roy LF, Villeneuve JP, Dumont A, Dufresne LR, Duran MA, Morin C, et al. Irreversible renal failure associated with triamterene. Am J Nephrol. 1991;11(6):486–8. Epub 1991/01/01.
27. Geller DS, Farhi A, Pinkerton N, Fradley M, Moritz M, Spitzer A, et al. Activating mineralocorticoid receptor mutation in hypertension exacerbated by pregnancy. Science. 2000;289(5476):119–23. Epub 2000/07/07.
28. Rossi GP, Bernini G, Caliumi C, Desideri G, Fabris B, Ferri C, et al. A prospective study of the prevalence of primary aldosteronism in 1,125 hypertensive patients. J Am Coll Cardiol. 2006;48(11):2293–300. Epub 2006/12/13.
29. Choi M, Scholl UI, Yue P, Bjorklund P, Zhao B, Nelson-Williams C, et al. K+ channel mutations in adrenal aldosterone-producing adenomas and hereditary hypertension. Science. 2011;331(6018):768–72. Epub 2011/02/12.
30. Boulkroun S, Beuschlein F, Rossi GP, Golib-Dzib JF, Fischer E, Amar L, et al. Prevalence, clinical, and molecular correlates of KCNJ5 mutations in primary aldosteronism. Hypertension. 2012;59(3):592–8. Epub 2012/01/26.
31. Geller DS, Zhang J, Wisgerhof MV, Shackleton C, Kashgarian M, Lifton RP. A novel form of human mendelian hypertension featuring nonglucocorticoid-remediable aldosteronism. J Clin Endocrinol Metab. 2008;93(8):3117–23. Epub 2008/05/29.
32. Scholl UI, Nelson-Williams C, Yue P, Grekin R, Wyatt RJ, Dillon MJ, et al. Hypertension with or without adrenal hyperplasia due to different inherited mutations in the potassium channel KCNJ5. Proc Natl Acad Sci U S A. 2012;109(7):2533–8. Epub 2012/02/07.
33. Scholl UI, Goh G, Stolting G, de Oliveira RC, Choi M, Overton JD, et al. Somatic and germline CACNA1D calcium channel mutations in aldosterone-producing adenomas and primary aldosteronism. Nat Genet. 2013;45(9):1050–4. Epub 2013/08/06.
34. Azizan EA, Poulsen H, Tuluc P, Zhou J, Clausen MV, Lieb A, et al. Somatic mutations in ATP1A1 and CACNA1D underlie a common subtype of adrenal hypertension. Nat Genet. 2013;45(9):1055–60. Epub 2013/08/06.
35. Beuschlein F, Boulkroun S, Osswald A, Wieland T, Nielsen HN, Lichtenauer UD, et al. Somatic mutations in ATP1A1 and ATP2B3 lead to aldosterone-producing adenomas and secondary hypertension. Nat Genet. 2013;45(4):440–4, 4e1–2. Epub 2013/02/19.
36. Speiser PW, White PC. Congenital adrenal hyperplasia. N Engl J Med. 2003;349(8):776–88. Epub 2003/08/22.
37. Speiser PW. Medical treatment of classic and nonclassic congenital adrenal hyperplasia. Adv Exp Med Biol. 2011;707:41–5. Epub 2011/06/22.
38. Gordon RD, Geddes RA, Pawsey CG, O'Halloran MW. Hypertension and severe hyperkalaemia associated with suppression of renin and aldosterone and completely reversed by dietary sodium restriction. Australas Ann Med. 1970;19(4):287–94. Epub 1970/11/01.
39. Mayan H, Vered I, Mouallem M, Tzadok-Witkon M, Pauzner R, Farfel Z. Pseudohypoaldosteronism type II: marked sensitivity to thiazides, hypercalciuria, normomagnesemia, and low bone mineral density. J Clin Endocrinol Metab. 2002;87(7):3248–54. Epub 2002/07/11.
40. Schambelan M, Sebastian A, Rector Jr FC. Mineralocorticoid-resistant renal hyperkalemia without salt wasting (type II pseudohypoaldosteronism): role of increased renal chloride reabsorption. Kidney Int. 1981;19(5):716–27. Epub 1981/05/01.
41. Wilson FH, Disse-Nicodeme S, Choate KA, Ishikawa K, Nelson-Williams C, Desitter I, et al. Human hypertension caused by mutations in WNK kinases. Science. 2001;293(5532):1107–12. Epub 2001/08/11.
42. Kahle KT, Wilson FH, Lalioti M, Toka H, Qin H, Lifton RP. WNK kinases: molecular regulators of integrated epithelial ion transport. Curr Opin Nephrol Hypertens. 2004;13(5):557–62. Epub 2004/08/10.
43. Rotin D, Staub O. Nedd4-2 and the regulation of epithelial sodium transport. Front Physiol. 2012;3:212. Epub 2012/06/28.
44. Alessi DR, Zhang J, Khanna A, Hochdorfer T, Shang Y, Kahle KT. The WNK-SPAK/OSR1 pathway: master regulator of cation-chloride cotransporters. Science signaling. 2014;7(334):re3. Epub 2014/07/17.

45. Boyden LM, Choi M, Choate KA, Nelson-Williams CJ, Farhi A, Toka HR, et al. Mutations in kelch-like 3 and cullin 3 cause hypertension and electrolyte abnormalities. Nature. 2012;482(7383):98–102. Epub 2012/01/24.
46. Pacak K, Linehan WM, Eisenhofer G, Walther MM, Goldstein DS. Recent advances in genetics, diagnosis, localization, and treatment of pheochromocytoma. Ann Intern Med. 2001;134(4):315–29. Epub 2001/02/22.
47. Tischler AS. Molecular and cellular biology of pheochromocytomas and extra-adrenal paragangliomas. Endocr Pathol. 2006;17(4):321–8. Epub 2007/05/26.
48. Juhlin CC, Stenman A, Haglund F, Clark VE, Brown TC, Baranoski J, et al. Whole-exome sequencing defines the mutational landscape of pheochromocytoma and identifies KMT2D as a recurrently mutated gene. Genes Chromosomes Cancer. 2015;54(9):542–54. Epub 2015/06/03.
49. Bilginturan N, Zileli S, Karacadag S, Pirnar T. Hereditary brachydactyly associated with hypertension. J Med Genet. 1973;10:253–9.
50. Toka HR, Bahring S, Chitayat D, Melby JC, Whitehead R, Jeschke E, et al. Families with autosomal dominant brachydactyly type E, short stature, and severe hypertension. Ann Intern Med. 1998;129(3):204–8. Epub 1998/08/08.
51. Schuster H, Wienker TF, Toka HR, Bahring S, Jeschke E, Toka O, et al. Autosomal dominant hypertension and brachydactyly in a Turkish kindred resembles essential hypertension. Hypertension. 1996;28(6):1085–92. Epub 1996/12/01.
52. Schuster H, Toka O, Toka HR, Busjahn A, Oztekin O, Wienker TF, et al. A cross-over medication trial for patients with autosomal-dominant hypertension with brachydactyly. Kidney Int. 1998;53(1):167–72. Epub 1998/02/07.
53. Jordan J, Toka HR, Heusser K, Toka O, Shannon JR, Tank J, et al. Severely impaired baroreflex-buffering in patients with monogenic hypertension and neurovascular contact. Circulation. 2000;102(21):2611–8. Epub 2000/11/22.
54. Naraghi R, Schuster H, Toka HR, Bahring S, Toka O, Oztekin O, et al. Neurovascular compression at the ventrolateral medulla in autosomal dominant hypertension and brachydactyly. Stroke. 1997;28(9):1749–54. Epub 1997/09/26.
55. Bahring S, Kann M, Neuenfeld Y, Gong M, Chitayat D, Toka HR, et al. Inversion region for hypertension and brachydactyly on chromosome 12p features multiple splicing and noncoding RNA. Hypertension. 2008;51(2):426–31. Epub 2007/12/19.
56. Maass PG, Aydin A, Luft FC, Schachterle C, Weise A, Stricker S, et al. PDE3A mutations cause autosomal dominant hypertension with brachydactyly. Nat Genet. 2015;47(6):647–53. Epub 2015/05/12.
57. Toka O, Tank J, Schachterle C, Aydin A, Maass PG, Elitok S, et al. Clinical effects of phosphodiesterase 3A mutations in inherited hypertension with brachydactyly. Hypertension. 2015;66(4):800–8. Epub 2015/08/19.
58. Wilson FH, Hariri A, Farhi A, Zhao H, Petersen KF, Toka HR, et al. A cluster of metabolic defects caused by mutation in a mitochondrial tRNA. Science. 2004;306(5699):1190–4. Epub 2004/10/23.
59. Mori T, Ogawa S, Cowely Jr AW, Ito S. Role of renal medullary oxidative and/or carbonyl stress in salt-sensitive hypertension and diabetes. Clin Exp Pharmacol Physiol. 2012;39(1):125–31. Epub 2011/12/14.
60. Yang Q, Kim SK, Sun F, Cui J, Larson MG, Vasan RS, et al. Maternal influence on blood pressure suggests involvement of mitochondrial DNA in the pathogenesis of hypertension: the Framingham Heart Study. J Hypertens. 2007;25(10):2067–73. Epub 2007/09/22.
61. DeStefano AL, Gavras H, Heard-Costa N, Bursztyn M, Manolis A, Farrer LA, et al. Maternal component in the familial aggregation of hypertension. Clin Genet. 2001;60(1):13–21. Epub 2001/09/05.
62. Hebert SC. Bartter syndrome. Curr Opin Nephrol Hypertens. 2003;12(5):527–32. Epub 2003/08/16.
63. Simon DB, Karet FE, Hamdan JM, DiPietro A, Sanjad SA, Lifton RP. Bartter's syndrome, hypokalaemic alkalosis with hypercalciuria, is caused by mutations in the Na-K-2Cl cotransporter NKCC2. Nat Genet. 1996;13(2):183–8. Epub 1996/06/01.

64. Simon DB, Karet FE, Rodriguez-Soriano J, Hamdan JH, DiPietro A, Trachtman H, et al. Genetic heterogeneity of Bartter's syndrome revealed by mutations in the K+ channel, ROMK. Nat Genet. 1996;14(2):152–6. Epub 1996/10/01.
65. Simon DB, Bindra RS, Mansfield TA, Nelson-Williams C, Mendonca E, Stone R, et al. Mutations in the chloride channel gene, CLCNKB, cause Bartter's syndrome type III. Nat Genet. 1997;17(2):171–8. Epub 1997/11/05.
66. Lee SE, Han KH, Jung YH, Lee HK, Kang HG, Moon KC, et al. Renal transplantation in a patient with Bartter syndrome and glomerulosclerosis. Korean J Pediatr. 2011;54(1):36–9. Epub 2011/03/02.
67. Estevez R, Boettger T, Stein V, Birkenhager R, Otto E, Hildebrandt F, et al. Barttin is a Cl-channel beta-subunit crucial for renal Cl- reabsorption and inner ear K+ secretion. Nature. 2001;414(6863):558–61. Epub 2001/12/06.
68. Vargas-Poussou R, Huang C, Hulin P, Houillier P, Jeunemaitre X, Paillard M, et al. Functional characterization of a calcium-sensing receptor mutation in severe autosomal dominant hypocalcemia with a Bartter-like syndrome. J Am Soc Nephrol. 2002;13(9):2259–66. Epub 2002/08/23.
69. Simon DB, Nelson-Williams C, Bia MJ, Ellison D, Karet FE, Molina AM, et al. Gitelman's variant of Bartter's syndrome, inherited hypokalaemic alkalosis, is caused by mutations in the thiazide-sensitive Na-Cl cotransporter. Nat Genet. 1996;12(1):24–30. Epub 1996/01/01.
70. Nicolet-Barousse L, Blanchard A, Roux C, Pietri L, Bloch-Faure M, Kolta S, et al. Inactivation of the Na-Cl co-transporter (NCC) gene is associated with high BMD through both renal and bone mechanisms: analysis of patients with Gitelman syndrome and Ncc null mice. J Bone Miner Res. 2005;20(5):799–808. Epub 2005/04/13.
71. Geller DS, Rodriguez-Soriano J, Vallo Boado A, Schifter S, Bayer M, Chang SS, et al. Mutations in the mineralocorticoid receptor gene cause autosomal dominant pseudohypoaldosteronism type I. Nat Genet. 1998;19(3):279–81. Epub 1998/07/14.
72. Chang SS, Grunder S, Hanukoglu A, Rosler A, Mathew PM, Hanukoglu I, et al. Mutations in subunits of the epithelial sodium channel cause salt wasting with hyperkalaemic acidosis, pseudohypoaldosteronism type 1. Nat Genet. 1996;12(3):248–53. Epub 1996/03/01.
73. Reichold M, Zdebik AA, Lieberer E, Rapedius M, Schmidt K, Bandulik S, et al. KCNJ10 gene mutations causing EAST syndrome (epilepsy, ataxia, sensorineural deafness, and tubulopathy) disrupt channel function. Proc Natl Acad Sci U S A.107(32):14490–5. Epub 2010/07/24.
74. Scholl UI, Choi M, Liu T, Ramaekers VT, Hausler MG, Grimmer J, et al. Seizures, sensorineural deafness, ataxia, mental retardation, and electrolyte imbalance (SeSAME syndrome) caused by mutations in KCNJ10. Proc Natl Acad Sci U S A. 2009;106(14):5842–7. Epub 2009/03/18.
75. Rozengurt N, Lopez I, Chiu CS, Kofuji P, Lester HA, Neusch C. Time course of inner ear degeneration and deafness in mice lacking the Kir4.1 potassium channel subunit. Hear Res. 2003;177(1–2):71–80. Epub 2003/03/06.
76. Schreiber R, Gubler MC, Gribouval O, Shalev H, Landau D. Inherited renal tubular dysgenesis may not be universally fatal. Pediatr Nephrol. 2010;25(12):2531–4. Epub 2010/07/08.
77. Gubler MC, Antignac C. Renin-angiotensin system in kidney development: renal tubular dysgenesis. Kidney Int. 2010;77(5):400–6. Epub 2009/11/20.
78. Sedman AB, Kershaw DB, Bunchman TE. Recognition and management of angiotensin converting enzyme inhibitor fetopathy. Pediatr Nephrol. 1995;9(3):382–5. Epub 1995/06/01.

Chapter 12
Drug-Induced Hypertension in Chronic Kidney Disease

Alfred A. Vichot and Mark A. Perazella

Introduction

Hypertension is a common condition representing both a risk factor and a consequence of CKD [1, 2]. Causal relationships between hypertension, CKD progression, and rising cardiovascular risk are well documented [3–5]. Hypertension's increasing prevalence as CKD [6] progresses is also well established [7–9]. The identification of factors that influence the onset and maintenance of hypertension is central to the management of CKD.

CKD is a highly prevalent disease with multiple comorbidities (pain, depression, anxiety, malignancy, etc.) and, by its nature, requires treatment with a number of medications that are prescribed or purchased over-the-counter. Many of these medications are associated with de novo hypertension and/or exacerbation of previously controlled hypertension. As such, drug-induced hypertension represents one such controllable factor that clinicians can modify.

Provider-prescribed and patient-initiated agents through over-the-counter purchase warrant scrutiny for their effects on blood pressure augmentation in the CKD patient population. It is critical that all clinicians and healthcare providers, not only nephrologists, recognize that CKD patients are vulnerable to the blood pressure raising effects of drugs. The goal of this chapter is to identify exogenous agents that induce or exacerbate hypertension in CKD patients, to characterize pertinent clinical

A.A. Vichot, MD
Department of Internal Medicine, Yale University, New Haven, CT, USA

M.A. Perazella, MD, MS (✉)
Department of Medicine, Section of Nephrology, Yale University School of Medicine
and Yale-New Haven Hospital, P.O. Box 208029, Boardman Building 122, 330 Cedar Street,
New Haven, CT 06520-8029, USA
e-mail: mark.perazella@yale.edu

© Springer Science+Business Media New York 2016
A.K. Singh, R. Agarwal (eds.), *Core Concepts in Hypertension in Kidney Disease*, DOI 10.1007/978-1-4939-6436-9_12

features associated with these agents, and to facilitate an understanding of how these agents affect blood pressure homeostasis in the setting of underlying CKD.

Blood Pressure Control and CKD

Mean arterial pressure (MAP) is classically defined as the product of systemic vascular resistance and cardiac output. Cardiac output is defined as the product of heart rate and stroke volume with the latter determined by the difference in end-diastolic volume (preload) and end-systolic volume (afterload and myocardial contractility).

The factors influencing cardiac output and systemic vascular resistance are well established and unknown. Baroreceptors, natriuretic peptides, the renin–angiotensin–aldosterone system (RAAS), the kinin–kallikrein system, the adrenergic receptor system, vascular endothelial growth factor signaling, and effectors of vasoconstriction and vasodilation all are known to interact with each other. Determining which of these factors actually contributes the most to blood pressure homeostasis is difficult because of the challenge in distinguishing primary responses from adaptive secondary responses [10].

Under normal physiologic conditions, the RAAS and SNS are known to activate each other [11–14] and this relationship is further intensified in the setting of CKD [15–17]. Calcium, uric acid, renalase, nitric oxide synthase inhibition, and vascular endothelial growth factor signaling have also been shown to influence blood pressure homeostasis in CKD [18–24]. Given the various causes of CKD, it is unclear which system is driving the hypertensive phenotype and how many systems are affected by the introduction of an exogenous agent.

Many medications have been implicated in hypertension such as decongestants, birth control pills, androgens, combination antiretroviral therapy [25], alcohol, and illicit substances such as cocaine, methamphetamines, and bath salts [26, 27]. To make this review a useful reference for the practicing clinician, this chapter will focus on common clinical conditions and the agents used in the practice of CKD management that are known to augment or exacerbate the hypertensive phenotype (Table 12.1).

Acute and Chronic Pain Syndromes

Acute and chronic pain are common symptoms experienced by patients with CKD [28, 29]. Although the effect of chronic pain on blood pressure elevation is not as clear as it is in the acute setting [30–32], the hypertensive effects of analgesics used for management of both forms of pain are well established, but not often recognized by most practitioners [33]. An understanding of the effects of the various analgesics prescribed to and self-administered by patients with CKD should be at the forefront of medical management and preventative care.

Table 12.1 Common conditions and therapies observed in CKD associated with hypertension	**Acute and chronic pain syndromes**
	Anthocyanins
	Non-steroidal anti-inflammatory drugs (NSAIDs)
	Anemia
	Erythropoiesis stimulating agents (ESAs)
	Inflammatory syndromes
	Calcineurin inhibitors (CNIs)
	Glucocorticosteroids
	Mood disorders
	Monoamine oxidase inhibitors (MAOIs)
	Noradrenergic and specific serotonergic antidepressants (NaSSAs)
	Serotonin-norepinephrine inhibitors (SNRIs)
	St. John's Wort (SJW)
	Tricyclic antidepressants (TCAs)
	Polypharmacy
	Serotonin syndrome
	Renal cell carcinoma
	Anti-VEGF antibodies
	Tyrosine kinase inhibitors (TKIs)
	Withdrawal syndromes
	Antihypertensive medications
	Alpha-2 receptor agonists
	Angiotensin-II receptors antagonists (ARBs)
	Beta-adrenergic antagonists
	Vasodilators

Non-Steroidal Anti-Inflammatory Drugs (NSAIDS)

NSAIDs are the foundation of pain management plans for headache, osteoarthritis, gout, and post-operative care [34–38]. In the setting of CKD, achievement of pain control with NSAIDs becomes a challenge because of their association with hypertension and a wide variety of renal syndromes (hyponatremia, hyperkalemia, metabolic acidosis, edema formation, acute and chronic papillary necrosis) [39–44]. As a result of differing opinions on the risk–benefit profile of NSAIDs in CKD, the reported prevalence and recommendations have been variable [45–48]. Although a discussion on the effects of NSAIDs on CKD progression is beyond the scope of this chapter, the effects of NSAIDs on blood pressure homeostasis in a patient group already predisposed to higher blood pressures will be discussed.

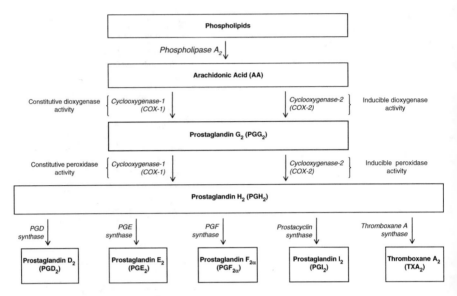

Fig. 12.1 Prostaglandin synthesis

Function

NSAIDs are a heterogeneous group of molecules that inhibit cyclooxygenase-mediated synthesis of prostaglandins from arachidonic acid (Fig. 12.1) [49]. Prostaglandins are local hormones with autocrine and paracrine function that are present in different tissues and, within the kidney, are known to influence autoregulation of renal blood flow, water excretion, and natriuresis. Prostaglandin (PG) synthesis is affected by NSAID type, time of onset, duration of action, and preference for cyclooxygenase-1 (COX-1) or cyclooxygenase-2 (COX-2) (Table 12.2).

Prostaglandin-mediated effects in the kidney are diverse [50]. The mechanisms by which NSAIDs augment hypertension are incompletely understood but are postulated to affect renal blood flow and natriuresis [51]. To provide an example, PGE_2 is a major product of prostaglandin synthesis in the renal medulla and has been implicated in the inhibition of chloride uptake in the thick ascending limb of Henle [52, 53]. A neonatal variant of Bartter's syndrome marked by hypotension and electrolyte wasting occurs in the setting of excess PGE_2 production and can be reversed with indomethacin [54]. Conversely, when PGE_2 synthesis is impaired or production is blocked with indomethacin, hypertension often occurs [51, 55–57].

Renal sodium retention promoted by NSAID use is most apparent in hypertensive subjects [51, 55–57], but NSAIDs do not constitutively result in an elevation of blood pressure. Inhibition of the PGH_2/TXA_2 pathway results in decreased peripheral myogenic constriction [58, 59] and the absence of the prostaglandin I_2 receptor, a promoter of renin release, results in decreased susceptibility to hypertension [60].

Table 12.2 Currently available NSAIDS classified by chemical structure and/or mechanism of action

Acetic acids	Propionic acids
Diclofenac	Dexibuprofen
Etodolac	Dexketoprofen
Indomethacin	Fenoprofen
Ketorolac	Flurbiprofen
Nabumetone	Ibuprofen
Sulindac	Ketoprofen
Tolmetin	Loxoprofen
	Naproxen
COX-2 inhibitors	Oxaprozin
Celecoxib	
Etoricoxib	**Salicylic acids**
	Aspirin
Enolic acids (Oxicams)	Diflunisal
Droxicam	Salicylic acid
Lornoxicam	Salsalate
Meloxicam	
Piroxicam	
Tenoxicam	
Fenamic acids	
Flufenamic acid	
Meclofenamic acid	
Mefenamic acid	
Tolfenamic acid	

Antihypertensive Medication Interactions

NSAIDs can strengthen or weaken the effects of antihypertensive medications by prostaglandin-mediated pathways and other undefined routes. Most studies demonstrate a tendency towards NSAID-induced antagonism of antihypertensive medications with either no change in blood pressure or a rise in blood pressure. The relationship between NSAIDs and several antihypertensive medication classes will be discussed below.

Loop Diuretics

NSAIDs, particularly indomethacin and sulindac, antagonize the effect of furosemide and bumetanide by reducing their natriuretic effect [61–64].

The mechanisms proposed for this effect are NSAID-loop diuretic competition for transport into the proximal tubule via the organic acid transporter pathway [63] and enhanced sodium uptake in the loop of Henle [62].

Thiazide Diuretics

NSAIDS, like indomethacin, ibuprofen, and sulindac, confer variable effects on blood pressure in the presence of thiazides [65–69]. The reason for these different observations is unclear with variability attributed possibly to NSAID type [66, 70] or thiazide clearance [67]. Antagonism of the antihypertensive effect is, however, more common.

Beta (β)-Blockers

NSAID effects on blood pressure also vary with different beta-blockers. Patients on indomethacin and piroxicam have been observed to increase blood pressure with pindolol, propranolol, oxprenolol, and atenolol [69, 71–74]. On the other hand, blood pressure control with propranolol was not affected by ibuprofen or sulindac [68, 74] nor was the effectiveness of atenolol attenuated by sulindac or flurbiprofen [73, 75]. The mechanisms mediating the rise in blood pressure in the setting of NSAID use with beta-blockers (BB) are also unclear. Weakened RAAS blockade and enhancement of alpha-mediated vascular tone have been proposed [76].

Angiotensin Converting Enzyme Inhibitors (ACEi)

Blood pressure effects in human subjects taking NSAIDs and ACEi have been studied. Indomethacin increases the blood pressure of subjects on captopril [77–80] while mildly attenuating the blood pressure control with lisinopril [81]. The reason for this variability is unclear.

Insights into the relationship between prostaglandin inhibition and ACE inhibition have come from Bartter's syndrome—a syndrome associated with hypotension and salt wasting. Patients with Bartter's syndrome typically have high plasma bradykinin, plasma renin activity (PRA), urinary kallikrein, and urinary prostaglandin E excretion [82]. Following the administration of indomethacin, plasma bradykinin, plasma renin, urinary kallikrein, and urinary prostaglandin E excretion are reduced with resolution of hypotension and salt wasting [82]. A relationship between prostaglandins, the pro-hypertensive renin–angiotensin pathway and pro-hypotensive kallikrein–kinin pathway is recognized, but the interplay is still not well understood [82, 83].

Vasodilators

Variable effects on blood pressure control are also observed with vasodilators.

Diclofenac has been shown to reduce the effect of dihydralazine [84]. Indomethacin, however, has been shown to attenuate the effects of hydralazine [85], but did not affect blood pressure control with pindacidil [86]. The mechanisms mediating this interaction are unclear.

Meta-Analyses of NSAIDs and Hypertension

As prostaglandins demonstrate pro-hypertensive and antihypertensive effects [87, 88] that can be strengthened or weakened by blood pressure medications, 2 meta-analyses were performed to evaluate NSAID effects on blood pressure [89, 90].

In the 1993 study by Pope et al., 54 studies with 123 NSAID treatment arms were evaluated and 92 % of the study subjects were determined to be hypertensive [89]. An elevation in blood pressure was found strictly in subjects with hypertension [89]. The NSAIDs determined to have the largest effect on blood pressure were indomethacin, naproxen, and piroxicam, which increased the mean arterial pressure (MAP) by 3.59, 3.74, and 0.49 mmHg, respectively. Conversely, ibuprofen, sulindac, and aspirin did not have a large effect on blood pressure and were actually noted to reduce it by 0.83, 0.16, and 1.76 mmHg, respectively [89].

In the 1994 study by Johnson et al., 38 randomized placebo-controlled trials and 12 randomized trials comparing 2 or more NSAIDs were evaluated [90]. Of the 50 independent trials evaluated, 76 % included antihypertensive therapy employed for 1 week or longer [90]. When all the randomized placebo-controlled studies were pooled, all sub-types of NSAIDs administered demonstrated an increase in the supine mean blood pressure [90]. The mean rise in supine blood pressure was 5.0 mmHg with the highest effect on blood pressure observed with piroxicam, indomethacin, and ibuprofen [90]. There was no notable effect on weight, urine sodium output, creatinine clearance, or urine prostaglandin secretion [90].

Another notable feature was that the NSAID-induced increase in blood pressure was higher in studies that involved antihypertensive therapy; a 4.7 mmHg increase in blood pressure was observed compared to the 1.8 mmHg increase observed in studies not involving antihypertensive medications [90]. NSAIDs antagonized beta-blockers, diuretics, and vasodilators to different degrees with the greatest pooled effect observed with beta-blockers: a 6.2 mmHg rise in blood pressure [90].

The studies noted above demonstrate that NSAIDs increased blood pressure in subjects with hypertension or on antihypertensive therapy. Although these studies are not generalizable to the CKD population because they excluded elderly subjects and subjects with hypertension, it can be inferred that NSAIDs would be expected to exacerbate the hypertensive phenotype in this population because of its higher prevalence of hypertension.

A conclusion on which NSAID sub-type has the greater effect on blood pressure cannot be made from either meta-analysis because the study sizes varied and confidence intervals were wide. Data stratifying subjects by duration of therapy, cumulative dosing, and by half-life of NSAID was also not robust enough to make inferences.

Cyclooxygenase-2 (COX-2) Inhibitors

Non-specific NSAIDs target the constitutive isoform of COX-1, an enzyme responsible for otherwise normal physiologic functions. Disruption of the COX-1 pathway can result in upper gastrointestinal (GI) complications, platelet dysfunction, and renal toxicity [91–93]. To bypass these complications of COX-1 inhibition and target the inducible COX isoform that mediates inflammation, COX-2 inhibitors were developed.

Similar to non-selective NSAIDs, COX-2 inhibitors also raise blood pressure. This effect was observed in several studies evaluating the incidence of GI complications when either non-selective NSAIDs or COX-2 inhibitors were used for pain control [94]. For example, the Celecoxib Long-Term Arthritis Safety Study (CLASS) study was designed to investigate the incidence of upper GI complications of celecoxib and other NSAIDs [94]. In this study, hypertension was observed in 1.7 % of patients on celecoxib and 2.3 % of patients on NSAIDs [94]. In the VIOXX Gastrointestinal Outcomes Research (VIGOR) study, 8.5 % of 4047 subjects in the rofecoxib treatment arm had hypertension compared to the 5.0 % of 4029 subjects in the naproxen treatment arm [95, 96]. On 50 mg of rofecoxib, the mean systolic blood pressure was 133.2 mmHg (an increase of 4.6 mmHg from baseline) while the mean systolic blood pressure on 1000 mg of naproxen was 128.8 mmHg (a 1.0 mmHg increase from baseline). In a post-hoc analysis of 50 separate studies involving more than 13,000 subjects enrolled in the celecoxib clinical trial program, complications from celecoxib were compared to NSAIDs or placebo [97]. In this study, hypertension was observed in 0.8 % subjects on celecoxib regardless of dose- or duration of therapy [97]. The Successive Celecoxib Efficacy and Safety Studies (SUCCESS) VI and VII studies in older hypertensive patients with patients with osteoarthritis found rofecoxib as more likely to increase systolic blood pressure than celecoxib at week 6 [98, 99].

While direct trial comparison is difficult due to design variation, subject characteristics, endpoints, agents selected for investigation, and method of blood pressure measurement, they still provide important information. Table 12.3 summarizes clinical studies [94–103] that have evaluated the effects of COX-2 inhibition on blood pressure.

Blood pressure elevation by COX-2 inhibitors is mostly observed in hypertensive states. Some authors have suggested that COX-2 inhibitors may cause hypertension by augmentation of angiotensin-II effects [104, 105]. Others have suggested the role of dietary sodium as a mediator of hypertension. For example, rofecoxib was administered to spontaneously hypertensive rats (SHR) and normotensive Wistar–Kyoto rat (WKY) sustained on normal- to high-salt diets or low-salt diets [106]. COX-2 inhibitors significantly elevated the blood pressure in both rat models fed normal- to high-salt diets and did not effect rats fed a low-salt diet [106]. The authors of the study did not propose a mechanism for this observed difference. They did, however, suggest that salt deprivation could prevent hypertension in the setting of chronic COX-2 inhibitor use as a rise in blood pressure was noted to be independent of genetic predisposition [106].

Antihypertensive Medication Interactions

COX-2 inhibitors are variable in their effect on antihypertensive medications.

In one trial that evaluated the effects of COX-2 inhibitors with antihypertensive monotherapy (ACEi, BB, calcium-channel blocker [CCB]) or antihypertensive dual

Table 12.3 Studies evaluating effects Of COX-2 inhibition on blood pressure control

Study (Year)	Study design	Enrollment	Duration	Incidence of hypertension
Catella-Lawson et al. [99] (1999)	Randomized, double-blind Controlled trial 1 center	36 subjects Ages: between 59 and 80 years Comorbidities: healthy	2 weeks	Mild BP increase in all groups: 12 subjects on Indomethacin 150 mg/day 12 subjects on Rofecoxib(MK-966) 50 mg/day 12 subjects on Placebo
Emery et al. [98] (1999)	Randomized, Parallel-Group, Double-blind, Double-dummy Trial 132 centers	655 subjects Ages: Age cut-off not defined Comorbidities: Adult onset RA	24 weeks	1 % of 222 subjects on Celecoxib 400 mg/day 2 % of 239 subjects on Diclofenac 150 mg/day
Simon et al. [101] (1999)	Randomized, Double-Blind, Placebo-Controlled Trial 79 centers	1149 subjects Ages: >18 years of age Comorbidities: RA	12 weeks	<1 % of 217 subjects on Celecoxib 800 mg/day <1 % of 235 subjects on Celecoxib 400 mg/day 0 % of 240 subjects on Celecoxib 200 mg/day <1 % of 225 subjects on Naproxen 1000 mg/day <1 % of 231 subjects on Placebo
CLASS [92] (2000)	Prospective, Randomized, Double-blind, Controlled Trial 386 centers	8059 subjects Ages: ≥18 years of age Comorbidities: OA or RA	6 months	1.7 % of 3987 subjects on Celecoxib 800 mg/day 2.3 % of 3981 subjects on NSAIDS 1985 subjects on Ibuprofen 2400 mg/day 1996 subjects on Diclofenac 150 mg/day
Whelton et al. [95] (2000)	Post-hoc analysis of 12 randomized controlled trials	3366 subjects with OA (3 studies) 2091 subjects with OA (4 studies⁑) 2250 subjects with RA (2 studies) 327 subjects with RA (1 study#) 1633 subjects with OA and RA (2 studies) Age: 62 years, range 18–93 (OA) Age: 55 years, range 20–92 (RA)	12 weeks ¶ 4 weeks ♯ 2–6 weeks	0.8 % of 5704 subjects on Celecoxib 50–800 mg/day 0.7 % of 2098 subjects on NSAIDs Diclofenac 100–150 mg/day Ibuprofen 2400 mg/day Naproxen 1000 mg/day 0.3 % of 1864 subjects on Placebo

therapy (diuretic plus ACEi, BB, or CCB), rofecoxib antagonized the effects of all hypertensive classes with a mean rise in systolic blood pressure [99]. The antagonistic effect of rofecoxib on CCBs was minimal, however, and was not statistically significant [99]. In the same trial, celecoxib augmented the effect of ACEi monotherapy and dual therapy (diuretic plus ACEi, BB, or CCB) by causing a reduction in systolic blood pressure while slightly increasing the blood pressure of subjects on BB or CCBs [99]. Celecoxib was observed to have no significant effect on the antihypertensive actions of ACEi in another study [107]. Although celecoxib had less of an effect with ACEi than rofecoxib, the reasons for this discrepancy are unclear.

Based on current studies, both non-selective COX inhibition and COX-2 selective inhibition have the potential to raise blood pressure and exacerbate hypertension in at-risk patients.

Anthocyanins

Antioxidants of plant origin are appealing form of medicinal therapy to some patients as they are free of synthetic compounds. Anthocyanins represent one class of these kinds of drugs. Anthocynanins provide the orange, red, and blue coloring to fruits, flower, and vegetables and also provide a natural remedy for suppression of inflammatory pain by way of cyclooxygenase inhibition [108, 109]. Several authors have suspected an improvement in blood pressure control as a result of the anti-inflammatory effect of anthocyanins and study results have been negative or equivocal to date [110, 111].

A case report demonstrating the potential harmful effects of cherry extract, an anthocynanin, in the setting of CKD implied an effect similar to that of NSAIDs [112]. Although this supposition is reasonable and hypertensive effects can be suspected, surveillance of compounds containing anthocyanins should be considered given their similarity to NSAIDs and the potential for augmenting blood pressures until more evidence supporting this effect accrues.

Treatment

Treatment of NSAID-induced hypertension is fairly straightforward: abstinence from NSAIDs and use of an alternate agent for acute and chronic pain. Unfortunately, there are no specific guidelines for management of pain in the CKD population. The acuity, location, and source of pain are factors to consider as well as the clearance of the parent agent and its metabolites. When underlying pain symptoms require NSAID therapy for analgesia, using the lowest effective drug dose is recommended. Hypertension can be treated with calcium channel antagonists, and the sodium retaining effect of NSAIDs can be targeted with diuretics. Diuretic use may, however, increase the risk of AKI. Renin angiotensin system (RAS) inhibitor therapy is risky in CKD patients taking NSAIDs due to the risk for both acute kidney injury (AKI) and hyperkalemia. Thus, this drug combination should be avoided or monitored very closely when employed.

Although acetaminophen has been associated with complications of acute liver failure, nephrotoxicity, and pyroglutamic (5-oxoproline) metabolic acidosis in the setting of malnutrition [113–115], it is generally regarded as a safer choice when dosed less than 4 g/day in the setting of CKD and the elderly [116–118].

Inflammatory Syndromes

The spectrum of inflammatory diseases affecting the glomerulus, tubulointerstitium, and systemic arteriovenous circulation is wide. From systemic lupus erthyematosus (SLE) to the humoral and cellular immune responses involved with transplantation, treatments aimed at reducing inflammation are common in CKD. With expanding insight into inflammation's role in CKD progression [119], the use of immunosuppressive strategies will continue to be frequently employed in the general and CKD population. Thus, an understanding of their hypertensive effects is paramount.

Glucocorticoids

Glucocorticoids are mainstays of anti-inflammatory and immunosuppressive management, especially in conditions often encountered in CKD: lupus nephritis, HIV nephropathy, IgA nephropathy, and transplantation [120–124]. These drugs are thought to reduce inflammation mainly by two pathways: genomic induction or repression of gene transcription or non-genomic pathways involving cytosolic and membrane-bound receptor interactions [125, 126] (Figs. 12.2 and 12.3).

As patients with CKD are predisposed to hypertension and glucocorticoids are implicated in causing hypertension, an understanding of glucocorticoid potency and mineralocorticoid activity is necessary to facilitate more widespread blood pressure surveillance and optimize blood pressure control.

Hypertension onset with corticosteroids is mediated by enhanced activity of the mineralocorticoid receptor. Under normal conditions, the mineralocorticoid receptor is activated by aldosterone and induces increased expression of the sodium chloride co-transporter (NCC) and epithelial sodium channel [ENaC] [41, 127, 128].

Activation of the mineralocorticoid receptor by cortisol represents an important pathway that mediates the development of hypertension. Although corticosteroids activate the glucocorticoid receptor, they also interact with the mineralocorticoid receptor setting in motion intracellular signaling pathways that promote sodium reabsorption via NCC and ENaC. Intracellular concentrations of corticosteroids are typically several folds higher than aldosterone and compete with aldosterone to bind

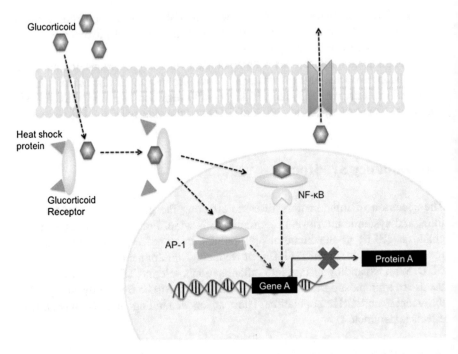

Fig. 12.2 Transcription inhibition, or transrepression, by glucocorticoids is considered to be the main anti-inflammatory action of glucocorticoids. Glucocorticoids enter the cell and bind to glucocorticoid receptors (GCR). On ligation, the GCR loses chaperone proteins including heat shock proteins. The Glucorticoid-GCR complex migrates into the nucleus and binds with transcription factors like AP-1 or NF-KB. This complex inhibits the transcription of target genes like IL-2. Excess glucocorticoids not metabolized by 11 beta-hydroxysteroid dehydrogenase are actively transported out of the cell by P-glycoprotein [125]

and activate the mineralocorticoid receptor. This does not occur, however, due to the activities of 11 beta-hydroxysteroid dehydrogenase (11B-HSD) which debulks intracellular cortisol by converting it to cortisone. When 11B-HSD is reduced in quantity, inhibited, or saturated, cortisol concentrations are not reduced and activate the mineralocorticoid receptor unopposed. This alteration is observed in conditions like apparent-mineralocorticoid excess (AME), licorice consumption, and Cushing's syndrome. High doses of exogenous glucocorticoids can overwhelm the capacity for 11B-HSD to metabolize the drug and protect the specificity of mineralocorticoid binding to the receptor. In addition, glucocorticoids possessing higher degrees of mineralocorticoid activity are larger effectors of hypertension through activation of this pathway.

Another pathway that glucocorticoids mediate hypertension is through potentiation of catecholamine-induced vasoconstriction. Interest in this pathway was mainly driven by studies of hypotension in the setting of acute adrenal insufficiency [129]. In human studies, greater pressor responses were seen with norepinephrine in the presence of glucocorticoids than in the absence of glucocorticoids [130, 131]. The

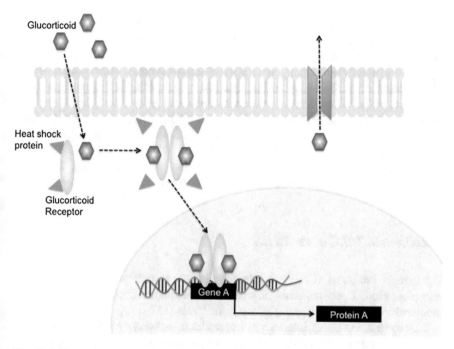

Fig. 12.3 Transcription activation, or transactivation, is considered to be the main pathway mediating the metabolic side effects of glucocorticoids. Glucocorticoids enter the cell and bind to glucocorticoid receptors (GCR). On ligation, the GCR loses chaperone proteins including heat shock proteins. The GC-GCR complex creates a homodimer and begins transcription of genes involved in metabolism and lipocortin 1 [125]

mechanisms underlying the vascular smooth muscle response to corticosteroids are unclear with some studies implicating 11B-HSD [132–134]

The prevalence, doses, and hypertensive effects of glucocorticoid use in different subpopulation of the CKD population are unknown. In one study, the hypertensive effects of dexamethasone and methylprednisolone were observed in the management of steroid resistant nephrotic syndrome in pediatric subjects with proteinuria, but otherwise normal renal function [135]. Transient hypertension or worsening of pre-existing hypertension was seen in 54.4% of patients with dexamethasone and 47.6% of subjects with methylprednisolone [135]. Although methylprednisolone has mineralocorticoid activity, the degree of blood pressure change caused by either agent was not included in the evaluation.

Treatment

Transplant recipients have provided a model for long-term management of hypertension with glucocorticoids, as steroid-free regimens are not always possible or practical. Lowering the dose of glucocorticoids is a first step, but there is no clear evidence supporting one dose or agent over another. Ponticelli and colleagues have suggested that a dose of prednisone less than 10 mg/day makes little contribution to hypertension post-transplant [136].

There is little evidence supporting a hypertensive agent of choice in the setting of escalation of immunosuppression with glucocorticoids. As the mechanism of glucocorticoid-mediated hypertension is by enhanced sodium and chloride uptake by NCC and ENaC, arguments can be made to use thiazide diuretics or potassium-sparing diuretics such as amiloride or triamterene. Calcium channel antagonists are frequently employed for hypertension in patients. They are effective and safe, although lower extremity edema can complicate therapy. Unfortunately, there is no evidence for this at this time to recommend a definitive drug regimen.

Calcineurin Inhibitors (CNIS)

Calcineurin inhibitors (CNI) are immunosuppressive therapeutic agents used in transplantation, lupus nephritis, idiopathic membranous nephropathy, and other glomerular diseases manifesting as nephrotic states [137–140].

Calcineurin inhibitors interfere in intracellular pathways mediating inflammation. Calcineurin is a serine/threonine protein phosphatase and plays a role in intracellular calcium-dependent signal transduction pathways [141]. Expression of IL-2, a stimulator of T-cell growth and differentiation, is regulated by NFAT (nuclear factor of activated T cells). Calcineurin dephosphorylates and thereby activates NFAT triggering the cascade which causes activation of T cells and cellular immunity [142]. The introduction of CNIs like cyclosporine and tacrolimus has revolutionized the field of transplantation by their ability to suppress T cell activation and prevent acute rejection, but they are not without risk.

CKD progression following transplant is a notable feature of both renal and non-renal transplants [143–150] and its association with CNIs has resulted in a pursuit of alternate strategies for long-term immunosuppression [151]. CNIs are also contributors to CKD progression via their promotion of risk factors like hypertension, diabetes and dyslipidemia [152–156].

Hypertensive physiology influenced by CNIs has been best observed in patients with liver disease that receive liver transplants. Patients with liver disease are typically characterized by reduced systemic vasoconstriction, increased cardiac output, and reduced mean arterial pressures. Following liver transplantation, portal hypertension is reversed, systemic vasoconstriction increases and cardiac output normalizes resulting in an improvement in hemodynamics and mean arterial pressures [157]. Despite the compensatory hemodynamic changes, more than 50 % of liver transplant patients develop hypertension within a year of transplant and this has been attributed to CNIs [157]. The contribution to hypertension from unrecognized CKD is another factor to consider. The prevalence of pre-transplant CKD in liver disease is likely underestimated given the decreased muscle mass and creatinine generation in this population [158, 159]

The pathways mediating CNI-induced hypertension are slowly becoming apparent [160, 161]. CNIs mediate salt-sensitive hypertension in a manner very similar to pseudohypoaldosteronism type II (PHA II, Gordon's syndrome) which causes constitutive NCC activation in the distal convoluted tubule [160]. In an elegant study performed by Hoorn et al., tacrolimus administration increased phosphorylated NCC and the NCC-regulatory kinases WNK3, WNK4, and SPAK. Tacrolimus effect was exaggerated in NCC-overexpressing mice, minimized in NCC-knockout mice, and the observed tacrolimus effect was reversed with the use of hydrochlorothiazide [160]. Thus, as with many forms of drug-induced hypertension, excessive sodium reabsorption ultimately promotes the elevation in blood pressure.

Top of Form The dose-related blood pressure responses to tacrolimus and cyclosporine in the setting of CKD have not been documented, but in a study of hypertensive liver transplant patients with normal renal function, cyclosporine had a greater effect on blood pressure than tacrolimus when administered with low-dose steroids [162]. The mean 24-h arterial blood pressure in cyclosporine treated patients was 99.4 versus 95.8 mmHg with tacrolimus [162]. As the actual doses were not documented, recommendations cannot be made regarding the superiority of tacrolimus or cyclosporine, as this study was not generalizable to the CKD population.

Treatment

The treatment of CNI-related hypertension has evolved over time. Verapamil once held promise because of its immunosuppressive effects and its ability to counter CNI-induced reductions in renal blood flow [163, 164]. While verapamil can potentially result in supra-therapeutic levels of cyclosporine through inhibition of the cytochrome p450 system [165, 166], providers saw this drug–drug interaction as an opportunity to reduce the total effective dose of cyclosporine and potentially reduce CNI-toxicity. Unfortunately, there was no evidence of benefit in preventing rejection or reducing cyclosporine nephrotoxicity in a controlled, double-blind, randomized trial in deceased donor transplant recipients co-administered verapamil and cyclosporine [167]. Current strategies now aim at blocking CNI effects in the kidney, with thiazide diuretics offering the most targeted approach to lowering blood pressure [160, 168]. Ultimately, CNI-related hypertension, as in other forms of hypertension, will likely require more than one antihypertensive agent after taking into account existing comorbidities, drug–drug interactions, and medication side-effect profiles.

Mood Disorders

Depression is a complex disease process commonly observed in patients with CKD [169–173]. Depression can be influenced by multiple stressors such as chronic pain, fatigue, itching, constipation, decreased appetite, restless legs, and erectile

Table 12.4 Common antidepressants associated with hypertension

Monoamine oxidase inhibitors (MAOIs)
Moclobemide
Selegiline (Eldepryl, Emsam, Zelapar)
Noradrenergic and specific serotonergic antidepressants (NaSSAs)
Mirtazapine (Remeron)
Serotonin-norepinephrine reuptake inhibitors (SNRIs)
Duloxetine (Cymbalta)
Milnacipran (Savella)
Venlafaxine (Effexor XR)
St. John's Wort
Tricyclic antidepressants (TCAs)
Amitriptyline (Elavil)
Doxepin (Silenor, Sinequan)
Imipramine (Tofranil)
Nortriptyline (Pamelor)
Trimipramine (Surmontil)

dysfunction; by dietary changes associated with sodium, potassium, and phosphate restriction; and, finally, by lifestyle changes associated with dialysis planning and renal replacement therapy [169–173].

The evidence supporting depression and hypertension risk has been mixed [174–177]. In one study, subjects meeting Diagnostic and Statistical Manual of Mental Disorders, Fourth Edition (DSM-IV) criteria for major depressive disorder and anxiety disorder were selected and grouped into those taking antidepressants, those not taking antidepressants, and then compared them with subjects without MDD or anxiety disorder [178]. In this study, subjects with depression that were not on medications had lower blood pressure and those subjects using tricyclic antidepressants (TCAs) or noradrenergic and serotonergic (NS) working antidepressants had increases in systolic and diastolic blood pressure [178].

Antidepressants

Hypertensive effects of varying severity have been reported for TCAs [179–181], monoamine oxidase inhibitors (MAOIs) [182], serotonin-norepinephrine inhibitors (SNRIs) [183, 184], noradrenergic and specific serotonergic antidepressants (NaSSAs) [185], and St. John's Wort (SJW) [186, 187] (Table 12.4). No documented case reports demonstrating augmented blood pressures isolated solely within the CKD population are available to review. There are, however, multiple

Table 12.5 Drugs commonly associated with serotonin syndrome

Analgesics	Antiemetics
Fentanyl	Granisetron
Meperidine	Metoclopramide
Pentazocine	Ondansetron
Tramadol	
	Antimigraines
Antibiotics	Sumatriptan
Linezolid[a]	
Ritonavir	**Cough and Cold**
	Dextromethorphan
Anticonvulsants	
Valproate	**Dietary supplements**
	Ginseng (Panax ginseng)
Antidepressants	St. John's Wort (Hypericum perforatum)
MAOIs	Tryptophan
Clorgiline	
Isocarboxazid	**Drugs of abuse**
Moclobemide	Ecstasy or Methylenedioxymethamphetamine
Phenelzine	Foxy Methoxy (5-methoxydiisopropyltryptamine)
SSRIs	LSD (Lysergic acid diethylamide))
Citalopram	Syrian rue[a]
Fluoxetine	
Fluvoxamine	**Other**
Paroxetine	Lithium
Sertraline	
Other	
Buspirone	
Clomipramine	
Nefazodone	
Trazodone	
Venlafaxine	

Adapted from Boyer E, Shannon M. The serotonin syndrome. N Engl J Med. 2005;352(11):1112–20
MAOIs monoamine oxidase inhibitors, *SSRIs* selective serotonin reuptake inhibitors
[a]Monoamine oxidase inhibitor properties

reports of serotonin-syndrome in the setting of acute kidney injury and end-stage renal disease [188–190] (Tables 12.5 and 12.6).

The mechanism of antidepressant mediated hypertension is unclear but could center on unopposed activation of adrenergic and dopaminergic receptors (Figs. 12.4 and 12.5). An example supporting this observation is serotonin syndrome, a condition classically composed of the clinical triad of mental status changes, autonomic

Table 12.6 Drug interactions associated with severe presentations serotonin syndrome

MAOIs
Phenelzine plus Meperidine (Analgesic)
Tranylcypromine plus Imipramine (TCA)
MAOIs Plus SSRIs
Phenelzine plus any SSRI
Moclobemide plus any SSRI
SSRIs
Citalopram plus Linezolid (Antibiotic)
Paroxetine plus Buspirone (Antidepressant, anxiolytic)
Other
Tramadol (Analgesic), Venlafaxine (SNRI) plus Mirtazapine (NaSSA)

Adapted from Boyer E, Shannon M. The serotonin syndrome. N Engl J Med. 2005;352(11):1112–20 *MAOIs* monoamine oxidase inhibitors, *SSRIs* selective serotonin reuptake inhibitors

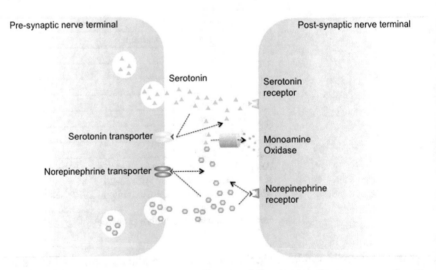

Fig. 12.4 Tricyclic antidepressants block the serotonin and norepinephrine transporters (and/or the norepinephrine receptor) resulting in an accumulation of serotonin and norepinephrine in the synaptic cleft

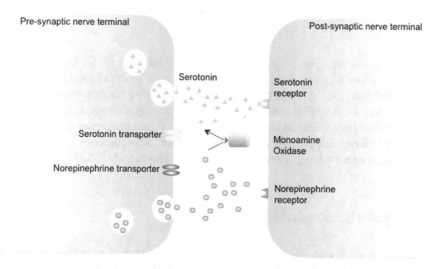

Fig. 12.5 Monoamine oxidase inhibitors prevent degradation of serotonin and norepinephrine resulting in an accumulation of serotonin and norepinephrine in the synaptic cleft

hyperactivity (such as hypertension, tachycardia, hyperhidrosis, and hyperthermia), and neuromuscular abnormalities (such as tremor, hyperreflexia, muscle rigidity, and myoclonus). Serotonin syndrome results from excess stimulation of the post-synaptic serotonin receptor [191]. Treatment of serotonin syndrome is focused on symptom control geared and reducing further serotonin receptor stimulation with cyproheptadine, a 5-HT2A antagonist [191].

The prevalence of serotonin syndrome is unknown because of its protean presentation and its association with medications that are not otherwise associated with depression management [191]. Given the medication burden associated with CKD, hypertension as a result of serotonin syndrome and inadvertent drug interactions should be considered before escalating antihypertensive therapy.

Treatment

Given the wide variety of anti-depressant and anxiolytic medications on the market and the unclear mechanism mediating hypertension in some patients, no evidence-based recommendations can be made to discontinue or pursue an alternative agent. That said, if a medication has an acceptable effect on mood control, then close surveillance of both blood pressures and weights would be warranted. If suspicion is present that hypertension is mediated directly or indirectly by an antidepressant, pursuit of alternate therapies that appropriately control mood without worsening blood pressure would be warranted. In addition to exercise and sodium reduction, a plan that would involve an antidepressant dose reduction, initiation of a new antihypertensive, or the selection of another antidepressant would be recommended following a discussion of patient expectations of mood and blood pressure control.

Anemia

Anemia is a common hematologic abnormality in patients with CKD, especially those with estimated glomerular filtration rates less than 30 ml/min and underlying diabetes mellitus [192]. Anemia in CKD is primarily due to a combination of endogenous erythropoietin (EPO) insufficiency, EPO hypo-responsiveness from inflammation, and true or functional iron deficiency [193]. Given the causes of anemia in this setting, therapeutic options typically involve oral or intravenous iron therapy, red blood cell transfusions, or erythropoiesis stimulating agents (ESAs).

Erythropoiesis Stimulating Agents (ESAs)

ESAs are a mainstay of anemia management in CKD. After observational studies suggested that CKD and ESRD patients would benefit from higher hemoglobin levels, use of ESAs in the CKD population expanded tremendously in the 1990s and 2000s. ESA use in the CKD population became more focused following several trials that demonstrate increased cardiovascular risk and a lack of benefit at higher hemoglobin targets, ESAs [194–198].

Adverse Drug Effects

In the Trial to Reduce Cardiovascular Events with Aranesp Therapy [199] study, 4038 patients with diabetes and CKD were targeted to a hemoglobin level of 13 g/dl with darbepoetin [198] as compared with a lower target (9.0 g/dl) with placebo. 632 patients died or had a cardiovascular event on darbepoetin and 602 patients died or had a cardiovascular event when targeted to a higher hemoglobin level with no significant difference detected [198]. Fatal or nonfatal stroke occurred in 101 patients on darbepoetin compared to 53 patients on placebo. There was no significant difference in systolic blood pressure between either group (median systolic blood pressure 134 mmHg), but the diastolic pressure was higher in the darbepoetin group compared to placebo (73 vs 71 mmHg, respectively). Although hypertension was not a primary end-point in these studies, it has become a well-established side effect of ESAs [200].

ESAs and Hypertension

The association between ESAs and hypertension is well documented [200–202], but the mechanisms mediating ESA-induced hypertension are unclear. Some studies have inferred that increased blood pressure is due to increased RBC mass and plasma volume [203, 204]. Other studies suggest that erythropoietin effects a variety of vasoactive substances to raise blood pressure such as augmented endothelin-1 [205, 206] and thromboxane A2 [207] production and suppressed nitric oxide [208] and prostacyclin [209] synthesis. These combinations of pressor effects at the level of the vasculature, and likely within the kidneys, lead to an increase in blood pressure and frank hypertension.

There are a lack of data examining the level of increase in blood pressure in CKD patients exposed to ESA therapy for anemia, but data are available in other groups treated with these drugs, such as the hemodialysis population. In one study of normotensive subjects, resting mean arterial pressure was found to increase in approximately 49 % subjects by 6 mmHg [204]. More robust data evaluating the hypertensive effects of ESAs are available from end-stage renal disease patients on hemodialysis [210–212]. A study that evaluated epoetin alfa in the dialysis population noted no blood pressure effects in groups of end-stage renal disease patients targeting both high and low hemoglobin levels [213]. However, routine monitoring of blood pressure may miss a hypertensionogenic effect of EPO.

Treatment

Recognition of the hypertensive effect of ESAs was recognized early and promoted the creation of administrative guidelines that recommend holding the ESA therapy when blood pressure is above the upper limit of normal. This approach limits development of severe and/or worsening hypertension in the CKD population. In addition, a slow increase in hemoglobin and hematocrit may limit development of hypertension. When hypertension develops on therapy, further drug ESA exposure is stopped until blood pressure is controlled with adjustment of the underlying antihypertensive medication regimen.

Renal Cell Carcinoma in CKD

Renal cell carcinoma (RCC) is a relatively common cancer comprising 2–3 % of all cancers in the USA with an incidence of 5–10 cases per 100,000 in the general population [214]. Patients with inherited and acquired cystic diseases and end-stage renal disease (ESRD) are all at a greater risk for RCC than the general population [214]. For this reason, providers should be aware of the need for surveillance of RCC in the CKD and ESRD population and of current medical treatments available. In addition, treatment of RCC with radical or partial nephrectomy often leads to the development or further progression of CKD [215–217] Thus, there is a bi-directional relationship between RCC and CKD. Medical management of RCC with certain drugs can induce or exacerbate hypertension in this group of patients. The drug class most commonly associated with hypertension is the anti-angiogenesis agents.

Anti-Angiogenic Therapy

Vascular endothelial growth factor (VEGF) is a key regulator of angiogenesis associated with tumor growth [218]. VEGF promotes growth of arterial, venous, and lymphatic endothelial cells [218] and has been shown to be variably expressed in multiple carcinomas (lung, breast, pancreas, ovary, and kidney) [219–223]. There are two main VEGF receptor tyrosine kinases (RTKs) known as VEGFR1 (Flt-1) [224, 225] and VEGFR2 (KDR) [226] with VEGFR2 acting as the major mediator of angiogenic effects of VEGF [218, 227].

Medications targeting angiogenesis have emerged as an important primary or adjunctive therapy for many malignancies including RCC [228, 229]. They include anti-vascular endothelial growth factor (VEGF) monoclonal antibody (bevacizumab), circulating VEGF decoy receptor molecule (aflibercept), and VEGF receptor tyrosine kinase inhibitors (sunitinib, sorafenib, axitinib, pazopanib, vandetanib) (Fig. 12.6) [228]. The anti-cancer efficacy of these agents is based on interruption of unregulated tumor angiogenesis mediated by the VEGF signaling pathway [228]. The anti-angiogenic effect is also effective in a number of non-malignant neo-vascular processes that are likely to be present in patients with underlying CKD. The beneficial effects of the agents are countered by dose-dependent nephrotoxicity, which includes hypertension, proteinuria, and renal lesions such as thrombotic microangiopathy [228].

The focus of this discussion will be on hypertension, both de novo and exacerbation of underlying hypertension, as a complication of these drugs in patients receiving these drugs.

Anti-VEGF Monoclonal Antibodies

Studies of bevacizumab, an anti-VEGF monoclonal antibody, have implicated its use as a cause of hypertension [230]. A rise in blood pressure has been noted in 20–30 % of bevacizumab-treated patients and 15–60 % of patients administered tyrosine kinase inhibitors [231].

The effect of bevacizumab on blood pressure is dose-dependent and the severity of hypertension appears to reflect the extent of target inhibition. A phase 2 study in patients with renal cell carcinoma (RCC) treated with placebo, bevacizumab (3 mg/kg), or bevacizumab (10 mg/kg) noted that the rate of hypertension was significantly higher in the high-dose group (36 %) compared with the low-dose group (3 %) [229]. A review of 7 clinical trials including 1850 patients described a significant increase in hypertension in patients receiving bevacizumab [232]. The relative risks for hypertension were dose dependent with 3.0 for low dose and 7.5 for high dose [232].

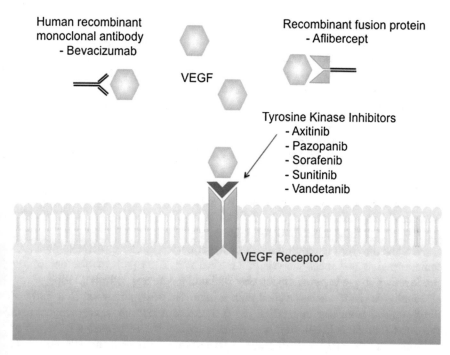

Fig. 12.6 Anti-angiogenesis medications work by preventing VEGF from interacting with VEGF receptor 1 or 2. Three main inhibitors are currently available: Bevacizumab, a human recombinant monoclonal antibody; Aflibercept, a recombinant fusion protein which contains the extracellular domain of VEGF1 and VEGF2 receptors with the Fc portion of IgG1; and the Tyrosine kinase inhibitors, Axitinib, Pazopanib, Sorafenib, Sunitinib, and Vandetanib, which block VEGF from interacting with the membrane-bound VEGF receptor

Tyrosine Kinase Inhibitors (TKIs)

Tyrosine kinase inhibitors (TKIs) have been implicated in hypertension, nephrotic-range proteinuria, reversible posterior leukoencephelopathy syndrome, and thrombotic microangiopathy [233–240]. The TKI effects on blood pressure have been shown to be dose-dependent [241]. A phase 1 study of sunitinib described hypertension in 5 of 28 patients, of which grade 3 or 4 hypertension developed in 2 patients treated at doses of >75 mg/day [242]. Hypertension occurred after approximately 3–4 weeks of treatment. A dose of 50 mg/day was associated with 5 % hypertension in a phase 2 study in patients with advanced renal cell carcinoma; supporting the dose dependency of hypertension [243]. A systematic review and meta-analysis revealed significant risk for hypertension with sunitinib [244]. The incidence of all-grade and high-grade hypertension were 21.6 % (95 % CI: 18.7–24.8 %) and 6.8 % (95 % CI: 5.3–8.8 %), respectively [244]. The risk varied with the sunitinib dosing schedule. Sunitinib was associated with a significantly increased risk of high-grade hypertension (RR = 22.72, 95 % CI: 4.48–115.29, $p < 0.001$) [244].

Sorafenib was associated with development of hypertension in 86 of 202 patients (43%) and antihypertensive therapy was needed in 46% of patients [245]. An increase in systolic blood pressure greater than 10 or 20 mmHg was reported in 75% (15 of 20) and 60% (12 of 20) of treated patients compared with their baseline after 3 weeks of therapy, respectively [246].

Pazopanib was found to significantly increase the risk of hypertension in a meta-analysis conducted by the same group that studied axitinib [247]. 13 clinical trials with 1651 subjects with solid tumors on pazopanib were studied and hypertension grading was defined as above [247]. The use of pazopanib was associated with all-grade hypertension in 35.9% of subjects with RCC and high-grade hypertension in 6.5% of subjects [247]. The risk of high-grade hypertension was similar to sorafenib and sunitinib, but the risk of all-grade hypertension was higher for pazopanib when compared to sorafenib (RR 1.99; 95%, CI: 1.73–2.29, $p=0.00$) and sunitinib (RR 2.20; 95%, CI: 1.92–2.52, $p=0.00$), respectively [247].

Vandetanib also increased the risk of hypertension in cancer patients. In a systematic review and meta-analysis of 11 trials with 3154 patients, the risk of all-grade and high-grade hypertension was 24.2 and 6.4%, respectively [248]

Finally, axitinib was associated with a high risk of hypertension in a study of 1908 subjects from 10 clinical trials [249]. The risk of axitinib was also higher than the other four TKIs [249]. In this systematic review and meta-analysis, the use of axitinib was associated with all-grade hypertension in 40.1% of subjects with RCC and high-grade hypertension in 13.1% of subjects [249].

Mechanisms of Hypertension

Patients with an underlying history of hypertension and CKD appear more prone to developing hypertension with VEGF receptor kinase inhibitors. Increased sympathetic activity, renalase deficiency, and oxidative stress typically present in CKD [19–24] exacerbate hypertension following exposure to anti-angiogenesis medications [250]. Recent studies have advanced our understanding of the pathophysiology of hypertension associated with this class of drugs.

VEGF modulates vascular contractility and blood pressure in humans (Fig. 12.7). An association between VEGF and blood pressure regulation was demonstrated by VEGF-induced nitric oxide (NO)-dependent relaxation in coronary arteries [251]. In a clinical trial examining the effect of VEGF on ischemia, a rapid decline in mean arterial pressure (~8–12 mmHg) was observed, in patients receiving an intravenous infusion of recombinant human $VEGF_{165}$ [252]. These data suggest that inhibition of the VEGF signaling pathway reduces NO production and increases blood pressure through increased vasoconstriction and vascular resistance. Anti-angiogenesis inhibitors may also increase blood pressure by pressor effects that result from inhibition of prostacyclin I2 (PGI2) production in the vascular endothelium [253].

Hypertension induced by anti-angiogenesis agents may also result from a structural reduction in the total number of arteries and arterioles, known as rarefaction. Both spontaneously hypertensive rats and rats fed a high-salt diet develop capil-

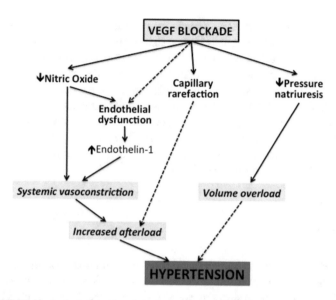

Fig. 12.7 VEGF blockade induces hypertension via several pathways including increased systemic vasoconstriction from decreased nitric oxide and increased endothelin-1 production; increased afterload which is augmented by increased SVR and capillary rarefaction; and finally decreased pressure natriuresis which results in volume overload

lary rarefaction early in the development of hypertension [254, 255]. In humans, microvascular rarefaction has been consistently observed in adults with hypertension [256]. VEGF signaling in endothelial cells is crucial to endothelial cell survival and inhibition is associated with apoptosis of these cells and the development of microvascular rarefaction [257]. In fact, this phenomenon has been shown in patients treated with VEGF inhibitors [258]. Although there is support for rarefaction as a pathway mediating hypertension [259], there are some that question rarefaction as a cause given the degree of blood pressure change and the amount of rarefaction that actually occurs [260].

Other mechanisms have also been speculated as causing blood pressure rise in patients treated with these drugs, including increased endothelin-1 activity and reduced pressure natriuresis, leading to hypervolemia [261]. Ultimately, this is a real phenomenon that occurs and must be recognized and treated by the healthcare provider.

Treatment

Hypertension management in patients with cancer and CKD is to maintain an acceptable blood pressure level to preserve continued but safe delivery of anti-angiogenesis therapy. Close monitoring of blood pressure and timely initiation or titration of hypertension medications are critical to achieve these goals. As there are data to suggest that hypertension associated with anti-angiogenesis drug therapy is a marker for tumor response, it is logical that continued drug treatment along with blood pressure control is warranted [262]. Hypertension can be controlled with standard oral hypertensive medications in most cases where therapeutic doses of these anti-VEGF agents are used. Non-dihydropyridine calcium-channel blockers and ACE-inhibitors/ARBs are acceptable and quite effective [263] Addition of a diuretic or escalation of the dose may be necessary in some patients. In patients who develop hypertensive crisis and posterior reversible encehalopathy syndrome [264] both described as a complication of therapy with these agents likely require permanent discontinuation of anti-VEGF therapy.

Summary

In summary, drug-induced hypertension is a fairly common condition in the setting of CKD. De novo hypertension or exacerbation of underlying hypertension occurs as a result of drug-induced systemic vasoconstriction or cardiac output, which either exacerbate or diminish compensatory mechanisms that occur in the setting of reduced renal mass or function. Knowledge of this physiology and adverse drug effect in this population is critical to proving care to these patients. As such, all healthcare providers should be cognizant of the medications and supplements that CKD patients are prescribed and over-the-counter medications that patients are self-administering. As hypertension represents a risk factor for progression of kidney disease, stroke, and heart disease, this represents a modifiable condition that can be identified and targeted for intervention.

References

1. Fox C, Larson M, Leip E, Culleton B, Wilson P, Levy D. Predictors of new-onset kidney disease in a community-based population. JAMA. 2004;291(7):844–50.
2. Kidney Disease: Improving Global Outcomes (KDIGO) Blood Pressure Work Group. KDIGO clinical practice guideline for the management of blood pressure in chronic kidney disease. Kidney Int. 2012;2:337–414.
3. Brazy P, Stead W, Fitzwilliam J. Progression of renal insufficiency: role of blood pressure. Kidney Int. 1989;35(2):670–4.
4. Oldrizzi L, Rugiu C, De Biase V, Maschio G. The place of hypertension among the risk factors for renal function in chronic renal failure. Am J Kidney Dis. 1993;21(5 Suppl 2):119–23.
5. U.S.R.D.S. USRDS 2013 Annual Data Report: Atlas of Chronic Kidney Disease and End-Stage Renal Disease in the United States. Bethesda: National Institutes of Health, National Institute of Diabetes and Digestive and Kidney Diseases; 2013.
6. Akerstrom T, Crona J, Delgado Verdugo A, Starker L, Cupisti K, Willenberg H, et al. Comprehensive re-sequencing of adrenal aldosterone producing lesions reveal three somatic mutations near the KCNJ5 potassium channel selectivity filter. PLoS One. 2012;7(7):e41926.

7. Buckalew V, Berg R, Wang S, Porush J, Rauch S, Schulman G. Prevalence of hypertension in 1,795 subjects with chronic renal disease: the modification of diet in renal disease study baseline cohort. Am J Kidney Dis. 1996;28(6):811–21.
8. K/DOQI clinical practice guidelines for chronic kidney disease: evaluation, classification, and stratification. Am J Kidney Dis. 2002;39(2 Suppl 1):S1–266.
9. Whaley-Connell A, Sowers J, Stevens L, McFarlane S, Shlipak M, Norris K, et al. CKD in the United States: Kidney Early Evaluation (KEEP) and National Health and Nutrition Examination Survery (NHANES) 1999–2004. Am J Kidney Dis. 2008;51(4 Suppl 2):S13–20.
10. Lifton R, Gharavi A, Geller D. Molecular mechanisms of human hypertension. Cell. 2001;104(4):545–56.
11. Davis J, Freeman R. Mechanisms regulating renin release. Physiol Rev. 1976;56(1):1–56.
12. Reid I, Morris B, Ganong W. The renin-angiotensin system. Annu Rev Physiol. 1978;40:377–410.
13. Matsukawa T, Gotoh E, Minamisawa K, Kihara M, Ueda S, Shioniri H, et al. Effects of intravenous infusions of angiotensin II on muscle sympathetic nerve activity in humans. Am J Physiol. 1991;261(3 Pt 2):R690–6.
14. Reid I. Interactions between ANG II, sympathetic nervous system, and baroreceptor reflexes in regulation of blood pressure. Am J Physiol. 1992;262(6 Pt 1):E763–78.
15. Neumann J, Ligtenberg G, Klein I, Koomans H, Blankestijn P. Sympathetic hyperactivity in chronic kidney disease: pathogenesis, clinical revelance, and treatment. Kidney Int. 2004;65(5):1568–76.
16. Anderson S, Rennke H, Brenner B. Therapeutic advantage of converting enzyme inhibitors in arresting progressive renal disease associated with systemic hypertension in the rat. J Clin Invest. 1986;77(6):1993–2000.
17. Meyer T, Anderson S, Rennke H, Brenner B. Reversing glomerular hypertension stabilizes established glomerular injury. Kidney Int. 1987;31(3):752–9.
18. Johnson R, Kang D, Feig D, Kivlighn S, Kanellis J, Watanabe S, et al. Is there a pathogenetic role for uric acid in hypertension and cardiovascular and renal disease? Hypertension. 2003;41(6):1183–90.
19. Xu J, Li G, Wang P, Velazquez H, Yao X, Li Y, et al. Renalase is a novel, soluble monoamine oxidase that regulates cardiac function and blood pressure. J Clin Invest. 2005;115(5):1275–80.
20. Nakagawa T. Uncoupling of the VEGF-endothelial nitric oxide axis in diabetic nephropathy: an explanation for the paradoxical effects of VEGF in renal disease. Am J Physiol Renal Physiol. 2007;292(6):F1665–72.
21. Doi K, Noiri E, Fujita T. Role of vascular endothelial growth factor in kidney disease. Curr Vasc Pharmacol. 2010;8(1):122–8.
22. Kang D, Joly A, Oh S, Hugo C, Kerjaschki D, Gordon K, et al. Impaired angiogenesis in the remnant kidney model: I. Potential role of vascular endothelial growth factor and thrombospondin-1. J Am Soc Nephrol. 2001;12(7):1434–47.
23. Brown K, Dhaun N, Goddard J, Webb D. Potential therapeutic role of phosphodiesterase type 5 inhibition in hypertension and chronic kidney disease. Hypertension. 2014;63(1):5–11.
24. Baylis C. Nitric oxide synthase derangements and hypertension in kidney disease. Curr Opin Nephrol Hypertens. 2012;21(1):1–6.
25. Collantes E, Curtis S, Lee K, Casa N, McCarthy T, Melian A, et al. A multinational randomized, controlled, clinical trial of etoricoxib in the treatment of rheumatoid arthritis. BMC Fam Pract. 2002;3:10.
26. Handler J. Drug-induced hypertension. J Clin Hypertens (Greenwich). 2003;5(1):83–5.
27. Grossman E, Messerli F. Drug-induced hypertension: an unappreciated cause of secondary hypertension. Am J Med. 2012;125(1):14–22.
28. Sandler D, Smith J, Weinberg C, Buckalew VJ, Dennis V, Blythe W, et al. Analgesic use and chronic renal disease. N Engl J Med. 1989;320(19):1238–43.

29. Pham P, Dewar K, Hashmi S, Toscano E, Pham P, Pham P, et al. Pain prevalence in patients with chronic kidney disease. Clin Nephrol. 2010;73(4):294–9.
30. Fagius J, Karhuvaara S, Sundlof G. The cold pressor test: effects on sympathetic nerve activity in human muscle and skin nerve fascicles. Acta Physiol Scand. 1989;137(3):325–34.
31. Nordin M, Fagius J. Effect of noxious stimulation on sympathetic vasoconstrictor outflow to human muscles. J Physiol. 1995;489(Pt 3):885–94.
32. Maixner W, Gracely R, Zuniga J, Humphrey C, Bloodworth G. Cardiovascular and sensory responses to forearm ischemia and dynamic hand exercise. Am J Physiol. 1990;259(6 Pt 2):R1156–63.
33. Chan C, Reid C, Aw T, Liew D, Haas S, Krum H. Do COX-2 inhibitors raise blood pressure more than nonselective NSAIDs and placebo? An updated meta-analysis. J Hypertens. 2009;27(12):2332–41.
34. Holland S, Silberstein S, Freitag F, Dodick D, Argoff C, Ashman E. Evidence-based guideline update: NSAIDs and other complementary treatments for episodic migraine prevention in adults: report of the Quality Standards Subcommittee of the American Academy of Neurology and the American Headache Society. Neurology. 2012;78(17):1346–53.
35. McAlindon T, Bannuru R, Sullivan M, Arden N, Berenbaum F, Bierma-Zeinstra S, et al. OARSI guidelines for the non-surgical management of knee osteoarthritis. Osteoarthritis Cartilage. 2014;22(3):363–88.
36. Khanna D, Khanna P, Fitzgerald J, Singh M, Bae S, Neogi T, et al. 2012 American College of Rheumatology guidelines for management of gout. Part 2: therapy and antiinflammatory prophylaxis of acute gouty arthritis. Arthritis Care Res. 2012;64(10):1447–61.
37. Moore R, Derry S, McQuay H, Wiffen P. Single dose oral analgesics for acute postoperative pain in adults. Cochrane Database Syst Rev. 2011;9:CD008659.
38. Nelson A, Allen K, Golightly Y, Goode A, Jordan J. A systematic review of recommendations and guidelines for the management of osteoarthritis: the chronic osteoarthritis management initiative of the U.S. bone and joint initiative. Semin Arthritis Rheum. 2014;2014(43):6.
39. De Broe M, Elseviers M. Over-the-counter analgesic use. J Am Soc Nephrol. 2009;20(10):2098–103.
40. Ingrasciotta Y, Sultana J, Giorgianni F, Caputi A, Arcoraci V, Tari D, et al. The burden of nephrotoxic drug prescription in patients with chronic kidney disease: a retrospective population-based study in Southern Italy. PLoS One. 2014;9(2):e89072.
41. Gooch K, Culleton B, Manns B, Zhang J, Alfonso H, Tonelli M, et al. NSAID use and progression of chronic kidney disease. Am J Med. 2007;120(3):280.e–17.
42. Kramer H, Glanzer K, Dusing R. Role of prostaglandins in the regulation of renal water excretion. Kidney Int. 1981;19(6):851–9.
43. Breyer M, Breyer R. Prostaglandin E receptors and the kidney. Am J Physiol Renal Physiol. 2000;279(1):F12–23.
44. Henrich W, Agodoa L, Barrett B, Bennett W, Blantz R, Buckalew VJ, et al. Analgesics and the kidney: summary and recommendations to the Scientific Advisory Board of the National Kidney Foundation from an Ad Hoc Committee of the National Kidney Foundation. Am J Kidney Dis. 1996;27(1):162–5.
45. Plantinga L, Grubbs V, Sarkar U, Hsu C, Hedgeman E, Robinson B, et al. Nonsteroidal anti-inflammatory drug use among persons with chronic kidney disease in the United States. Ann Fam Med. 2011;9(5):423–30.
46. Patel K, Diamantidis C, Zhan M, Hsu V, Walker L, Gardner J, et al. Influence of creatinine versus glomerular filtration rate on non-steroidal anti-inflammatory drug prescriptions in chronic kidney disease. Am J Nephrol. 2012;36(1):19–26.
47. Nderitu P, Doos L, Jones P, Davies S, Kadam U. Non-steroidal anti-inflammatory drugs and chronic kidney disease progression: a systematic review. Fam Pract. 2013;30(3):247–55.
48. Ruilope L, Garcia Robles R, Paya C, Alcazar J, Miravalles E, Sancho-Rof J, et al. Effects of long-term treatment with indomethacin on renal function. Hypertension. 1986;8(8):677–84.
49. Smith W. Prostanoid biosynthesis and mechanisms of action. Am J Physiol. 1992;263(2 Pt 2):F181–91.

50. Nasrallah R, Clark J, Hebert R. Prostaglandins in the kidney: developments since Y2K. Clin Sci (Lond). 2007;113(7):297–311.
51. Smith M, Dunn M. The role of prostaglandins in human hypertension. Am J Kidney Dis. 1985;5(4):A32–9.
52. Stokes J. Effect of prostaglanding E2 on chloride transport across the rabbit thick ascending limb of Henle. Selective inhibitions of the medullary portion. J Clin Invest. 1979;64(2):495–502.
53. Hebert S, Andreoli T. Control of the NaCl transport in the thick ascending limb. Am J Physiol. 1984;246(6 Pt 2):F745–56.
54. Seyberth H, Rascher W, Schweer H, Kuhl P, Mehls O, Schärer, K. Congenital hypokalemia with hypercalciuria in pre-term infants: a hyperprostaglandinuric tubular syndrome different from Bartter syndrome. J Pediatr. 1985;107(5):694–701.
55. Tan S, Bravo E, Mulrow P. Impaired renal prostaglandin E2 biosynthesis in human hypertensive states. Prostaglandins Med. 1978;1(1):76–85.
56. Dunn M, Grone H. The relevance of prostaglandins in human hypertension. Adv Prostaglandin Thromboxane Leukot Res. 1985;13:179–87.
57. Trimarco B, De Simone A, Cuocolo A, Ricciardelli B, Volpe M, Patrignani P, et al. Role of prostaglandins in the renal handling of a salt load in essential hypertension. Am J Cardiol. 1985;55(1):116–21.
58. Ungvari Z, Koller A. Endothelin and prostaglandin H(2)/thromboxane A (2) enhance myogenic constriction in hypertension by increasing Ca(2+) sensitivity of arteriolar smooth muscle. Hypertension. 2000;2000(36):5.
59. Huang A, Koller A. Endothelin and prostaglandin H2 enhance arteriolar myogenic tone in hypertension. Hypertension. 1997;30(5):1210–5.
60. Fujino T, Nakagawa N, Yuhki K, Hara A, Yamada T, Takayama K, et al. Decreased susceptibility to renovascular hypertension in mice lacking the prostaglandin I2 receptor IP. J Clin Invest. 2004;114(6):805–12.
61. Brater D. Analysis of the effect of indomethacin on the response to furosemide in man: effect of dose of furosemide. J Pharmacol Exp Ther. 1979;210(3):386–90.
62. Favre L, Glasson P, Riondel A, Vallotton M. Interaction of diuretics and non-steroidal anti-inflammatory drugs in man. Clin Sci (Lond). 1983;64(4):407–15.
63. Chennavasin P, Seiwell R, Brater D. Pharmacokinetic-dynamic analysis of the indomethacin-furosemide interaction in man. J Pharmacol Exp Ther. 1980;215(1):77–81.
64. Skinner M, Mutterperl R, Zeitz H. Sulindac inhibits bumetanide-induced sodium and water excretion. Clin Pharmacol Ther. 1987;42(5):542–6.
65. Koopmans P, Thien T, Thomas C, Van den Berg R, Gribnau F. The effects of sulindac and indomethacin on the anti-hypertensive and diuretic action of hydrochlorothiazide in patients with mild to moderate essential hypertension. Br J Clin Pharmacol. 1986;21(4):417–23.
66. Steiness E, Waldorff S. Different interactions of indomethacin and sulindac with thiazides in hypertension. Br Med J (Clin Res Ed). 1982;285(6356):1702–3.
67. Koopmans P, Kateman W, Tan Y, van Ginneken C, Gribnau F. Effects of indomethacin and sulindac on hydrochlorothiazide kinetics. Clin Pharmacol Ther. 1985;37(6):625–8.
68. Davies J, Rawlins D, Busson M. Effect of ibuprofen on blood pressure control by propranolol and bendrofluazide. J Int Med Res. 1988;16(3):173–81.
69. Watkins J, Abbot E, Hensby C, Webster J, Dollery C. Attenuation of hypotensive effect of propranolol and thiazide diuretics by indomethacin. Br Med J. 1980;281(6242):702–5.
70. Salvetti A, Pedrinelli R, Alberici P, Magagna A, Abdel-Haq B. The influence of indomethacin on some pharmacological actions of atenolol in hypertensive patients. Br J Clin Pharmacol. 1984;17 Suppl 1:108S–11.
71. Durao V, Prata M, Goncalves L. Modification of antihypertensive effect of beta-adrenoceptor-blocking agents by inhibition of endogenous prostaglandin synthesis. Lancet. 1977;2(8046):1005–7.
72. Lopez-Ovejero J, Weber M, Drayer J, Sealery J, Laragh J. Effects of indomethacin alone and during diuretic or beta-adrenoreceptor-blockade therapy on blood pressure and the renin system in essential hypertension. Clin Sci Mol Med Suppl. 1978;4:203s–5s.

73. Salvetti A, Arzilli F, Pedrinelli R, Beggi P, Motolese M. Interaction between oxprenolol and indomethacin on blood pressure in essential hypertensive patients. Eur J Clin Pharmacol. 1982;22(3):197–201.

74. Ebel D, Rhymer A, Stahl E, Tipping R. Effect of Clinoril (sulindac, MSD), piroxicam and placebo on the hypotensive effect of propranolol in patients with mild to moderate essential hypertension. Scand J Rheumatol Suppl. 1986;62:41–9.

75. Webster J, Petrie J, McLean I, Hawksworth G. Flurbiprofen interaction with single doses of atenolol and propranolol. Br J Clin Pharmacol. 1984;18(6):861–6.

76. Sahloul M, al-Kiek R, Ivanovich P, Mujais S. Nonsteroidal anti-inflammatory drugs and anti-hypertensives. Cooperative malfeasance. Nephron. 1990;56(4):345–52.

77. Witzgall H, Hirsch F, Scherer B, Weber P. Acute haemodynamic and hormonal effects of captopril are diminished by indomethacin. Clin Sci (Lond). 1982;62(6):611–5.

78. Moore T, Crantz F, Hollenberg N, Koletsky R, Leboff M, Swartz S, et al. Contribution of prostaglandins to the antihypertensive action of captopril in essential hypertension. Hypertension. 1981;3(2):168–73.

79. Fujita T, Yamashita N, Yamashita K. Effect of indomethacin on antihypertensive action of captopril in hypertensive patients. Clin Exp Hypertens. 1981;3(5):939–52.

80. Salvetti A, Pedrinelli R, Sassano P, Arzilli F, Turini F. Effects of prostaglandins inhibition on changes in active and inactive renin induced by antihypertensive drugs. Clin Exp Hypertens. 1982;4(11–12):2435–48.

81. Heeg J, de Jong P, Vriesendrop R, de Zeeuw D. Additive antiproteinuric effect of the NSAID indomethacin and the ACE inhibitor lisinopril. Am J Nephrol. 1990;10 Suppl 1:94–7.

82. Vinci J, Gill JJ, Bowden R, Pisano J, Izzo JJ, Radfar N, et al. The kallikrein-kinin system in Bartter's syndrome and its response to prostaglandin synthetase inhibition. J Clin Invest. 1978;61(6):1671–82.

83. Katori M, Majima M. Roles of the renal kallikrein-kinin system in salt-sensitive hypertension. Hypertension. 2004;44(6):e12.

84. Reimann I, Ratge D, Wisser H, Frolich J. Are prostaglandins involved in the antihypertensive effect of dihydralazine? Clin Sci (Lond). 1981;61 Suppl 7:319s–21s.

85. Cinquegrani M, Liang C. Indomethacin attenuates the hypotensive action of hydralazine. Clin Pharmacol Ther. 1986;39(5):564–70.

86. Cinquegrani M, Liang C. Antihypertensive effects of pinacidil in patients with and without indomethacin pretreatment. Clin Exp Hypertens A. 1988;10(3):411–31.

87. Nasjletti A, Arthur C. Corcoran Memorial Lecture. The role of eicosanoids in angiotensin-dependent hypertension. Hypertension. 1998;31(1 Pt 2):194–200.

88. Mistry M, Nasjletti A. Prostanoids as mediators of prohypertensive and antihypertensive mechanisms. Am J Med Sci. 1988;295(4):263–7.

89. Pope J, Anderson J, Felson D. A meta-analysis of the effects of nonsteroidal anti-inflammatory drugs on blood pressure. Arch Intern Med. 1993;153(4):477–84.

90. Johnson A, Nguyen T, Day R. Do nonsteroidal anti-inflammatory drugs affect blood pressure? A meta-analysis. Ann Int Med. 1994;121(4):289–300.

91. Gabriel S, Jaakkimainen L, Bombardier C. Risk for serious gastrointestinal complications related to use of nonsteroidal anti-inflammatory drugs. A meta-analysis. Ann Int Med. 1991;115(10):787–96.

92. Schafer A. Effects of nonsteroidal antiinflammatory drugs on platelet function and systemic hemostasis. J Clin Pharmacol. 1995;35(3):209–19.

93. Clive D, Stoff J. Renal syndromes associated with nonsteroidal antiinflammatory drugs. N Engl J Med. 1984;310(9):563–72.

94. Silverstein F, Faich G, Goldstein J, Simon L, Pincus T, Whelton A, et al. Gastrointestinal toxicity with celecoxib vs nonsteroidal anti-inflammatory drugs for osteoarthritis and rheumatoid arthritis: the CLASS study: a randomized controlled trial. Celecoxib Long-Term Arthritis Study. JAMA. 2000;284(10):1247–55.

95. Rofecoxib: FDA Advisory Committee Background Information 2001 [March 26, 2015]. Available from: http://www.fda.gov/ohrms/dockets/ac/01/briefing/3677b2_01_merck.pdf.

96. Bombardier C, Laine L, Reicin A, Shapiro D, Burgos-Vargas R, Davis B, et al. Comparison of upper gastrointestinal toxicity of rofecoxib and naproxen in patients with rheumatoid arthritis. VIGOR Study Group. N Engl J Med. 2000;343(21):1520–8.
97. Whelton A, Maurath C, Verburg K, Geis G. Renal safety and tolerability of celecoxib, a novel cyclo-oxygenase-2 inhibitor. Am J Ther. 2000;7(3):159–75.
98. Whelton A, Fort J, Puma J, Normandin D, Bello A, Verburg K. Cyclooxygenase-2--specific inhibitors and cardiorenal function: a randomized, controlled trial of celecoxib and rofecoxib in older hypertensive osteoarthritis patients. Am J Ther. 2001;8(2):85–95.
99. Whelton A, White W, Bello A, Puma J, Fort J. Effects of celecoxib and rofecoxib on blood pressure and edema in patients > or =65 years of age with systemic hypertension and osteoarthritis. Am J Cardiol. 2002;90(9):959–63.
100. Emery P, Zeidler H, Kvien T, Guslandi M, Naudin R, Stead H, et al. Celecoxib versus diclofenac in long-term management of rheumatoid arthritis: randomised double-blind comparison. Lancet. 1999;354(9196):2106–11.
101. Catella-Lawson F, McAdam B, Morrison B, Kapoor S, Kujubu D, Antes L, et al. Effects of specific inhibition of cyclooxygenase-2 on sodium balance, hemodynamics, and vasoactive eicosanoids. J Pharmacol Exp Ther. 1999;289(2):735–41.
102. Geba G, Weaver A, Polis A, Dixon M, Schnitzer T. Efficacy of rofecoxib, celecoxib, and acetaminophen in osteoarthritis of the knee: a randomized trial. JAMA. 2002;287(1):64–71.
103. Simon L, Weaver A, Graham D, Kivitz A, Lipsky P, Hubbard R, et al. Anti-inflammatory and upper gastrointestinal effects of celecoxib in rheumatoid arthritis: a randomized controlled trial. JAMA. 1999;282(20):1921–8.
104. Qi Z, Hao C, Langenbach R, Breyer R, Redha R, Morrow J, et al. Opposite effects of cyclooxygenase-1 and -2 activity on the pressor response to angiotensin II. J Clin Invest. 2002;110(1):61–9.
105. Qi Z, Cai H, Morrow J, Breyer M. Differentiation of cyclooxygenase 1- and 2-derived prostanoids in mouse kidney and aorta. Hypertension. 2006;48(2):323–8.
106. Hocherl K, Endemann D, Kammerl M, Grobecker H, Kurtz A. Cyclo-oxygenase-2 inhibition increases blood pressure in rats. Br J Pharmacol. 2002;2002(136):8.
107. White W, Kent J, Taylor A, Verburg K, Lefkowith J, Whelton A. Effects of celecoxib on ambulatory blood pressure in hypertensive patients on ACE inhibitors. Hypertension. 2002;39(4):929–34.
108. Seeram N, Momin R, Nair M, Bourquin L. Cyclooxygenase inhibitory and antioxidant cyanidin glycosides in cherries and berries. Phytomedicine. 2001;8(5):362–9.
109. Tall J, Seeram N, Zhao C, Nair M, Meyer R, Raja S. Tart cherry anthocyanins suppress inflammation-induced pain behavior in rat. Behav Brain Res. 2004;153(1):181–8.
110. Mykkanen O, Huotari A, Herzig K, Dunlop T, Mykannen H, Kirjavainen P. Wild blueberries (Vaccinium myrtillus) alleviate inflammation and hypertension associated with developing obesity in mice fed with a high-fat diet. PLoS One. 2014;9(12):e114790.
111. Takemura S, Yoshimasu K, Fukumoto J, Mure K, Nishio N, Kishida K, et al. Safety and adherence of Umezu polyphenols in the Japanese plum (Prunus mume) in a 12-week double-blind randomized placebo-controlled pilot trial to evaluate antihypertensive effects. Environ Health Prev Med. 2014;19(6):444–51.
112. Luciano R. Acute kidney injury from cherry concentrate in a patient with CKD. Am J Kidney Dis. 2014;63(3):503–5.
113. Mazer M, Perrone J. Acetaminophen-induced nephrotoxicity: pathophysiology, clinical manifestations, and management. J Med Toxicol. 2008;4(1):2–6.
114. Lancaster E, Hiatt J, Zarrinpar A. Acetaminophen hepatotoxicity: an updated review. Arch Toxicol. 2015;89(2):193–9.
115. Emmett M. Acetaminophen toxicity and 5-oxoproline (pyroglutamic acid): a tale of two cycles, one an ATP-depleting futile cycle and the other a useful cycle. Clin J Am Soc Nephrol. 2014;9(1):191–200.
116. Kurella M, Bennett W, Chertow G. Analgesia in patients with ESRD: a review of available evidence. Am J Kidney Dis. 2003;42(2):217–28.

117. Pharmacological management of persistent pain in older persons. J Am Geriatr Soc. 2009;57(8):1331–46.
118. Tawfic Q, Bellingham G. Postoperative pain management in patients with chronic kidney disease. J Anaesthesiol Clin Pharmacol. 2015;31(1):6–13.
119. Kinsey G. Macrophage dynamics in AKI to CKD progression. J Am Soc Nephrol. 2014;25(2):209–11.
120. Henderson L, Masson P, Craig J, Flanc R, Roberts M, Strippoli G, et al. Treatment for lupus nephritis. Cochrane Database Syst Rev. 2012;12:CD002922.
121. Montero N, Webster A, Royuela A, Zamora J, Crespo Barrio M, Pascual J. Steroid avoidance or withdrawal for pancreas and pancrease with kidney transplant recipients. Cochrane Database Syst Rev. 2014;9:CD007669.
122. Yahaya I, Uthman O, Uthman M. Interventions for HIV-associated nephropathy. Cochrane Database Syst Rev. 2013;1:CD007183.
123. Lv J, Xu D, Perkovic V, Ma X, Johnson D, Woodward M, et al. Corticosteroid therapy in IgA nephropathy. J Am Soc Nephrol. 2012;23(6):1108–16.
124. Knight S, Morris P. Steroid avoidance or withdrawal after renal transplantation increases the risk of acute rejection but decreases cardiovascular risk. A meta-analysis. Transplantation. 2010;89(1):1–14.
125. Luijten R, Fritsch-Stork R, Bijlsma J, Derksen R. The use of glucocorticoids in systemic lupus erythematosus. After 60 years still more an art than science. Autoimmun Rev. 2013;12(5):617–28.
126. Stahn C, Buttgereit F. Genomic and nongenomic effects of glucocorticoids. Nat Clin Pract Rheumatol. 2008;4(10):525–33.
127. Ko B, Mistry A, Hanson L, Mallick R, Wynne B, Thai T, et al. Aldosterone acutely stimulates NCC activity via a SPAK-mediated pathway. Am J Physiol Renal Physiol. 2013;305(5):F645–52.
128. Chen S, Bhargava A, Mastroberardino L, Meijer O, Wang J, Buse P, et al. Epithelial sodium channel regulated by aldosterone-induced protein sgk. Proc Natl Acad Sci U S A. 1999;96(5):2514–9.
129. Fritz I, Levine R. Action of adrenal cortical steroids and nor-epinephrine on vascular responses of stress in adrenalectomized rats. Am J Physiol. 1951;165(2):456–65.
130. Whitworth J, Connell J, Lever A, Fraser R. Pressor responsiveness in steroid-induced hypertension in man. Clin Exp Pharmacol Physiol. 1986;13(4):353–8.
131. Pirpiris M, Sudhir K, Yeung S, Jennings G, Whitworth J. Pressor responsiveness in corticosteroid-induced hypertension in humans. Hypertension. 1992;6 Pt 1:567–74.
132. Funder J, Pearce P, Smith R, Campbell J. Vascular type I aldosterone binding sites are physiological mineralocorticoid receptors. Endocrinology. 1989;125(4):2224–6.
133. Walker B, Yau J, Brett L, Seckl J, Monder C, Williams B, et al. 11 beta-hydroxysteroid dehydrogenase in vascular smooth muscle and heart: implications for cardiovascular responses to glucocorticoids. Endocrinology. 1991;129(6):3305–12.
134. Brem A, Bina R, King T, Morris D. Bidirectional activity of 11 beta-hydroxysteroid dehydrogenase in vascular smooth muscle cells. Steroids. 1995;60(5):406–10.
135. Hari P, Bagga A, Mantan M. Short term efficacy of intravenous dexamethasone and methylprednisolone therapy in steroid resistant nephrotic syndrome. Indian Pediatr. 2004;41(10):993–1000.
136. Ponticelli C, Cucchiari D, Graziani G. Hypertension in kidney transplant recipients. Transpl Int. 2011;24(6):523–33.
137. Pascual J, Quereda C, Zamora J, Hernandez D. Steroid withdrawal in renal transplant patients on triple therapy with a calcineurin inhibitor and mycophenolate mofetil: a meta-analysis of randomized, controlled trials. Transplantation. 2004;78(10):1548–56.
138. Hofstra J, Fervenza F, Wetzels J. Treatment of idiopathic membranous nephropathy. Nat Rev Nephrol. 2013;9(8):443–58.
139. Boyer O, Niaudet P. Nephrotic syndrome: Rituximab in childhood steroid-dependent nephrotic syndrome. Nat Rev Nephrol. 2013;9(10):562–3.

140. Chan T. Treatment of severe lupus nephritis: the new horizon. Nat Rev Nephrol. 2015;11(1):46–61.
141. Rusnak F, Mertz P. Calcineurin: form and function. Physiol Rev. 2000;80(4):1483–521.
142. Shibasaki F, Price E, Milan D, McKeon F. Role of kinases and the phosphatase calcineurin in the nuclear shuttling of transcription factor NF-AT4. Nature. 1996;382(6589):370–3.
143. Goldstein D, Zuech N, Sehgal V, Weinberg A, Drusin R, Cohen D. Cyclosporine-associated end-stage nephropathy after cardiac transplantation: incidence and progression. Transplantation. 1997;63(5):664–8.
144. Ishani M, Erturk S, Hertz M, Matas A, Savik K, Rosenberg M. Predictors of renal function following lung or heart-lung transplantation. Kidney Int. 2002;61(6):2228–34.
145. Ojo A, Held P, Port F, Wolfe R, Leichtman A, Young E, et al. Chronic renal failure after transplantation of a nonrenal organ. N Engl J Med. 2003;349(10):931–40.
146. Bloom R, Doyle A. Kidney disease after heart and lung transplantation. Am J Transplant. 2006;6(4):671–9.
147. Ellis M, Parikh C, Inrig J, Kanbay M, Patel U. Chronic kidney disease after hematopoietic cell transplantation: a systematic review. Am J Transplant. 2008;8(11):2378–90.
148. Solez K, Vincenti F, Filo R. Histopathologic findings from 2-year protocol biopsies from a U.S. multicenter transplant trial comparing tacrolimus versus cyclosporine: a report of the FK506 Kidney Transplant Study Group. Transplantation. 1998;66(12):1736–40.
149. Bloom R, Reese P. Chronic kidney disease after nonrenal solid-organ transplantation. J Am Soc Nephrol. 2007;18(12):3031–41.
150. Karthikeyan V, Karpinski J, Nair R, Knoll G. The burden of chronic kidney disease in renal transplant recipients. Am J Transplant. 2004;4(2):262–9.
151. Yan H, Zong H, Cui Y, Li N, Zhang Y. Calcineurin inhibitor avoidance and withdrawal for kidney transplantation: a systematic review and meta-analysis of randomized controlled trials. Transplant Proc. 2014;46(5):1302–13.
152. Marin M, Renoult E, Bondor C, Kessler M. Factors influencing the onset of diabetes mellitus after kidney transplantation: a single French center experience. Transplant Proc. 2005;37(4):1851–6.
153. Gnatta D, Keitel E, Heineck I, Cardoso B, Rodrigues A, Michel K, et al. Use of tacrolimus and the development of posttransplant diabetes mellitus: a Brazilian single-center, observational study. Transplant Proc. 2010;42(2):475–8.
154. Prokai A, Fekete A, Pasti K, Rusai K, Banki N, Reusz G, et al. The importance of different immunosuppressive regimens in the development of posttransplant diabetes mellitus. Pediatr Diabetes. 2012;13(1):81–91.
155. Pereira M, Palming J, Rizell M, Aureliano M, Carvalho E, Svensson M, et al. The immunosuppressive agents rapamycin, cyclosporin A and tacrolimus increase lipolysis, inhibit lipid storage and alter expression of genes involved in lipid metabolism in human adipose tissue. Mol Cell Endocrinol. 2013;365(2):260–9.
156. Koomans H, Ligtenberg G. Mechanisms and consequences of arterial hypertension after renal transplantation. Transplantation. 2001;72(6 Suppl):S9–12.
157. Textor S, Taler S, Canzanello V, Schwartz L, Augustine J. Posttransplantation hypertension related to calcineurin inhibitors. Liver Transpl. 2000;6(5):521–30.
158. Borrows R, Cockwell P. Measuring renal function in solid organ transplant recipients. Transplantation. 2007;83(5):529–31.
159. Nair S, Verma S, Thuluvath P. Pretransplant renal function predicts survival in patients undergoing orthotopic liver transplantation. Hepatology. 2002;35(5):1179–85.
160. Hoorn E, Walsh S, McCormick J, Furstenberg A, Yang C, Roeschel T, et al. The calcineurin inhibitor tacrolimus activates the renal sodium chloride cotransporter to cause hypertension. Nat Med. 2011;17(10):1304–9.
161. Hoorn E, Walsh S, McCormick J, Zietse R, Unwin R, Ellison D. Pathogenesis of calcineurin inhibitor-induced hypertension. J Nephrol. 2012;25(3):269–75.
162. Dikow R, Degenhard M, Kraus T, Sauer P, Schemmer P, Uhl W, et al. Blood pressure profile and treatment quality in liver allograft recipients-benefit of tacrolimus versus cyclosporine. Transplant Proc. 2004;36(5):1512–5.

163. Weir M, Klassen D, Shen S, Sullivan D, Buddemeyer E, Handwerger B. Acute effects of intravenous cyclosporine on blood pressure, hemodynamics, and urine prostaglandin production of healthy humans. Transplantation. 1990;49(1):41–7.

164. McMillen M, Tesi R, Baumgarten W, Jaffe B, Wait R. Potentiation of cyclosporine by verapamil in vitro. Transplantation. 1985;40(4):444–6.

165. Sabate I, Grino J, Castelao A, Ortola J. Evaluation of cyclosporin-verapamil interaction, with observations on parent cyclosporin and metabolites. Clin Chem. 1988;34(10):2151.

166. Lindholm A, Henricsson S. Verapamil inhibits cyclosporin metabolism. Lancet. 1987;1(8544):1262–3.

167. Pirsch J, D'Alessandro A, Roecker E, Knechtle S, Reed A, Sollinger H, et al. A controlled, double-blind, randomized trial of verapamil and cyclosporine in cadaver renal transplant patients. Am J Kidney Dis. 1993;1993(21):2.

168. Moes A, Hesselink D, Zietse R, van Schaik R, van Gelder T, Hoorn E. Calcineurin inhibitors and hypertension: a role for pharmacogenetics? Pharmacogenomics. 2014;15(9):1243–51.

169. Tsai Y, Chiu Y, Hung C, Hwang S, Tsai J, Wang S, et al. Association of depression with progression of CKD. Am J Kidney Dis. 2012;60(1):54–61.

170. Palmer S, Vecchio M, Craig J, Tonelli M, Johnson D, Nicolucci A, et al. Prevalence of depression in chronic kidney disease: systematic review and meta-analysis of observational studies. Kidney Int. 2013;84(1):179–91.

171. Cukor D, Fruchter Y, Ver Halen N, Naidoo S, Patel A, Saggi S. A preliminary investigation of depression and kidney functioning in patients with chronic kidney disease. Nephron Clin Pract. 2012;122(3–4):139–45.

172. Hedayati S, Minhajuddin A, Toto R, Morris D, Rush A. Validation of depression screening scales in patients with CKD. Am J Kidney Dis. 2009;54(3):433–9.

173. Vecchio M, Palmer S, Tonelli M, Johnson D, Strippoli G. Depression and sexual dysfunction in chronic kidney disease: a narrative review of the evidence in areas of significant unmet need. Nephrol Dial Transplant. 2012;27(9):3420–8.

174. Rutledge T, Hogan B. A quantitative review of prospective evidence linking psychological factors with hypertension development. Psychosom Med. 2002;64(5):758–66.

175. Scherrer J, Xian H, Bucholz K, Eisen S, Lyons M, Goldberg J, et al. A twin study of depression symptoms, hypertension, and heart disease in middle-aged men. Psychosom Med. 2003;65(4):548–57.

176. Paterniti S, Alperovitch A, Ducimetiere P, Dealberto M, Lepine P, Bisserbe J. Anxiety but not depression is associated with elevated blood pressure in a community group of French elderly. Psychosom Med. 1999;61(1):77–83.

177. Yan L, Liu K, Matthews K, Daviglus M, Ferguson T, Kiefe C. Psychosocial factors and risk of hypertension: the Coronary Artery Risk Development in Young Adults (CARDIA) study. JAMA. 2003;290(16):2138–48.

178. Licht C, de Geus E, Seldenrijk A, van Hout H, Zitman F, van Dyck R, et al. Depression is associated with decreased blood pressure, but antidepressant use increases the risk for hypertension. Hypertension. 2009;53(4):631–8.

179. Messerli F, Frohlich E. High blood pressure. A side effect of drugs, poisons, and food. Arch Intern Med. 1979;139(6):682–7.

180. Prange AJ, McCurdy R, Cochrane C. The systolic blood pressure response of depressed patients to infused norepinephrine. J Psychiatr Res. 1967;5(1):1–13.

181. Adler L, Angrist B, Lautin A, Rotrosen J. Differential effects of tricyclic antidepressants on mean arterial pressure in a hypertensive patient. J Clin Psychopharmacol. 1983;3(2):122.

182. Fenvez A, Ram C. Drug treatment of hypertensive urgencies and emergencies. Semin Nephrol. 2005;25(4):272–80.

183. Degner D, Grohmann R, Kropp S, Ruther E, Bender S, Engel R, et al. Severe adverse drug reactions of antidepressants: results of the German multicenter drug surveillance program AMSP. Pharmacopsychiatry. 2004;37 Suppl 1:S39–45.

184. Westanmo A, Gayken J, Haight R. Duloxetine: a balanced and selective norepinephrine- and serotonin-reuptake inhibitor. Am J Health Syst Pharm. 2005;62(23):2481–90.

185. Hernandez J, Ramos F, Infante J, Rebollo M, Gonzalez-Macias J. Severe serotonin syndrome induced by mirtazapine monotherapy. Ann Pharmacother. 2002;36(4):641–3.
186. Patel S, Robinson R, Burk M. Hypertensive crisis associated with St. John's Wort. Am J Med. 2002;112(6):507–8.
187. Brown T, Acute S. John's wort toxicity. Am J Emerg Med. 2000;18(2):231–2.
188. Cheng P, Hung S, Lin L, Chong C, Lau C. Amantadine-induced serotonin syndrome in a patient with renal failure. Am J Emerg Med. 2008;26(1):112.e5–6.
189. Rajapakse S, Abeynaike L, Wickramarathne T. Venlafaxine-associated serotonin syndrome causing severe rhabdomyolysis and acute renal failure in a patient with idiopathic Parkinson disease. J Clin Psychopharmacol. 2010;30(5):620–2.
190. Chander W, Singh N, Mukhiya G. Sertononin syndrome in maintenance haemodialysis patients following sertraline treatment for depression. J Indian Med Assoc. 2011;109(1):36–7.
191. Boyer E, Shannon M. The serotonin syndrome. N Engl J Med. 2005;352(11):1112–20.
192. Covic A, Nistor I, Donciu M, Dumea R, Bolignano D, Goldsmith D. Erythropoiesis-stimulating agents (ESA) for preventing the progression of chronic kidney disease: a meta-analysis of 19 studies. Am J Nephrol. 2014;40(3):263–79.
193. van der Putten K, Braam B, Jie K, Gaillard C. Mechanisms of Disease: erythropoietin resistance in patients with both heart and kidney failure. Nat Clin Pract Nephrol. 2008;4(1):47–57.
194. Singh A, Szczech L, Tang K, Barnhart H, Sapp S, Wolfson M, et al. Correction of anemia with epoetin alfa in chronic kidney disease. N Engl J Med. 2006;355(20):2085–98.
195. Drueke T, Locatelli F, Clyne N, Echardt K, Macdougall I, Tsakiris D, et al. Normalization of hemoglobin level in patients with chronic kidney disease and anemia. N Engl J Med. 2006;355(20):2071–84.
196. Palmer S, Navaneethan S, Craig J, Johnson D, Tonelli M, Garg A, et al. Meta-analysis: erythopoiesis-stimulating agents in patients with chronic kidney disease. Ann Intern Med. 2010;153(1):23–33.
197. Kidney Disease: Improving Global Outcomes (KDIGO) Anemia Work Group. KDIGO clinical practice guideline for anemia in chronic kidney disease. Kidney Int Suppl. 2012;2(4):279–335.
198. Pfeffer M, Burdmann E, Chen C, Cooper M, de Zeeuw D, Eckardt K, et al. A trial of darbepoetin alfa in type 2 diabetes and chronic kidney disease. N Engl J Med. 2009;361(21):2019–32.
199. Chobanian A, Bakris G, Black H, Cushman W, Green L, Izzo JJ, et al. The Seventh Report of the Joint National Committee on Prevention, Detection, Evaluation, and Treatment of High Blood Pressure: the JNC 7 report. JAMA. 2003;289(19):2560–72.
200. Boyle S, Berns J. Erythropoietin and resistant hypertension in CKD. Semin Nephrol. 2014;34(5):540–9.
201. Maschio G. Erythropoietin and systemic hypertension. Nephrol Dial Transplant. 1995;10 Suppl 2:74–9.
202. Krapf R, Hulter H. Arterial hypertension induced by erythropoietin and erythropoiesis-stimulating agents (ESA). Clin J Am Soc Nephrol. 2009;4(2):470–80.
203. Schwartz A, Prior J, Mintz G, Kim K, Kahn S. Cardiovascular hemodynamic effects of correction of anemia of chronic renal failure with recombinant-human erythropoietin. Transplant Proc. 1991;23(2):1827–30.
204. Lundby C, Thomsen J, Boushel R, Koskolou M, Warberg J, Calbet J, et al. Erythropoietin treatment elevates haemoglobin concentration by increasing red cell volume and depressing plasma volume. J Physiol. 2007;578(Pt 1):309–14.
205. Takahashi K, Totsune K, Imai Y, Sone M, Nozuki M, Murakami O, et al. Plasma concentrations of immunoreactive-endothelin in patients with chronic renal failure treated with recombinant human erythropoietin. Clin Sci (Lond). 1993;84(1):47–50.
206. Carlini R, Dusso A, Obialo C, Alvarez U, Rothstein M. Recombinant human erythropoietin (rHuEPO) increases endothelin-1 release by endothelial cells. Kidney Int. 1993;43(5):1010–4.
207. Wu X, Richards N, Johns E. The influence of erythropoietin on the vascular responses of rat resistance arteries. Exp Physiol. 1999;84(5):917–27.

208. Ruschitzka F, Wenger R, Stallmach T, Quaschning T, de Wit C, Wagner K, et al. Nitric oxide prevents cardiovascular disease and determines survival in polyglobulic mice overexpressing erythropoietin. Proc Natl Acad Sci U S A. 2000;97(21):11609–13.

209. Bode-Boger S, Boger R, Kuhn M, Radermacher J, Frolich J. Recombinant human erythropoietin enhances vasoconstrictor tone via endothelin-1 and constrictor prostanoids. Kidney Int. 1996;50(4):1255–61.

210. Eschbach J, Abdulhadi M, Browne J, Delano B, Downing M, Egrie J, et al. Recombinant human erythropoietin in anemic patients with end-stage renal disease. Results of a phase III multicenter clinical trial. Ann Intern Med. 1989;111(12):992–1000.

211. Baskin S, Lasker N. Erythropoietin-associated hypertension. N Engl J Med. 1990;323(14):999–1000.

212. Sundal E, Kaeser U. Correction of anaemia of chronic renal failure with recombinant human erythropoietin: safety and efficacy of one year's treatment in a European multicentre study of 150 haemodialysis-dependent patients. Nephrol Dial Transplant. 1989;4(11):979–87.

213. Parfrey P, Foley R, Wittreich B, Sullivan D, Zagari M, Frei D. Double-blind comparison of full and partial anemia correction in incident hemodialysis patients without symptomatic heart disease. J Am Soc Nephrol. 2005;16(7):2180–9.

214. Bosnib S. Renal cystic diseases and renal neoplasms: a mini-review. Clin J Am Soc Nephrol. 2009;4(12):1998–2007.

215. Li L, Lau W, Rhee C, Harley K, Kovesdy C, Sim J, et al. Risk of chronic kidney disease after cancer nephrectomy. Nat Rev Nephrol. 2014;10(3):135–45.

216. Canter D, Kutikov A, Sirohi M, Street R, Viterbo R, Chen D, et al. Prevalence of baseline chronic kidney disease in patients presenting with solid renal tumors. Urology. 2011;77(4):781–5.

217. Huang W, Levey A, Serio A, Snyder M, Vickers A, Raj G, et al. Chronic kidney disease after nephrectomy in patients with renal cortical tumours: a retrospective cohort study. Lancet Oncol. 2006;7(9):735–40.

218. Ferrara N, Hillan K, Gerber H, Novotny W. Discovery and development of bevacizumab, an anti-VEGF antibody for treating cancer. Nat Rev Drug Discov. 2004;3(5):391–400.

219. Volm M, Koornagl R, Mattern J. Prognostic value of vascular endothelial growth factor and its receptor Flt-1 in squamous cell lung cancer. Int J Cancer. 1997;74(1):64–8.

220. Yoshiji H, Gomez D, Shibuya M, Thorgeirsson U. Expression of vascular endothelial growth factor, its receptor, and other angiogenic factors in human breast cancer. Cancer Res. 1996;56(9):2013–6.

221. Ellis L, Takahashi Y, Fenoglio C, Cleary K, Bucana C, Evans D. Vessel counts and vascular endothelial growth factor expression in pancreatic adenocarcinoma. Eur J Cancer. 1998;34(3):337–40.

222. Sowter H, Corps A, Evans A, Clark D, Charnock-Jones D, Smith S. Expression and localization of the vascular endothelial growth factor family in ovarian epithelial tumors. Lab Invest. 1997;77(6):607–14.

223. Tomisawa M, Tokunaga T, Oshika Y, Tsuchida T, Kukushima Y, Sato H, et al. Expression pattern of vascular endothelial growth factor isoform is closely correlated with tumour stage and vascularisation in renal cell carcinoma. Eur J Cancer. 1999;35(1):133–7.

224. de Vries C, Escobedo J, Ueno H, Houck K, Ferrara N, Williams L. The fms-like tyrosine kinase, a receptor for vascular endothelial growth factor. Science. 1992;255(5047):989–91.

225. Shibuya M, Yamaguchi S, Yamane A, Ikeda T, Tojo A, Matsuchime H, et al. Nucleotide sequence and expression of a novel human receptor-type tyrosine kinase gene (flt) closely related to the fms family. Oncogene. 1990;5(4):519–24.

226. Terman B, Dougher-Vermazen M, Carrion M, Dimitrov D, Armellino D, Godspodarowicz D, et al. Identification of the KDR tyrosine kinase as a receptor for vascular endothelial cell growth factor. Biochem Biophys Res Commun. 1992;187(3):1579–86.

227. Ferrara N. Vascular endothelial growth factor: basic science and clinical progress. Endocr Rev. 2004;25(4):581–611.

228. Vasudev N, Reynolds A. Anti-angiogenic therapy for cancer: current progress, unresolved questions and future directions. Angiogenesis. 2014;17(3):471–94.
229. Yang J, Haworth L, Sherry R, Hwu P, Schwartzentruber D, Topalian S, et al. A randomized trial of bevacizumab, an anti-vascular endothelial growth factor antibody, for metastatic renal cancer. N Engl J Med. 2003;349(5):427–34.
230. Sica D. Angiogenesis inhibitors and hypertension: an emerging issue. J Clin Oncol. 2006;24(9):1329–31.
231. Verheul H, Pinedo H. Possible molecular mechanisms involved in the toxicity of angiogenesis inhibition. Nat Rev Cancer. 2007;7(6):475–85.
232. Zhu X, Wu S, Dahut W, Parikh C. Risks of proteinuria and hypertension with bevacizumab, an antibody against vascular endothelial growth factor: systematic review and meta-analysis. Am J Kidney Dis. 2007;49(2):186–93.
233. Chen Y, Chen C, Wang J. Nephrotic syndrome and acute renal failure apparently induced by sunitinib. Case Rep Oncol. 2009;2(3):172–6.
234. Jha P, Vankalakunti M, Siddini V, Bonu R, Prakash G, Babu K, et al. Sunitinib induced nephrotic syndrome and thrombotic microangiopathy. Indian J Nephrol. 2013;23(1):67–70.
235. Patel T, Morgan J, Demetri G, George S, Maki R, Quigley M, et al. A preeclampsia-like syndrome characterized by reversible hypertension and proteinuria induced by the multitargeted kinase inhibitors sunitinib and sorafenib. J Natl Cancer Inst. 2008;100(4):282–4.
236. Wallace E, Lyndon W, Chumley P, Jaimes E, Fatima H. Dasatinib-induced nephrotic range proteinuria. Am J Kidney Dis. 2013;61(6):1026–31.
237. Turan N, Benekli M, Ozturk S, Inal S, Memis L, Guz G, et al. Sunitinib- and sorafenib-induced nephrotic syndrome in a patient with gastrointestinal stromal tumor. Ann Pharmacother. 2012;46(10):e27.
238. Bollee G, Patey N, Cazajous G, Robert C, Goujon J, Fahouri F, et al. Thrombotic microangiopathy secondary to VEGF pathway inhibition by sunitinib. Nephrol Dial Transplant. 2009;24(2):682–5.
239. Frangie C, Lefaucheur C, Medioni J, Jacquot C, Hill G, Nochy D. Renal thrombotic microangiopathy caused by anti-VEGF-antibody treatment for metastatic renal-cell carcinoma. Lancet Oncol. 2007;8(2):177–8.
240. Kapiteijn E, Brand A, Kroep J, Gelderblom H. Sunitinib induced hypertension, thrombotic microangiopathy and reversible posterior leukencephalopathy syndrome. Ann Oncol. 2007;18(10):1745–7.
241. Maitland M, Moshier K, Imperial J, Kasza K, Karrison T, Elliott W, et al. Blood pressure (BP) as a biomarker for sorafenib (S), an inhibitor of the vascular endothelial growth factor (VEGF) signaling pathway. J Clin Oncol 2006 ASCO Annual Meeting Proceedings. 2006;24(18):2035.
242. Faivre S, Delbaldo C, Vera K, Robert C, Lozahic S, Lassau N, et al. Safety, pharmacokinetic, and antitumor activity of SU11248, a novel oral multitarget tyrosine kinase inhibitor, in patients with cancer. J Clin Oncol. 2006;24(1):25–35.
243. Motzer R, Michaelson M, Redman B, Hudes G, Wilding G, Figlin R, et al. Activity of SU11248, a multitargeted inhibitor of vascular endothelial growth factor receptor and platelet-derived growth factor receptor, in patients with metastatic renal cell carcinoma. J Clin Oncol. 2006;24(1):16–24.
244. Zhu X, Stergiopoulos K, Wu S. Risk of hypertension and renal dysfunction with an angiogenesis inhibitor sunitinib: systematic review and meta-analysis. Acta Oncol. 2009;48(1):9–17.
245. Ratain M, Eisen T, Stadler W, Flaherty K, Kaye S, Rosner G, et al. Phase II placebo-controlled randomized discontinuation trial of sorafenib in patients with metastatic renal cell carcinoma. J Clin Oncol. 2006;24(16):2505–12.
246. Veronese M, Mosenkis A, Flaherty K, Gallager M, Stevenson J, Townsend R, et al. Mechanisms of hypertension associated with BAY 43-9006. J Clin Oncol. 2006;24(9):1363–9.
247. Qi W, Lin F, Sun Y, Tang L, He A, Yao Y, et al. Incidence and risk of hypertension with pazopanib in patients with cancer: a meta-analysis. Cancer Chemother Pharmacol. 2013;71(2):431–9.

248. Qi W, Shen Z, Lin F, Sun Y, Min D, Tang L, et al. Incidence and risk of hypertension with vandetanib in cancer patients: a systematic review and meta-analysis of clinical trials. Br J Clin Pharmacol. 2013;75(4):919–30.
249. Qi W, He A, Shen Z, Yao Y. Incidence and risk of hypertension with a novel multi-targeted kinase inhibitor axitinib in cancer patients: a systematic review and meta-analysis. Br J Clin Pharmacol. 2013;76(3):348–57.
250. Zhu X, Perazella M. Anti-vascular endothelial growth factor (VEGF) therapy: a new cause of hypertension. Curr Hypertens Rev. 2007;3(2):149–55.
251. Ku D, Zaleski J, Liu S, Brock T. Vascular endothelial growth factor induces EDRF-dependent relaxation in coronary arteries. Am J Physiol. 1993;265(2 Pt 2):H586–92.
252. Eppler S, Combs D, Henry T, Lopez J, Ellis S, Yi J, et al. A target-mediated model to describe the pharmacokinetics and hemodynamic effects of recombinant human vascular endothelial growth factor in humans. Clin Pharmacol Ther. 2002;72(1):20–32.
253. Wheeler-Jones C, Abu-Ghazaleh R, Cospedal R, Houliston R, Martin J, Zachary I. Vascular endothelial growth factor stimulates prostacyclin production and activation of cytosolic phospholipase A2 in endothelial cells via p42/p44 mitogen-activated protein kinase. FEBS Lett. 1997;420(1):28–32.
254. Hutchins P, Lynch C, Cooney P, Curseen K. The microcirculation in experimental hypertension and aging. Cardiovasc Res. 1996;32(4):772–80.
255. Hansen-Smith F, Morris L, Greene A, Lombard J. Rapid microvessel rarefaction with elevated salt intake and reduced renal mass hypertension in rats. Circ Res. 1996;79(2):324–30.
256. Prasad A, Dunnill G, Mortimer P, MacGregor G. Capillary rarefaction in the forearm skin in essential hypertension. J Hypertens. 1995;13(2):265–8.
257. Lee S, Chen T, Barber C, Jordan M, Murdock J, Desai S, et al. Autocrine VEGF signaling is required for vascular homeostasis. Cell. 2007;130(4):691–703.
258. Steeghs N, Gelderblom H, Roodt J, Christensen O, Rajagopalan P, Hovens M, et al. Hypertension and rarefaction during treatment with telatinib, a small molecule angiogenesis inhibitor. Clin Cancer Res. 2008;14(11):3470–6.
259. Greene A, Tonellato P, Lui J, Lombard J, Cowley AJ. Microvascular rarefaction and tissue vascular resistance in hypertension. Am J Physiol. 1989;256(1 PT 2):H126–31.
260. Lankhorst S, Saleh L, Danser A, van den Meiracker A. Etiology of angiogenesis inhibition-related hypertension. Curr Opin Pharmacol. 2014;21:7–13.
261. Humphreys B, Sanders P. Cancer and the Kidney. NephSAP. Am Soc Nephrol. 2013;12(1).
262. Bono P, Elfving H, Utriainen T, Osterlund P, Saarto T, Alanko T, et al. Hypertension and clinical benefit of bevacizumab in the treatment of advanced renal cell carcinoma. Ann Oncol. 2009;20(2):393–4.
263. Lankhorst S, Kappers M, van Esch J, Smedts F, Sleijfer S, Methijssen R, et al. Treatment of hypertension and renal injury induced by the angiogenesis inhibitor sunitinib: preclinical study. Hypertension. 2014;64(6):1282–9.
264. Tiemsani C, Mir O, Boudou-Rouquette P, Huillard O, Maley K, Ropert S, et al. Posterior reversible encephalopathy syndrome induced by anti-VEGF agents. Target Oncol. 2011;6(4):253–8.

Chapter 13
Diagnosis and Management of Hypertension in Children with Chronic Kidney Disease

Susan M. Halbach and Joseph T. Flynn

Background

Hypertension is a leading cause and risk factor for chronic kidney disease (CKD) among adults in the USA [1]. The appropriate management of hypertension influences both cardiovascular outcomes and the progression of kidney disease [2–4]. While hypertensive kidney disease, per se, is exceedingly rare in childhood, the influence of blood pressure (BP) on both the progression of CKD in children and development of early cardiovascular disease is proving to be as significant as in adults. Treatment of hypertension, therefore, remains one of the few available interventions that can influence the course of CKD in children. Over the past 10–20 years, the organization of registries and multicenter research studies has contributed greatly to our understanding of the prevalence of hypertension in pediatric CKD, its relationship to markers of cardiovascular disease, and approaches to therapy. Managing hypertension in children with CKD requires familiarity with important differences in diagnostic and measurement techniques, complications that are associated with hypertension in pediatric CKD and guidelines for pharmacotherapy.

Definition of Hypertension

Because blood pressure (BP) is closely related to age and body size, using a single threshold value in diagnosing hypertension in children from birth to 18 years is not feasible [5, 6]. In addition, the time needed to correlate childhood BP values with

S.M. Halbach, MD, MPH • J.T. Flynn, MD, MS (✉)
Department of Pediatrics, University of Washington, Seattle Children's Hospital, Seattle, WA, USA

Division of Nephrology, Seattle Children's Hospital, Seattle, WA, USA
e-mail: joseph.flynn@seattlechildrens.org

© Springer Science+Business Media New York 2016
A.K. Singh, R. Agarwal (eds.), *Core Concepts in Hypertension in Kidney Disease*, DOI 10.1007/978-1-4939-6436-9_13

Table 13.1 Definition of hypertension in children and adolescents

| | SBP or DBP percentile[a] | |
	4th Report [7]	KDIGO [8]
Normal	<90th	≤90th
Pre-hypertension	90th to <95th or >120/80 even if <90th up to <95th	n/a
Stage 1 hypertension	95th to 99th + 5 mmHg	>90th
Stage 2 hypertension	>99th + 5 mmHg	n/a

SBP systolic blood pressure, *DBP* diastolic blood pressure, *KDIGO* Kidney Disease: Improving Global Outcomes
[a]BP should be obtained by auscultation on at least 3 separate occasions; classification should be based on the higher reading if SBP and DBP fall into different categories

hard outcomes, such as mortality or major cardiovascular events, is sufficiently long as to preclude its use as an indicator of desirable BP targets in childhood. Given this, the normative BP values for children currently in use are taken from population surveys of healthy children, and BP targets for treatment are based upon expert opinion, rather than upon data from clinical trials [7].

Per consensus guidelines, a child is considered hypertensive when the average BP is >95th percentile for age, sex, and height percentile on 3 separate occasions (see Table 13.1) [7]. An average BP between the 90th–95th percentiles is classified as pre-hypertensive, although in one recent consensus document, it was recommended that BP values in this range in children with CKD should be considered hypertensive [8]. Recently there have been several studies linking these BP targets with intermediate outcomes, such as CKD progression, proteinuria, and other early markers of cardiovascular disease, but additional investigation is certainly needed. In addition, the increasing use of ambulatory BP monitoring (ABPM) has provided valuable information in identifying children with CKD and hypertension who might otherwise have been missed, as it captures children with masked hypertension, many of whom may have nocturnal hypertension only.

Prevalence of Hypertension and Controlled BP Among Children with CKD

Although the prevalence of primary pediatric hypertension has increased somewhat in recent years, it remains a relatively uncommon condition among children and adolescents, with rates in screening studies ranging from 3 to 5% [9, 10]. In the pediatric CKD population, however, elevated BP is quite common (Table 13.2). An early study characterizing hypertension among children with CKD was based on data from the NAPRTCS (North American Pediatric Renal Trials and Collaborative Studies) registry. Using casual measurements obtained in the clinical setting (including both oscillometric and auscultatory BPs), data on 3861 children with CKD enrolled from 1994 to 2001 demonstrated that hypertension was present in 28–41% of patients [11].

Table 13.2 Prevalence of HTN among children with CKD and ESRD

	Study population	Method of BP measurement	Definition of HTN	% Hypertensive	% Controlled
CKD					
Mitsnefes (2003) [11]	NAPRTCS (*n*=3861)	cBP	BP >95th percentile	28–41 % (BP only) 67 % (BP and/or meds)	33 %
Flynn (2008) [12]	CKiD (*n*=432)	cBP	BP >90th percentile +/- meds or history of HTN	54 %	53 %
Samuels (2012) [13]	CKiD (*n*=332)	ABPM	Mean BP ≥95th percentile OR loads ≥25 %	52 % abnormal ABPM	Not reported
ESRD					
Chavers (2009) [18]	USRDS (*n*=624)	cBP	BP>95th percentile or meds	79 %	26 %
Halbach (2012) [17]	NAPRTCS (*n*=3447)	cBP	BP>95th percentile or meds	81–84 %	15–26 %
Kramer (2011) [19]	ESPN/ ERA-EDTA (*n*=1315)	cBP	BP>95th percentile or meds	68–70 %	26–45 %
Transplant					
Sorof (1999) [20]	NAPRTCS (*n*=4821)	n/a	Medication use	60 %	n/a
Sinha (2012) [21]	Multicenter UK (*n*=564)	cBP	BP>95th percentile or meds	56–66 %	67 %
Seeman (2006) [22]	Single-center Czech Republic (*n*=36)	ABPM	BP >95th percentile or meds	89 %	47 %
Gulhan (2014) [23]	Single-center Turkey (*n*=29)	ABPM	BP>95th percentile or meds	93 %	18.5 %

ABPM ambulatory blood pressure monitoring, *BP* blood pressure, *cBP* casual blood pressure, *CKD* chronic kidney disease, *CKiD* Chronic Kidney Disease in Children Study, *ESPN/ERA-EDTA* European Society of Pediatric Nephrology/European Renal Association-European Dialysis and Transplant Association, *ESRD* end-stage renal disease, *HTN* hypertension, *NAPRTCS* North American Pediatric Renal Trials and Collaborative Studies, *UK* United Kingdom, *USRDS* United States Renal Data System

Among the patients with BPs in the normotensive range, approximately one-third had been prescribed antihypertensive medications. Taken together, patients with either controlled hypertension (normal BP and on medication), uncontrolled hypertension (elevated BP and on medication) or undiagnosed hypertension (elevated BP and not on medication) comprised 67 % of this cohort. Additionally, among the hypertensive children, only one-third had a controlled BP, suggesting that hypertension was both common and undertreated. While valuable, these data are limited by a lack of standardized BP measurements.

The CKiD (Chronic Kidney Disease in Children) study, a multicenter prospective observational study of children with CKD in North America, has provided a more rigorous characterization of BP in children with CKD. Baseline data using casual BPs (cBP) obtained by auscultation according to standardized procedures were published in 2008 [12]. The definition of hypertension in this analysis was more inclusive and captured patients with elevated BP (>90th percentile), hypertensive BP (>95th percentile), and those with controlled hypertension (antihypertensive medications, personal history of elevated BP and normal BP). Applying this definition to the 432 children with available baseline study data, 54 % were classified as hypertensive. It is important to note that of the hypertensive patients, just under half (47 %) had either undiagnosed or uncontrolled hypertension, which represents one-quarter of the patients in the study.

Additional information regarding BP status in pediatric CKD comes from a later CKiD analysis based upon ambulatory BP monitoring (ABPM) data [13]. ABPM recordings at 1 year after study entry were available on 332 children. Encouragingly, almost half of the subjects (42 %) had a normal recording, consistent with either normotension or controlled hypertension, and a small number had white-coat hypertension (4 %). Among the children in this category, the majority (~75 %) had been prescribed antihypertensive medications. The percentage of study subjects with newly diagnosed confirmed hypertension (defined as an elevated casual BP as well as abnormal ABPM recording) was actually fairly low, at 15 %. What was surprising was the significant number of children observed to have masked hypertension, defined as a normal casual BP but abnormal ABPM recording. 116 children, or 35 % of the study subjects, were in this group, with a significant proportion having abnormal sleep BP. It is important to note that this study was conducted prior to the publication of updated AHA criteria for BP classification on ABPM in pediatric patients [14]. The earlier classification scheme did not specifically address how to incorporate either diastolic pressures or isolated nocturnal hypertension into the diagnosis. The CKiD investigators considered an ABPM recording as abnormal if the mean sleeping or wake BP was ≥95th percentile or if sleeping or awake BP loads were ≥25 %. The rationale for this broader definition of hypertension (to include children who might otherwise be classified as pre-hypertensive) is to account for the fact that children with CKD are at higher cardiovascular risk and their BP treatment goals are lower (≤90th percentile vs. ≤95th percentile) [8, 15, 16]. Using these criteria, those with masked hypertension, confirmed hypertension and controlled hypertension (normal ABPM recording but history of hypertension) comprised nearly two-thirds (73 %) of the CKiD study cohort.

Although it is difficult to draw direct comparisons between the CKiD and NAPRTCS studies due to differing definitions of hypertension and methods of measuring BP, they both illustrate several features of hypertension among children with CKD. First, the overall prevalence is high, and likely higher than is commonly appreciated. Second, there is a sizeable portion of children with undiagnosed hypertension, either because the patient has masked hypertension and the elevated BPs are not being captured, or because they are simply not recognized as being elevated. Lastly, even among children with treated hypertension, many remain uncontrolled.

The prevalence of hypertension in pediatric CKD is even higher in those with ESRD, either on dialysis or with a kidney transplant. Multiple large studies of the pediatric dialysis population have documented high rates of hypertension and poor BP control, both in the USA and in Europe [17–19]. In these large registry studies, between 70 and 80% of children meet criteria for hypertension based on reported casual BPs and antihypertensive use. Among those patients on antihypertensive medications, the majority had uncontrolled BPs (52–74%). In the transplant population, reported rates of hypertension vary based on the definition used and method of measuring BP (ABPM or cBP). An early study using NAPTRCS data, where no BPs were available and hypertension was defined only by the use of antihypertensive medications, reported a prevalence of approximately 60% by 5-years posttransplant [20]. Newer studies, though smaller, have been more detailed in capturing the characteristics of hypertension after transplant. Recently published data from a large cohort of children transplanted in the United Kingdom showed a similar prevalence of hypertension (66% at 1-year and 56% at 5-years post-transplant) based on BP measurements and antihypertensive medication use [21]. Of the treated patients, approximately one-third were uncontrolled. Single-center studies using both ABPM and clinical criteria for hypertension (specifically antihypertensive use) report the highest prevalence—up to 90% [22, 23]. Studies using ABPM have also demonstrated that nocturnal hypertension is relatively common among pediatric renal transplant recipients [24].

Risk Factors for Hypertension Among Children with CKD

There are several characteristics that have been identified as carrying a higher risk for hypertension in children with CKD (Table 13.3). Some of these risk factors are consistent with those associated with primary hypertension in both children and adults, such as obesity and black race [12]. Other factors are more specifically related to CKD. Longer duration of CKD and the presence of glomerular disease (versus nonglomerular disease, such as structural abnormalities) had a higher risk for both hypertension and uncontrolled BP in the CKiD cohort. Male sex was associated with uncontrolled BP among known hypertensive children but not hypertension in general. Interestingly, some factors that may be assumed to influence BP status, such as GFR and age, were not significant predictors of either hypertension or controlled

Table 13.3 Risk factors for hypertension in children with CKD

CKD	Dialysis	Transplant
Age	Age	Immunosuppressive medications
Race	Race	Time since transplant
Obesity	Glomerular disease	
Glomerular disease	Shorter time on dialysis	
Shorter duration of CKD		

CKD chronic kidney disease

BP. Parental history of hypertension and low birth weight, characteristics known to be associated with primary hypertension in otherwise healthy children and adults, were also not predictive of hypertension in this cohort. Common risk factors reported to be associated with hypertension in pediatric dialysis patients include glomerular disease, younger age, and shorter time on dialysis [17, 18]. Among pediatric transplant recipients, risk factors that appear to affect the risk for hypertension include immunosuppressive medications, time since transplant and donor type (deceased versus living donor [22, 23]).

Proteinuria has emerged recently as an important factor not only associated with CKD progression in children, but control of BP as well. Historically, the relationship was felt to be the opposite after several large adult trials demonstrated that controlling hypertension reduced proteinuria, independent of the anti-proteinuric effects of medications such as ACE inhibitors. In part because of this relationship, most adult guidelines recommend lower BP treatment goals for adults with significant proteinuria [8, 25]. Recently published longitudinal data from the CKiD study, however, show that the relationship between hypertension and proteinuria in the progression of CKD may be more complex. Kogon et al. observed that, over time, the presence of proteinuria was predictive of poorer BP control, even though the mean SBP decreased in the study cohort as a whole [26]. The investigators hypothesized that proteinuria may alter vascular physiology thus making hypertension more difficult to treat in such patients. A separate analysis of the contributions of BP and proteinuria to CKD progression among children with non-glomerular disease showed both to be independent risk factors. Among children with normal BP, proteinuria contributed to a faster rate of GFR decline, while among children with elevated BP, GFR declined at all levels of proteinuria, suggesting that these two variables may not necessarily be additive in this population [27]. These findings demonstrate that there is more to be learned about the relationship between proteinuria and BP in children with CKD.

Pathophysiology

The pathophysiology of hypertension in children with CKD is similar to that in adults with CKD, though the vast majority of children do not have pre-existing primary hypertension prior to diagnosis with CKD. In the simplest terms, the two major mechanisms by which the BP is elevated are volume excess and activation of the renin–angiotensin–aldosterone system (RAAS). Impaired salt and water excretion leads to volume expansion and thereby increases cardiac output. RAAS activation contributes to hypertension via direct effects, such as vasoconstriction, and indirectly via actions of the sympathetic nervous system and decreased local production of vasodilatory substances. Similar mechanisms are operative in children with end-stage renal disease. Volume overload is probably the major contributing factor to hypertension in pediatric dialysis patients; neurohumoral mechanisms are also important. For a more thorough discussion of hypertension in CKD and ESRD, the interested reader is encouraged to consult more comprehensive reviews [28].

Diagnosis

Measurement Methods

There are several factors to consider when assessing BP in children in the clinical setting. Access to the appropriate equipment is extremely important to obtain reliable BP measurements. A range of cuff sizes should be available, from infant to large adult and thigh cuff, and the correct one selected based on the mid-arm circumference [29]. In the event that a child is between cuff sizes, the larger cuff should be used, as the potential for a falsely low reading with a larger cuff is much lower than that of a falsely high reading with a cuff that is too small. As with standard recommendations for BP measurements in adults, the child should be calmly resting in a seated position with foot support for several minutes prior to cuff inflation and the arm should be supported at approximately the level of the heart. By convention and to eliminate the possibility of a falsely low BP in the rare case of coarctation of the aorta, the right arm is preferred. Auscultatory measurements are preferred and considered the gold standard method of BP measurement in pediatric CKD [30]. An auscultated BP in a child should correspond to the first Korotkoff sound for systolic BP and the 5th Korotkoff sound for diastolic BP. Often the 5th Korotkoff sound can be heard all the way to zero mmHg; in such cases, the 4th Korotkoff sound should be used to estimate diastolic BP.

Although auscultation is recommended, oscillometric devices may be more commonly available in some settings. The principal disadvantage to these devices is that they are indirect measurements of BP and may not correspond to auscultated BP [31]. Oscillometric devices measure mean arterial pressure (MAP) and through proprietary algorithms that differ by manufacturer, calculate systolic and diastolic BP. The advantages to oscillometric devices include consistent repeated measurements, elimination of bias, and ease of use [32]. They may also be the only way to obtain BP readings in infants and very young children, as it can be extremely difficult to measure BP by auscultation in this age group.

Ambulatory Blood Pressure Monitoring (ABPM)

As ABPM devices have become more commonly available for use in children, they are becoming part of the standard evaluation for children with elevated BP. This is particularly pertinent to children with CKD who, as mentioned above, appear to have a fairly high prevalence of both nocturnal and masked hypertension. It is recommended that children and adolescents undergoing ABPM do so at a center with experience and the ability to interpret the readings according to age, sex, and height-specific norms. Dedicated pediatric equipment is necessary, with the application of the appropriate cuff size prior to initiating the test. Education of both parent and child is important and a diary should be kept with sleep and wake times along with periods of activity and timing of medications. One limitation of ABPM is the need for the child to be able to cooperate with the test, generally this occurs around age 6–8 years. Children with developmental delays or other neurocognitive impairments may not tolerate wearing the ABPM device at any age. As mentioned above, modified consensus guidelines on the interpretation of ABPM were published in 2014 [14]. Using data from ABPM and casual BPs, a child is classified as having sustained hypertension, white-coat hypertension, masked hypertension, or pre-hypertension (Table 13.4).

Normative Values

Because of the large variation in BP by age, sex, and height in children, reference tables are necessary to interpret BP readings in children, both for casual BPs and in interpreting ABPM. Normative values for casual BP are elaborated in the *4th Report* and are derived from data on over 63,000 healthy children in the USA from ages 1–17 years, including the National Health and Nutrition Examination Survey

Table 13.4 Revised classification for interpreting ABPM in children

	Office BP	Mean ambulatory SBP or DBP[a]	SBP or DBP load, %[a]
Normal	<90th percentile	<95th percentile	<25
White-coat hypertension	≥95th percentile	<95th percentile	<25
Pre-hypertension	≥90th percentile or >120/80	<95th percentile	≥25
Masked hypertension	<95th percentile	>95th percentile	≥25
Ambulatory hypertension	>95th percentile	>95th percentile	25–50
Severe ambulatory hypertension	>95th percentile	>95th percentile	>50

Adapted from Flynn et al. [14]
ABPM ambulatory blood pressure monitoring, *BP* blood pressure, *SBP* systolic blood pressure, *DBP* diastolic blood pressure
[a]Applies to either sleep or wake period (or both)

(NHANES) [7]. It is important to note that NHANES specifically seeks to over-sample minority racial groups in the USA, so the diversity of this reference population makes the normative values applicable to a wide range of patient groups. The reference values used for ABPM interpretation are less robust. Due to the more resource-intense nature of performing ABPM, obtaining such large, population-level sample sizes is much more difficult. The best available data, and those currently recommended by consensus guidelines, are derived from a population of predominantly Caucasian children from Central Europe [14, 33, 34]. Secondly, in addition to the lack of diversity in patient selection, the data on diastolic BP norms have long been considered problematic. Despite the knowledge that both systolic and diastolic BP vary with age and height, the survey data in this reference group resulted in a very little differences in diastolic BP norms for a very wide range of heights. Finally, it has been noted that the reference population for this study included very few children who were shorter (<140 cm), a feature that may be of some importance when using these data to interpret ABPM studies in children with CKD [35].

Additional Testing: When Hypertension Is the Presenting Symptom

Occasionally, a child may have undiagnosed CKD and only come to medical attention due to elevated BP. Among children with secondary hypertension, renal disease is the most common etiology. After establishing a diagnosis of sustained hypertension, additional studies may be required to better elucidate the etiology of the kidney disease. Congenital anomalies of the kidneys and urinary tract (CAKUT) such as renal hypodysplasia, obstructive uropathy, or reflux nephropathy can often be identified on ultrasound, which should also include imaging of the bladder. Other imaging that may be needed to obtain a diagnosis includes a voiding cystourethrogram to evaluate for vesicoureteral reflux or nuclear medicine studies, such as DMSA scan or MAG-3 renogram. Consultation with a pediatric urologist may be valuable in such cases.

Additional Testing: Evaluating for Target Organ Damage

Hypertensive target organ damage in children is less common and often more subtle than in adults. In cases of severe elevations in BP, children can have seizures, hypertensive encephalopathy, and cardiac dysfunction [36]. Because outcomes such as death, myocardial infarction and stroke, either directly related to or in the setting of hypertension, are rare in children, research efforts have focused primarily on identifying other early markers of developing cardiovascular disease. Some of these markers, including carotid intima-media thickness and pulse wave velocity are still primarily used as research tools and have not yet been adopted for clinical use [37–39].

The most common site for target organ damage among children with chronic hypertension is the heart, where there is a well-documented association between BP and both left ventricular hypertrophy (LVH) and elevated left ventricular mass index (LVMI) [40, 41]. Echocardiograms are widely available and should be performed on children with confirmed hypertension. The information obtained on echocardiogram should include both a subjective assessment of ventricular function and size, but also accurate measurements of LVMI by experienced technicians. The LVMI in children actually decreases from infancy until adulthood and interpretation should use pediatric reference values, which have been obtained from healthy children [42]. An LVMI >95th percentile for age and sex would be considered elevated and suggestive of sustained, uncontrolled hypertension.

Sequelae of Hypertension in Pediatric CKD (Table 13.5)

CKD Progression

The association between hypertension and CKD progression has been well established in adults for almost two decades, through both observational and interventional studies [2, 3]. Although hypertension as a primary cause of CKD in children is extremely rare, it appears to be a major contributor to progression in pediatric patients with established CKD. Early data examining this relationship comes from one of the few multicenter trials in the pediatric CKD population [43]. The trial was designed to test the effects on CKD progression of a low-protein versus conventional diet over a period of 2–3 years, while simultaneously examining other factors, including BP. The 284 enrolled patients from 25 centers were ages 2–18 with stages 3–4 CKD. The results demonstrated that protein restriction had no adverse effects on growth but did also not affect glomerular filtration rate (GFR) decline. In a multivariate analysis, only hypertension (defined as SBP >120 mmHg) and proteinuria (24-h urine protein >50 mg/kg) were independently correlated with GFR decline. Although this study was not designed to determine causality between these factors and CKD progression, the results were among the first to suggest a key role for BP.

Table 13.5 Complications of hypertension in children with CKD

Cardiovascular
• LVH
• Increased cIMT
• Decreased HRV
• Increased BPV
Neurocognitive deficits
Accelerated progression of CKD

CKD chronic kidney disease, *LVH* left ventricular hypertrophy, *cIMT* carotid intimal-media thickness

At least 2 large studies using data from the NAPRTCS registry have also reported hypertension to be an independent risk factor for CKD progression in children [11, 44]. An analysis by Mitsnefes et al. reported that, among those children with a starting eGFR (estimated GFR) between 50–75 mL/min/1.73 m^2, hypertensive children progressed significantly faster to the study endpoint (either renal replacement therapy or a decline in eGFR by 10 mL/min/1.73 m^2) than normotensive children. A multivariate analysis also demonstrated systolic hypertension to be an independent risk factor for GFR decline, along with African-American race, glomerular disease and older age. This association was confirmed by a later retrospective analysis of 4166 children in the NAPTRCS registry with CKD stages II–IV and a small, single-center, retrospective study from Poland [44, 45].

Evidence supporting the impact of hypertension on CKD progression is also provided by prospective data from the CKiD study. Although the study is ongoing, data examining changes in GFR over a 1-year period from study enrollment suggest that annualized GFR decline is faster among patients with an abnormal ABPM compared to those with a normal ABPM, though the relationship was not statistically significant [13]. BP appears to be an independent risk factor for GFR decline in children with non-glomerular disease as well as a significant factor among children with rapid disease progression (defined as a decrease in GFR by 50% or renal replacement therapy over a 1 year period) with both glomerular and non-glomerular disease [27, 46].

Future analyses with longer follow-up time should be helpful in characterizing this relationship in more detail, but until then, it is important to recognize that appropriate treatment of hypertension remains one of the few interventions available for practitioners in slowing the progression of CKD.

Left Ventricular Hypertrophy (LVH)

LVH is an important cardiovascular risk factor for adults and is not uncommon among children with CKD. Young adults diagnosed with CKD and ESRD during childhood have a dramatically elevated mortality rate compared to the general population, with the majority of deaths due to cardiovascular disease [16]. In general, reported rates of LVH in mild to moderate CKD (Stages 2–4) range from approximately 20–50%, with some variation due to methodology [47–51]. Some reports of LVH in pediatric CKD, including the earliest study from 1996, have not observed an association between BP and increased LVMI or abnormal cardiac geometry. In these studies, other factors such as GFR, sex, age, and evidence of anemia or inflammation were instead reported to be significant predictors of LVH [47, 48]. Other studies have contradicted these findings. Sinha et al. published data in 2011 on 49 children with non-hypertensive CKD from a single center and reported that 33% had LVH. The authors also observed a positive association between LVMI and systolic BP, even within the "normal" range [49]. A cross-sectional analysis from the CKiD study, published in 2010, used both echocardiographic and ABPM data to evaluate predictors of LVH. The authors reported that both confirmed (OR 4.3) and masked (OR 4.1) hypertension were the strongest independent predictors of LVH and that GFR was not significant [50].

Two prospective studies provide additional information on how BP may be related to LVH in children with CKD. The ESCAPE trial, a randomized, multicenter trial that examined intensive (<50th percentile) versus conventional (<90th percentile) BP goals during treatment with ACE inhibition, collected echocardiographic data on 84 patients at baseline, 1-year, and 2-years [52]. The overall prevalence of LVH decreased from 38 to 25% for the entire study cohort and LVMI decreased among those patients who had LVH at baseline, but not in patients without LVH. Treatment to intensive BP goals did not appear to have an effect on LVMI, but was significantly associated with improved systolic function, suggesting an independent drug effect on cardiac remodeling. Longitudinal data from the CKiD study looking at the effects of BP on LVMI and LVH were published in 2014 [53]. In this observational study, the prevalence of LVH also decreased over time. Significant predictors of LVMI included SBP, anemia, and antihypertensive use with agents other than ACE/ARB. Taken together, these studies suggest that BP likely plays a role in the development/regression of LVH, but that other factors may be contributing as well.

Carotid Intimal Media Thickness (cIMT)

To evaluate the presence and development of atherosclerosis, another major risk factor for cardiovascular disease, intermediate markers of vasculopathy have been examined in children with CKD. These include arterial calcification, intimal media thickness (IMT), and measures of arterial stiffness. Several studies have documented an increase in cIMT among children with CKD compared to healthy controls. A 2005 single-center study by Mitsnefes examined cIMT and other measures of cardiac function in healthy controls and children with either CKD or ESRD and their relationship to markers of calcium-phosphorus metabolism [54]. The authors observed that cIMT was increased in the CKD group compared to the control group and increased even further among patients on dialysis. The prevalence of hypertension increased from normal to CKD to dialysis, but BP was not examined as a predictor of cIMT in this analysis. To examine the evolution of vascular disease over time, a prospective study of 56 children from two centers in Europe looked at comparisons of vascular markers across the spectrum of CKD, from stages 2 to 5, including both dialysis and transplant, over a 1-year period [55]. cIMT was elevated above normal in all groups and found to worsen over time in both the CKD and dialysis groups. By contrast, renal transplant recipients showed improvement in cIMT measurements. Focusing solely on CKD stages 2–4, a cross-sectional analysis from the CKiD study was published in 2012, looking at a subset of study participants in comparison with healthy controls [38]. Again, median cIMT was observed to be significantly higher in the children with CKD. A multivariate analysis demonstrated that hypertension and dyslipidemia were significant predictors of increased cIMT, whereas markers of calcium and phosphorus metabolism were not.

Other Markers of Cardiovascular Dysfunction

Using ABPM data from the CKiD study, investigators have demonstrated that among children with CKD, those with hypertension have increased BP variability (BPV) and decreased heart rate variability (HRV) compared to those with normal BP [56]. All children in the analysis were untreated, thus removing any potential influence of antihypertensive medications. A low HRV has been reported in adult patients with ESRD, and correlates with an increased risk of cardiac death [57]. Increased BPV, a risk factor associated with adverse cardiovascular and cerebrovascular outcomes in hypertensive patients, has also been noted in the adult CKD population [58, 59]. Replicating these associations in children with CKD further illustrates that many aspects of cardiovascular risk are developing quite early in these patients.

Neurocognitive Function

While evidence of neurocognitive deficits among adults with mild hypertension compared to normal controls was identified over 25 years ago, it is only recently that similar studies have been conducted in pediatric patients with elevated BP. Using data from the NHANES III survey, Lande et al. demonstrated that children with elevated BP (defined as $BP \geq$ 90th percentile) had decreased performance on several cognitive measures compared to those with normal BP [60]. The same group published a series of smaller studies looking at changes after treatment with antihypertensive medications in children with primary hypertension. They observed that hypertensive children scored lower on parental reports of executive function and higher on measures of "internalizing" behaviors (such as depression and anxiety) compared to healthy controls [61]. After 1 year, parent ratings of executive functioning improved (as did BP) in the hypertensive children, but there was no significant change for the control group, suggesting that elevated BP could have subtle neurologic target organ changes [62].

Extensive neurocognitive testing is also a component of the CKiD study and data collected at baseline were published in 2011 [63, 64]. Although the average test performances were in the normal range for the study group as a whole, a substantial proportion of participants scored at least one SD below the mean on several of the tests, including intelligence quotient (IQ) and executive functioning. Higher GFR was associated with lower risk of poor scores on tests of executive functioning. A multivariate analysis also demonstrated that elevated BP was independently associated with a lower performance IQ score. Although these studies are not definitive, they suggest that elevated BP may have early and subtle effects on neurocognitive functioning in children. The long-term effects of these deficits are unknown, but they add further impetus to achieving control of hypertension in children with CKD. Additional research in this area will be important as the life expectancy of patients with childhood onset CKD continues to improve.

Treatment

Goals of Therapy

There have been several clinical practice guidelines published over the past decade that include recommended treatment goals for children with CKD (Table 13.6). Perhaps the best known is the previously mentioned 4th Task Force Report, published in 2004, which provided updated BP norms based on height, sex, and age [7]. The 4th Report recommends treatment of hypertension in children with CKD be targeted to <90th percentile. Guidelines from the Kidney Disease Outcomes Quality Initiative (K/DOQI) were also issued in 2004 and specify similar treatment goals: BP should be <90th percentile or <130/80, whichever is lower [25]. Both of these guidelines are based partly on extrapolated data from adult evidence-based guidelines for the treatment of hypertension, specifically the JNC-7 report [65].

Clinical trial evidence provided from the ESCAPE study led to the publication of updated guidelines by the European Society of Hypertension (ESH) in 2009 [66, 67]. This study was a randomized controlled trial in children with CKD undergoing treatment with a fixed dose of ramipril. Participants were assigned to either conventional BP (MAP by ABPM at the 50–90th percentile) or "intense" BP control (MAP by ABPM <50th percentile). Additional agents not targeting the renin–angiotensin system were prescribed to achieve target BP. The investigators observed that those in the intensified arm of the study had slower rates of CKD progression than those in the conventional treatment arm, particularly in cases of proteinuria. In part because of these findings, the ESH guidelines from 2009

Table 13.6 Summary of clinical guidelines for treatment of hypertension in children with CKD

	BP measurement method	Target BP
4th Report (2004) [7]	Auscultated cBP	<90th percentile
K/DOQI (2004) [25]	Auscultated cBP	<90th percentile or 130/80
ESH (2009) [68]	ABPM	<75th percentile MAP or <50th percentile if proteinuria
KDIGO (2012) [8]	Auscultated cBP	≤50th percentile

CKD chronic kidney disease, *BP* blood pressure, *cBP* casual blood pressure, *K/DOQI* Kidney Disease Outcomes Quality Initiative, *ESH* European Society of Hypertension, *KDIGO* Kidney Disease Improving Global Outcomes, *MAP* mean arterial pressure stipulate that, among children with CKD, BP should be targeted to less than the 50th percentile by ABPM in those children with proteinuria and less than the 75th percentile in those without proteinuria.

The most recent guidelines were issued by the Kidney Disease Improving Global Outcomes (KDIGO) initiative in 2012 [8]. Their first recommendation states that anti-hypertensive treatment should be initiated when BP is >90th percentile in children with CKD, which is a departure from all prior guidelines where no threshold is explicitly stated above which to start pharmacologic therapy. Additionally, treatment goals in these guidelines are more stringent and state that casual BP should be lowered to less than the 50th percentile, unless achieving this target is precluded by symptoms of hypotension. Notably, this recommendation received a grade of "low" quality of evidence because it is based on a single trial (ESCAPE) and a single observational study (CKiD data). It is also complicated by the fact that the ESCAPE results were based upon ABPM, whereas the recommendation itself specifies a casual BP target.

While it is encouraging that the past decade has seen the publication of more studies, including one large clinical trial, there is currently no consensus on the preferred guideline for the management of hypertension in children with CKD. Indeed, large clinical trials in adults that have been designed to identify the optimal threshold BP that will slow CKD progression have not yielded a definitive answer to date. There are also emerging data looking at various measures of hypertension beyond casual BP measurements, including parameters of ABPM as well as pulse pressure and non-invasive measurements of central BP and how they relate to clinical outcomes [68–70]. Some evidence suggests that these measures may be more accurate prognostic indicators for such outcomes as cerebrovascular events, cardiovascular events, and CKD progression [71, 72]. More research is clearly needed in the pediatric population to elucidate the best BP target that will both minimize CKD progression and also future cardiovascular disease risk.

Non-Pharmacologic Recommendations

In children and adults with primary hypertension, non-pharmacologic interventions are typically recommended as an adjunct therapy to medications [65]. These often include increased physical activity, weight loss, and a low-sodium diet. In children with hypertension secondary to CKD, such measures may not always be appropriate. While the prevalence of obesity among children with CKD is higher than previously thought, it is much lower than in the general pediatric population and may not be a primary contributor to elevated BP [73]. Similarly, some children with CKD secondary to dysplasia and/or obstructive nephropathy may be polyuric, with both salt and water wasting. Sodium restriction in these cases should be considered carefully in conjunction with a nutritionist to ensure that the child's growth is not impacted. The relative contribution to BP reduction from non-pharmacologic interventions (such as increased physical activity or a specific total daily sodium intake) in children with CKD is unknown. Currently the recommendation would be to implement such changes on a case-by-case basis and as the clinical situation indicates.

Medications

Until recently, there were very few antihypertensive medications whose safety and efficacy had been studied in specifically in children. Since passage of the Food and Drug Administration Modernization Act (1997) and Best Pharmaceuticals for Children Act (2002) in the USA, enough data has been generated for most classes of antihypertensive medications to permit approval and labeling for pediatric use [74]. What is still lacking, however, are comparative prospective trials demonstrating superiority of one particular class of agent over another. Consensus guidelines currently recommend treating with a single agent to maximum dose, then adding additional agents if BP control has not been achieved [7]. Dosing recommendations for medications commonly used to treat pediatric hypertension are shown in Table 13.7. Based on physiologic mechanism and available data from both clinical trials and observational studies, agents that act on the renin–angiotensin–aldosterone system (RAAS) are currently recommended as first-line therapy for hypertension in children with CKD [74, 75]. This approach is supported by data from the CKiD study, which demonstrated that children receiving RAAS agents had better BP control than those receiving other classes of antihypertensives [12]. The impressive effects of the RAAS agent-based regimen used in the ESCAPE trial add further weight to the recommendations favoring this class of drugs in children with CKD [66].

Additional agents are frequently required to achieve adequate BP control and selection is typically guided by clinical considerations. Evidence-based information is now available for children on dosing, safety, and efficacy for most classes of antihypertensive medications. Dual therapy with both ARB and ACE inhibitor may have additive effects on both BP and proteinuria, but recent publication of safety concerns with this combination in adults precludes making this a standard approach in children [76]. Beta-blockers have been reported to have both anti-renin and anti-proteinuric effects in adults, in addition to their BP-lowering effects [77]. These agents should be avoided in children with reactive airways disease and diabetes, but are otherwise generally well tolerated. In patients with a component of volume overload, diuretics can be a helpful addition as second-line agents. Those with significant proteinuria or reduced GFR may require higher doses to achieve an appropriate clinical response, and loop diuretics are likely to be more effective than thiazides.

Previously, dihydropyridine calcium-channel blockers (DHP CCBs) tended to be prescribed as first-line therapy in children with CKD, but their lack of an anti-proteinuric effect makes them less desirable as monotherapy for many patients with CKD. Other classes of antihypertensive medications that have been used successfully in children include direct vasodilators, such as hydralazine or minoxidil, and central alpha-agonists. Aliskiren, a direct renin inhibitor, has been shown to be effective at lowering BP in adults and in one small pediatric study [78]. However, its clinical use is currently somewhat limited as adult trials have reported a significant incidence of worsening renal function, hypotension, and hyperkalemia in patients with CKD [79]. There are currently several trials in process to assess the efficacy and long-term safety of aliskiren in pediatric patients with hypertension. Given the

Table 13.7 Antihypertensive medications and dosing in children and adolescents

Class	Drug	Starting dose	Interval	Maximum dose[a]
ARAs	Eplerenone	25 mg/day	QD – BID	100 mg/day
	Spironolactone[b]	1 mg/kg/day	QD – BID	3.3 mg/kg/day up to 100 mg/day
ARBs	Candesartan[b]	1–6 yrs: 0.2 mg/kg/day;	QD	1–6 yrs: 0.4 mg/kg/day;
		6–17 yrs: <50 kg 4–8 mg QD		6–17 yrs: < 50 kg 16 mg daily
		>50 kg 8–16 mg QD		>50 kg 32 mg daily
	Losartan[b]	0.75 mg/kg/day (up to 50 mg QD)	QD	1.4 mg/kg/day (max 100 mg QD)
	Olmesartan[b]	20–35 kg: 10 mg QD	QD	20–35 kg: 20 mg QD
		≥35 kg: 20 mg QD		≥35 kg: 40 mg QD
	Valsartan[b]	<6 yrs: 5–10 mg/day	QD	<6 yrs: 80 mg QD
		6–17 yrs: 1.3 mg/kg/day		6–17 yrs: 2.7 mg/kg/day
		(up to 40 mg QD)		(up to 160 mg QD)
ACE inhibitors	Benzepril[b]	0.2 mg/kg/day (up to 10 mg/day)	QD	0.6 mg/kg/day (up to 40 mg/day)
	Captopril[b]	0.3–0.5 mg/kg/dose	BID – TID	0.6 mg/kg/day (up to 450 mg/day)
	Enalapril[c]	0.08 mg/kg/day	QD – BID	0.6 mg/kg/day (up to 40 mg/day)
	Fosinopril	0.1 mg/kg/day (up to 10 mg/day)	QD	0.6 mg/kg/day (up to 40 mg/day)
	Lisinopril[b]	0.07 mg/kg/day (up to 5 mg/day)	QD	0.6 mg/kg/day (up to 40 mg/day)
	Quinapril	5–10 mg/day	QD	80 mg/day
α- and β-Adrenergic antagonists	Carvedilol[b]	0.1 mg/kg/dose (up to 6.25 mg BID)	BID	0.5 mg/kg/dose up to 25 mg BID
	Labetalol[b]	2–3 mg/kg/day	BID	10–12 mg/kg/day (up to 1.2 g/day)
β-Adrenergic antagonists	Atenolol[b]	0.5–1 mg/kg/day	QD	2 mg/kg/day up to 100 mg day
	Bisoprolol/HCTZ	2.5/6.25 mg daily	QD	10/6.25 mg daily
	Metoprolol	1–2 mg/kg/day	BID	6 mg/kg/day (up to 200 mg/day)
	Propranolol[c]	1 mg/kg/day	BID – QID	8 mg/kg/day (up to 640 mg/day)

(continued)

Table 13.7 (continued)

Class	Drug	Starting dose	Interval	Maximum dose[a]
CCBs	Amlodipine[b]	0.06 mg/kg/day	QD	0.3 mg/kg/day (up to 10 mg/day)
	Felodipine	2.5 mg/day	QD	10 mg/day
	Isradipine[b]	0.05–0.15 mg/kg/dose	TID – QID	0.8 mg/kg/day up to 20 mg/day
	Extended-release nifedipine	0.25–0.5 mg/kg/day	QD – BID	3 mg/kg/day (up to 120 mg/day)
Central a-agonist	Clonidine[b]	5–20 mcg/kg/day	QD – BID	25 mcg/kg/day (up to 0.9 mg/day)
Diuretics	Amiloride	5–10 mg/day	QD	20 mg/day
	Chlorthalidone	0.3 mg/kg/day	QD	2 mg/kg/day (up to 50 mg/day)
	Furosemide[c]	0.5–2 mg/kg/dose	QD – BID	6 mg/kg/day
	HCTZ	0.5–1 mg/kg/day	QD	3 mg/kg/day (up to 50 mg/day)
Vasodilators	Hydralazine	0.25 mg/kg/dose	TID – QID	7.5 mg/kg/day (up to 200 mg/day)
	Minoxidil	0.1–0.2 mg/kg/day	BID – TID	1 mg/kg/day (up to 50 mg/day)

ARA aldosterone receptor antagonist, *ACE* angiotensin converting enzyme, *ARB* angiotensin receptor blocker, *BID* twice daily, *CCB* calcium channel blocker, *HCTZ* hydrochlorothiazide, *QD* once daily, *QID* four times daily, *TID* three times daily
[a]The maximum recommended adult dose should not be exceeded
[b]Information on preparation of a stable extemporaneous suspension is available for these agents
[c]Available as a FDA approved commercially supplied oral solution

available evidence in children with CKD, it seems clear that the first-line agents should be ACE inhibitors and ARBs, then consideration of beta-blockers, CCBs and/or diuretics if clinically appropriate and finally expanding medication choice to other classes of antihypertensives if additional BP control is needed.

Summary/Conclusion

The past two decades have greatly advanced our knowledge of the prevalence, risk factors, complications and treatment of hypertension in pediatric CKD. Newer clinical and research techniques have expanded our ability to detect evidence of early cardiovascular disease in this population and more studies characterizing the effects of antihypertensive medications in children have been published. The consistently high prevalence rates confirm that detection and treatment of elevated BP should be a top priority for practitioners caring for children with CKD. Additional research correlating specific treatment goals with clinical outcomes will be an important future step in this area.

References

1. U.S. Renal Data System, USRDS 2013 Annual Data Report: Atlas of Chronic Kidney Disease and End-Stage Renal Disease in the United States. Bethesda: National Institutes of Health, National Institute of Diabetes and Digestive and Kidney Diseases; 2013. Available at: http://www.usrds.org/adr.aspx. Accessed 25 June 2015
2. Klag MJ, Whelton PK, Randall BL, et al. Blood pressure and end-stage renal disease in men. N Engl J Med. 1996;34:13–8.
3. Peterson JC, Adler S, Burkart JM, et al. Blood pressure control, proteinuria, and the progression of renal disease. The Modification of Diet in Renal Disease Study. Ann Intern Med. 1995;123:754–62.
4. Prospective Studies Collaboration. Age-specific relevance of usual blood pressure to vascular mortality: a meta-analysis of individual data for one million adults in 61 prospective studies. Lancet. 2002;360:1913–20.
5. Rosner B, Prineas RJ, Loggie JMH, et al. Blood pressure nomograms for children and adolescents, by height, sex and age, in the United States. J Pediatr. 1993;123:871–86.
6. Giliam RF, Prineas RJ, Horibe H. Maturation vs age: assessing blood pressure by height. J Nat Med Assoc. 1982;74:43–6.
7. National High Blood Pressure Education Program Working Group on High Blood Pressure in Children and Adolescents. The fourth report on the diagnosis, evaluation, and treatment of high blood pressure in children and adolescents. Pediatrics 2004;114:555–576
8. Becker GJ, Wheeler DC. KDIGO clinical practice guideline for the management of blood pressure in chronic kidney disease. Kidney Int. 2012;2:S337–414.
9. Din-Dzietham R, Liu Y, Bielo MV, et al. High blood pressure trends in children and adolescents in national surveys, 1963 to 2002. Circulation. 2007;116:1488–96.
10. McNiece KL, Poffenbarger TS, Turner JL, et al. Prevalence of hypertension and pre-hypertension among adolescents. J Pediatr. 2007;150:640–4.
11. Mitsnefes M, Ho P-L, McEnery PT. Hypertension and progression of chronic renal insufficiency in children: a report of the North American Pediatric Renal Transplant Cooperative Study (NAPRTCS). J Am Soc Nephrol. 2003;14:2618–22.
12. Flynn JT, Mitsnefes M, Pierce C, et al. Blood pressure in children with chronic kidney disease. Hypertension. 2008;52:631–7.
13. Samuels J, Ng D, Flynn JT, et al. Ambulatory blood pressure patterns in children with chronic kidney disease. Hypertension. 2012;60:43–50.
14. Flynn JT, Daniels SR, Hayman LL, et al. Update: Ambulatory blood pressure monitoring in children and adolescents: a scientific statement from the American Heart Association. Hypertension. 2014;63:1116–35.
15. Kavey RW, Allade V, Daniels SR, et al. Cardiovascular risk reduction in high-risk pediatric patients: a scientific statement from the American Heart Association Expert Panel on Population and Prevention Science: The Councils on Cardiovascular Disease in the Young, Epidemiology and Prevention, Nutrition, Physical Activity and Metabolism, High Blood Pressure Research, Cardiovascular Nursing, and the Kidney in Heart Disease; and the Interdisciplinary Working Group on Quality of Care and Outcomes Research: Endorsed by the American Academy of Pediatrics. Circulation 2006;114:2710–2738
16. Parekh RS, Carroll CE, Wolfe RA, et al. Cardiovascular mortality in children and young adults with end-stage kidney disease. J Pediatr. 2002;141:191–7.
17. Halbach SM, Martz K, Mattoo T, et al. Predictors of blood pressure and its control in pediatric patients receiving dialysis. J Pediatr. 2012;160:621–5.
18. Chavers BM, Solid CA, Daniels FX, et al. Hypertension in pediatric long-term hemodialysis patients in the United States. Clin J Am Soc Nephrol. 2009;4:1363–9.
19. Kramer AM, van Stralen KJ, Jager KJ, et al. Demographics of blood pressure and hypertension in children on renal replacement therapy in Europe. Kidney Int. 2011;80:1092–8.

20. Sorof JM, Sullivan EK, Tejani A, et al. Antihypertensive mediation and renal allograft failure: A North American Renal Transplant Cooperative Study report. J Am Soc Nephrol. 1999;10:1324–30.
21. Sinha MD, Kerecuk L, Gilg J, et al. Systemic arterial hypertension in children following renal transplantation: prevalence and risk factors. Nephrol Dial Transplant. 2012;27:3359–68.
22. Seeman T, Simkova E, Kreisinger J, et al. Control of hypertension in children after renal transplant. Pediatr Transplant. 2006;10:316–22.
23. Gulhan B, Topaloglu R, Karabulut E, et al. Post-transplant hypertension in pediatric kidney transplant recipients. Pediatr Nephrol. 2014;29:1075–80.
24. McGlothan KR, Wyatt RJ, Ault BH, et al. Predominance of nocturnal hypertension in pediatric renal allograft recipients. Pediatr Transplant. 2006;10:558–64.
25. National Kidney Foundation. KDOQI Clinical practice guidelines on hypertension and antihypertensive agents in chronic kidney disease. Am J Kidney Dis. 2004;43:S1–290
26. Kogon AJ, Pierce CB, Cox C, et al. Nephrotic-range proteinuria is strongly associated with poor blood pressure control in pediatric chronic kidney disease. Kidney Int. 2014;85: 938–44.
27. Fatallah-Shaykh SA, Flynn JT, Pierce CB, et al. Progression of pediatric CKD of nonglomerular origin in the CKiD cohort. Clin J Am Soc Nephrol. 2015;10:571–7.
28. Hadstein C, Schaefer F. Hypertension in children with chronic kidney disease: pathophysiology and management. Pediatr Nephrol. 2008;23:363–71.
29. Gomez-Marin O, Prineas RJ, Rastam L. Cuff bladder width and blood pressure measurement in children and adolescents. J Hypertens. 1992;10:1235–41.
30. Flynn JT, Pierce CB, Miller ER, et al. Reliability of resting blood pressure measurement and classification using an oscillometric device in children with chronic kidney disease. J Pediatr. 2012;160:434–40.
31. Park MK, Menard SW, Yuan C. Comparison of auscultatory and oscillometric blood pressures. Arch Pediatr Adolesc Med. 2001;155:50–3.
32. Butani L, Morgenstern BZ. Are pitfalls of oscillometric blood pressure measurements preventable in children? Pediatr Nephrol. 2003;18:313–8.
33. Wuhl E, Witte K, Soergel M, et al. German Working Group on Pediatric Hypertension. Distribution of 24-h ambulatory blood pressure in children: normalized reference values and role of body dimensions. J Hypertens. 2002;20:1995–2007.
34. Soergel M, Kirschstein M, Busch C, et al. Oscillometric twenty-four-hour ambulatory blood pressure values in children and adolescents: a multicenter trial including 1141 subjects. J Pediatr. 1997;130:178–84.
35. Flynn JT. Ambulatory blood pressure monitoring in children: imperfect yet essential. Pediatr Nephrol. 2011;26:2089–94.
36. Baracco R, Mattoo TK. Pediatric hypertensive emergencies. Curr Hypertens Rep. 2014;16:456.
37. Shroff R, Degi A, Kerti A, et al. Cardiovascular risk assessment in children with chronic kidney disease. Pediatr Nephrol. 2013;28:875–84.
38. Brady TM, Schneider MF, Flynn JT, et al. Carotid intima-media thickness in children with CKD: results from the CKiD study. Clin J Am Soc Nephrol. 2012;7:1930–7.
39. Lindblad YT, Axelsson J, Balzano R, et al. Left ventricular diastolic dysfunction by tissue Doppler echocardiography in pediatric chronic kidney disease. Pediatr Nephrol. 2013;28:2003–13.
40. Hanevold C, Waller J, Daniels S, et al. The effects of obesity, gender and ethnic group on left ventricular hypertrophy and geometry in hypertensive children: a collaborative study of the International Pediatric Hypertension Association. Pediatrics. 2004;113:328–33.
41. Daniels SR, Loggie JM, Khoury P, et al. Left ventricular geometry and severe left ventricular hypertrophy in children and adolescents with essential hypertension. Circulation. 1998;97: 1907–11.
42. Khoury PR, Mitsnefes M, Daniels SR, et al. Age-specific reference intervals for indexed left ventricular mass in children. J Am Soc Echocardiogr. 2009;22:709–14.
43. Wingen AM, Fabian-Bach C, Schaefer F, et al. Randomized multi-centre study of a low-protein diet on the progression of chronic renal failure in children. Lancet. 1997;349:1117–23.

44. Staples AO, Greenbaum LA, Smith JM, et al. Association between clinical risk factors and progression of chronic kidney disease in children. Clin J Am Soc Nephrol. 2010;5:2172–9.
45. Ksiazek A, Klosowska J, Sygulla K, et al. Arterial hypertension and progression of chronic kidney disease in children during 10-year ambulatory observation. Clin Exp Hypertens. 2013;35:424–9.
46. Warady BA, Abraham AG, Schwartz GJ, et al. Predictors of rapid progression of glomerular and nonglomerular kidney disease in children and adolescents: The Chronic Kidney Disease in Children (CKiD) Cohort. Am J Kidney Dis. 2015;65:878–88.
47. Johnstone LM, Jones CL, Grigg LE, et al. Left ventricular abnormalities in children, adolescents and young adults with renal disease. Kidney Int. 1996;50:998–1006.
48. Matteucci MC, Wuhl E, Picca S, et al. Left ventricular geometry in children with mild to moderate chronic renal insufficiency. J Am Soc Nephrol. 2006;17:218–26.
49. Sinha MD, Tibby SM, Rasmussen P, et al. Blood pressure control and left ventricular mass in children with chronic kidney disease. Clin J Am Soc Nephrol. 2011;6:543–51.
50. Mitsnefes M, Flynn J, Cohn S, et al. Masked hypertension associates with left ventricular hypertrophy in children with CKD. Clin J Am Soc Nephrol. 2010;21:137–44.
51. Simpson JM, Savis A, Rawlins D, et al. Incidence of left ventricular hypertrophy in children with kidney disease: impact of method of indexation of left ventricular mass. Eur J Echocardiogr. 2010;11:271–7.
52. Matteucci MC, Chinali M, Rinelli G, et al. Change in cardiac geometry and function in CKD children during strict BP control: A randomized study. Clin J Am Soc Nephrol. 2013;8:203–10.
53. Kupferman JC, Friedman LA, Cox C, et al. BP control and left ventricular hypertrophy regression in children with CKD. J Am Soc Nephrol. 2014;25:167–74.
54. Mitsnefes MM, Kimball TR, Kartal J, et al. Cardiac and vascular adaptation in pediatric patients with chronic kidney disease: role of calcium-phosphorus metabolism. J Am Soc Nephrol. 2005;16:2796–803.
55. Litwin M, Wuhl E, Jourdan C, et al. Evolution of large-vessel arteriopathy in paediatric patients with chronic kidney disease. Nephrol Dial Transplant. 2008;23:2552–7.
56. Barletta GM, Flynn J, Mitsnefes M, et al. Heart rate and blood pressure variability in children with chronic kidney disease: a report from the CKiD study. Pediatr Nephrol. 2014;29:1059–65.
57. Fukuta H, Hayano J, Ishihara S, et al. Prognostic value of heart rate variability in patients with end-stage renal disease on chronic haemodialysis. Nephrol Dial Transplant. 2003;18:318–25.
58. Gorostidi M, Sarafidis P, Sierra Ade L, et al. Blood pressure variability increases with advancing chronic kidney disease stage (abstract). A cross-sectional analysis of 14,382 hypertensive patients from Spain. J Hypertens. 2015;33 Suppl 1:e40
59. Tanner RM, Shimbo D, Dreisbach AW, et al. Association between 24-hour blood pressure variability and chronic kidney disease: a cross-sectional analysis of African Americans participating in the Jackson heart study. BMC Nephrol. 2015;16:84.
60. Lande MB, Kaczorowski JM, Auinger P, et al. Elevated blood pressure and decreased cognitive function among school-age children and adolescents in the United States. J Pediatr. 2003;143:720–4.
61. Lande MB, Adams H, Falkner B, et al. Parental assessments of internalizing and externalizing behavior and executive function in children with primary hypertension. J Pediatr. 2009;154:207–12.
62. Lande MB, Adams H, Falkner B, et al. Parental assessment of executive function and internalizing and externalizing behavior in primary hypertension after anti-hypertensive therapy. J Pediatr. 2010;157:114–9.
63. Hooper SR, Gerson AC, Butler RW, et al. Neurocognitive functioning of children and adolescents with mild-to-moderate chronic kidney disease. Clin J Am Soc Nephrol. 2011;6:1824–30.
64. Lande MB, Gerson AC, Hooper SR, et al. Casual blood pressure and neurocognitive function in children with chronic kidney disease: a report of the children with chronic kidney disease cohort study. Clin J Am Soc Nephrol. 2011;6:1831–7.
65. Chobanian AV, Bakris GL, Black HR, et al. Joint National Committee on Prevention, Detection, Evaluation and Treatment of High Blood Pressure; National Heart, Lung and Blood Institute;

National High Blood Pressure Education Program Coordinating Committee. Seventh report of the Joint National Committee on Prevention, Detection. Hypertension. 2003;42:1206–52.

66. The ESCAPE Trial Group. Strict blood-pressure control and progression of renal failure in children. N Engl J Med. 2009;361:1639–50.
67. Lurbe E, Cifkova R, Cruickshank JK, et al. Management of high blood pressure in children and adolescents: recommendations of the European Society of Hypertension. J Hypertens. 2009;27:1719–42.
68. Gorostidi M, Sarafidis PA, de la Sierra A, et al. Differences between office and 24-hour blood pressure control in hypertensive patients with CKD: a 5693-patient cross-sectional analysis from Spain. Am J Kidney Dis. 2013;62:285–94.
69. Cha RH, Kim S, Ae YS, et al. Association between blood pressure and target organ damage in patients with chronic kidney disease and hypertension: results of the APrODiTe study. Hypertens Res. 2013;37:172–8.
70. Gabbai FB, Rahman M, Hu B, et al. Relationship between ambulatory BP and clinical outcomes in patients with hypertensive CKD. Clin J Am Soc Nephrol. 2012;7:1770–6.
71. Fedecostante M, Spannella F, Cola G, et al. Chronic kidney disease is characterized by "double trouble" higher pulse pressure plus night-time systolic blood pressure and more severe cardiac damage. PLoS One. 2014;9(1):e86155.
72. Yano Y, Bakris GL, Matsushita K, et al. Both chronic kidney disease and nocturnal blood pressure associate with strokes in elderly. Am J Nephrol. 2013;38:195–203.
73. Wilson AC, Schneider MF, Cox C, et al. Prevalence and correlates of multiple cardiovascular risk factors in children with chronic kidney disease. Clin J Am Soc Nephrol. 2011;6:2759–65.
74. Ferguson M, Flynn JT. Rational use of antihypertensive medications in children. Pediatr Nephrol. 2014;29:979–88.
75. Gartenmann AC, Fossali E, von Vigier RO, et al. Better renoprotective effect of angiotensin II antagonist compared to dihydropyridine calcium channel blocker in childhood. Kidney Int. 2003;64:1450–4.
76. The ONTARGET Investigators. Telmisartan, ramipril or both in patients at high risk for vascular events. N Engl J Med. 2008;358:1547–59.
77. Wright Jr JT, Bakris G, Greene T, et al. African American study of kidney disease and hypertension: effect of blood pressure lowering and antihypertensive drug class on progression of hypertensive kidney disease: results from the AASK trial. JAMA. 2003;288:2421–31.
78. Sullivan JE, Keefe D, Zhou Y, et al. Pharmacokinetics, safety profile, and efficacy of aliskiren in pediatric patients with hypertension. Clin Pediatr. 2013;52:599–607.
79. Harel Z, Gilbert C, Wald R, et al. The effect of combination treatment with aliskiren and blockers of the renin-angiotensin system on hyperkalemia and acute kidney injury: systematic review and meta-analysis. BMJ. 2012;344:e42.

Chapter 14
Devices to Treat Hypertension in Chronic Kidney Disease

George Thomas

Hypertension and Chronic Kidney Disease

High blood pressure (BP) is seen in up to 85–95 % of patients with chronic kidney disease (CKD), and can be a cause or consequence of CKD [1]. Resistant hypertension (defined as BP that is not at goal despite the use of at least 3 antihypertensive medication classes including a diuretic, or BP that is at goal but requires 4 or more medications) [2] is associated with CKD. The prevalence of resistant hypertension has been estimated to be as high as 23 % in patients with CKD [3], and adverse cardiovascular and renal outcomes have been reported in patients with resistant hypertension compared to those without resistant hypertension [4–6]. Additionally, the prevalence of resistant hypertension has been reported to increase with decreasing kidney function (from 15.8 % in those with eGFR $\geq$ 60 ml/min/1.73 m^2 to 33.4 % in those with eGFR < 45 ml/min/1.73 m^2) [7].

Optimal BP control is one of the most important targets that must be achieved for cardiovascular protection and to prevent adverse renal outcomes in CKD. A stepwise combination of lifestyle modifications and pharmacologic therapy is the cornerstone of management of hypertension in these patients, with individualization of BP targets and choice of pharmacologic agents depending on age, comorbidities, and side effect profile or tolerance to medications. Data available from the 2007–2012 NHANES analysis reported in the 2014 USRDS Annual Report show that despite increasing awareness and treatment of hypertension, only about 27 % of patients with CKD have BP at target [8].

Recent interest in device therapies for hypertension management as potential complementary or alternative treatments to pharmacologic therapy has increased due to suboptimal control rates of hypertension, and due to the possibility that in

G. Thomas, MD, FACP (✉)
Department of Nephrology and Hypertension, Glickman Urological and Kidney Institute,
Cleveland Clinic, Cleveland, OH, USA
e-mail: thomasg3@ccf.org

© Springer Science+Business Media New York 2016
A.K. Singh, R. Agarwal (eds.), *Core Concepts in Hypertension
in Kidney Disease*, DOI 10.1007/978-1-4939-6436-9_14

many cases effective pharmacologic treatment may be limited by inadequate doses or inappropriate combinations of antihypertensive medications, concurrent use of agents that raise BP, noncompliance with dietary restrictions, and side effects that result in poor compliance with medications. Additionally, although some novel molecules are being studied, there has only been a modest advance in pharmacologic options for hypertension management.

This chapter discusses the use of catheter-based renal denervation and carotid baroreceptor stimulation therapies for hypertension management, including their pathophysiological basis and results of clinical trials using these devices. Other device therapies (including central arteriovenous anastomosis and the use of carotid implant devices) are briefly reviewed. It should be noted that at the time of writing this chapter, these devices and techniques have not been approved by the Food and Drug Administration (FDA) in the USA for routine clinical use; use of these devices and techniques is limited to investigational purposes only in the USA.

Catheter-Based Renal Denervation

Pathophysiology

A variety of evidence suggests that hyperactivation of the sympathetic nervous system plays a major role in initiating and maintaining hypertension. For example, drugs that inhibit the sympathetic drive at various levels have a blood pressure-lowering effect, providing indirect evidence of the importance of sympathetic mechanisms in hypertension. Furthermore, microneurographic measurements show a high level of muscle sympathetic nerve activity (MSNA) in hypertensive patients, which is the centrally originated postganglionic sympathetic nerve activity directed towards the resistance vasculature; as well as have high levels of regional norepinephrine (NE) spillover, which is the amount of transmitter that escapes neuronal uptake and local metabolism and thus "spills over" into the circulation [7].

The kidneys have a dense network of postganglionic sympathetic nerve fibers that end in the efferent and afferent renal arterioles, the juxtaglomerular apparatus, and the renal tubular system [9]. An increase in efferent signals to the kidney leads to renal vasoconstriction and decreased renal blood flow (via α (alpha)1A receptor activation), stimulation of renin release (via β (beta)1 receptor activation) (with subsequent activation of the renin–angiotensin–aldosterone pathway), and increased tubular sodium retention (via α (alpha)1B receptor activation). Afferent renal sympathetic nerves originate mostly from the renal pelvic wall, with mechanoreceptors and chemoreceptors that respond to stretch and ischemia, respectively. Afferent signals from the kidney, which are increased in states of renal parenchymal injury, hypoxia, and renal ischemia (as in CKD) modulate central sympathetic outflow, leading to increased sympathetic efferent discharge to the kidneys, heart, and peripheral blood vessels. This enhanced sympathetic outflow can play a role in subsequent target-organ damage such as left ventricular hypertrophy, congestive heart failure, and progressive renal damage [9–13].

Studies of renal denervation in animals, using surgical and chemical techniques, have further helped to establish the role of renal sympathetic nerves in hypertension. In a rat model of CKD, the increase in BP associated with five-sixths nephrectomy is prevented by interrupting afferent sensory signals. The increased secretion of norepinephrine from the posterior hypothalamic nuclei in this rat model is preventable by dorsal rhizotomy (which is a procedure that specifically severs the afferent renal nerve fibers at the entrance to the ganglionic dorsal root). Progression of renal disease was also prevented by dorsal rhizotomy in this model. These observations suggest that afferent signals from diseased kidneys to central integrative vasomotor centers in the brain cause increased central sympathetic efferent discharge and contribute to hypertension and deterioration of renal function [14].

In DOCA-salt rat models, a model wherein uni-nephrectomized rats are given salt and deoxycorticosterone acetate, which has mineralocorticoid activity, there is a rise in BP that plateaus at about 3 weeks of DOCA-salt administration; in this model, subsequent renal denervation increased natriuresis and attenuates hypertension compared to a sham group that did not get denervation, suggesting that these responses result from, at least in part, loss of efferent renal nerve activity [15].

Technique

The concept of sympathetic denervation for blood pressure control is not new. More than a half century ago, surgical sympathectomy (including thoracolumbar sympathectomy, splanchnicectomy, and celiac ganglionectomy) was sometimes performed to control blood pressure in patients with malignant hypertension. This was effective but caused debilitating side effects including postural hypotension, erectile dysfunction, and syncope. Smithwick and Thompson reported that in 1266 hypertensive patients who underwent this procedure, the 5-year mortality rates were 19%, compared to 54% in 467 medically treated controls. Forty-five percent of those who survived the surgery had significantly lower blood pressure afterward, and the antihypertensive effect lasted 10 years or more [16]. The procedure fell out of favor due to the morbidity associated with this nonselective approach and with increased availability of antihypertensive drug therapy.

Catheter-based renal denervation is a more selective and less invasive technique that interrupts the afferent and efferent renal nerves which run together in a mesh like network in the adventitial layer of the renal arteries. The location of the nerves in the renal arteries is conducive to an approach with a specially designed catheter that is inserted percutaneously through the femoral artery and advanced into the renal arteries. Renal denervation in humans has been achieved by delivery of radiofrequency energy or norepinephrine depleting pharmaceuticals through the catheter, and applied to the endoluminal surface of the artery; thereby selectively targeting renal sympathetic nerves without affecting the abdominal, pelvic, or lower-extremity nerves [17, 18]. While several renal denervation systems of varying designs have been in use outside the USA, this review will be limited to studies using Medtronic's SYMPLICITY renal denervation system (Medtronic, Inc., Mountain View, CA), which has the vast majority of clinical data to date.

The SYMPLICITY studies used a unipolar platinum electrode mounted on the flexible tip of a non-occlusive catheter, delivering radiofrequency energy at 5–8 W (lower than that used for cardiac electrophysiologic procedures) to the wall of the renal artery. The procedure is performed on both renal arteries, with 4–6 sites ablated in a longitudinal distal-to-proximal and rotational manner in 2-min treatments at each site (with a distance of at least 5 mm between sites to avoid overlapping lesions) to cover the full circumference of the artery. The system is designed to automatically shut off after the designated ablation time or if the impedance or temperature exceeds pre-programmed safety limits. The procedure does not require general anesthesia and there is no device implantation involved; intravenous pain medications and sedatives are needed for pain management during the procedure. Median procedure time is reported to be about 38 min. Patients with renovascular abnormalities were not enrolled in the SYMPLICITY trials [19–21]. While it is known from prior anatomic studies that renal nerve density tends to increase from the proximal to distal end of the artery and that most nerves are located ≤2.5 mm from the lumen, the nerves are not imaged or mapped before or after treatment [22]; therefore, it is not known whether all ablation sites along the renal artery produce the same degree of denervation.

Studies using optical coherence tomography (OCT) have shown that radiofrequency energy delivered by the renal denervation catheter causes transmural tissue necrosis and loss of endothelium, along with local thrombus formation and renal artery spasm [23]. Smaller vessels are felt to be more prone to spasm, however, persistent flow-limiting spasm appears to be rare. Patches of edema along the artery are common, and are referred to as "denervation notching," which are reported to resolve without issues [24]. It is unclear whether these acute injury responses have any long-term impact.

Histologic data from pre-clinical studies in pigs, in which renal vessels that underwent denervation using the SYMPLICITY catheter were examined at 6 months, indicated radiofrequency energy induced renal nerve injury (with thickening and fibrosis of the perineural sheath in the nerve from treated vessel, along with a hypercellular appearance of the nerve bundle), and showed complete healing of the renal artery [25].

In a study in 25 patients who underwent renal denervation and had significant BP reduction at follow-up, multi-unit MSNA was moderately decreased, and all properties of single-unit MSNA including firing rates of individual vasoconstrictor fibers, firing probability, and multiple firing incidence of single units within a cardiac cycle were substantially reduced at follow-up. No changes were noted in a control group of ten patients. This would suggest that modulation of renal sympathetic nerve activity is the primary mechanism by which denervation reduces BP [26]. In contrast to this, however, another study in 13 patients who underwent denervation showed no change in MSNA, despite BP-lowering effect (the authors specifically noted variable effects of denervation on BP in individual patients). There was no relationship between the effect on BP and the effect on MSNA [27]. This raises questions regarding variable efficacy of denervation and variable effects on MSNA even if the procedure effectively disrupted the function of renal nerves.

Therapeutic Effectiveness and Safety

SYMPLICITY HTN-1 and SYMPLICITY HTN-2

SYMPLICITY HTN-1 was a proof-of-principle (first in man) study with an initial cohort of 45 patients, which was later expanded to 153 patients. Office BP, which was the primary endpoint, was reduced by an average of 27/17 mmHg at 12 months, and final follow-up at 36 months showed persistent BP reduction by an average of 32/14 mmHg in 88 patients. Heart rate did not change significantly from baseline to 36 months. According to the investigators, there were no major procedure-related or device-related complications. One patient had a new angiographically confirmed 80 % stenosis 24 months after denervation, which was successfully stented [19, 28].

SYMPLICITY HTN-2 was the first randomized controlled trial in renal denervation, and it enrolled patients who had a systolic BP of 160 mmHg or higher (or 150 mmHg or higher in patients with type 2 diabetes). Compared to control group ($n=54$) who continued treatment with antihypertensive medications alone, office BP in the denervation group ($n=52$) at the end of 6 months reduced by an average of 32/12 mmHg compared with average change of 1/0 mmHg in control group. The results were less striking in 20 patients who also had 24 h ambulatory blood pressure monitoring done in SYMPLICITY HTN-2, which showed an average reduction of only 11/7 mmHg post denervation. The large discrepancy between office BP and ABPM responses raises the possibility that a substantial effect of renal denervation is reduction in the "white-coat effect." Long-term follow-up in 40 of the 52 patients who initially had denervation reported sustained BP reduction by an average of 33/14 mmHg at 36 months. 85 % of these patients achieved an SBP reduction of ≥10 mmHg (defined as "responders"). Per trial design, patients in the control group were eligible to get renal denervation at the end of 6 months—this cross over group had an average systolic BP reduction of 33 mmHg at 30 months post denervation. There was a mean decrease in heart rate of 4 beats per minute, which persisted through 36 months of follow-up. No serious procedure-related or device-related complications were reported, and the occurrence of adverse events did not differ between groups at the time of primary analysis. No renal vascular events were reported [20, 29].

SYMPLICITY HTN-3

SYMPLICITY HTN-3 was the largest double-blinded randomized controlled trial in renal denervation, and randomized 535 patients in the USA in a 2:1 ratio to undergo denervation or a sham procedure. In an effort to minimize possible white-coat resistant hypertension, eligibility criteria included 24 h ABPM systolic BP $\geq$ 135 mmHg in addition to office systolic BP $\geq$ 160 mmHg on full and stable doses of at least 3 antihypertensive medications including a diuretic. A small design change in the catheter used in SYMPLICITY HTN-3 was that it was more flexible compared to the stiffer earlier version. In contrast to the dramatic results from earlier SYMPLICITY trials, SYMPLICITY HTN-3 showed only a 2.3 mmHg systolic BP difference between the denervation group and the sham procedure group ($p=0.26$), and the between-group difference did not meet the superiority margin of 5 mmHg. Additionally, the change in 24 h ABPM, which was a major secondary endpoint, showed only a difference of 1.9 mmHg between the groups ($p=0.98$). Follow-up at 12 months indicated that in denervation subjects, the office systolic BP change was greater than that observed at 6 months (-15.5 ± 24.1 mmHg vs. -18.9 ± 25.4 mmHg, respectively; $p=0.025$), but the 24 h systolic BP change was not significantly different at 12 months ($p=0.229$). There were no significant differences in safety between the groups at 6 months and 12 months [30, 31].

The results of SYMPLICITY HTN-3 have brought into question whether the efficacy of renal denervation has been overestimated. The reasons for the discrepancy in results between the earlier trials and SYMPLICITY HTN-3 have been extensively discussed in the literature, including the difference in patient characteristics (more African Americans in SYMPLICITY HTN-3), catheter design, experience of operators and the possibility of a learning curve with possible procedural shortcomings (post hoc analysis indicated that 253 of the participants randomized to the active treatment arm of the study did not have circumferential ablation of both renal arteries) [32–35]. It should be noted that there are currently no consistent or reliable predictors of response to renal denervation (other than that those with higher baseline blood pressures tend to show more response). Measurement of MSNA and norepinephrine spillover on a routine basis is not feasible in clinical practice. Although the incidence of de-novo renal artery stenosis attributable to the procedure is reportedly low, longer term follow-up is needed to assess this more carefully. The long-term evaluation of renal function is discussed in the next section.

Renal Function and Hemodynamics

The final 3-year report of SYMPLICITY HTN-1 noted that mean eGFR had decreased from 83.6 ml/min/1.73 m^2 to 74.3 ml/min/1.73 m^2—28 patients had a decrease in eGFR by more than 25 % at 1 or more time points during follow-up (of which decreases were transient in 16 patients). No significant change in renal function was reported in SYMPLICITY HTN-2 (in the final 36-month follow-up report) or SYMPLICITY HTN-3 (in the 6-month primary end point report) [28–30].

A study in 88 patients who underwent renal denervation examined renal resistive index in the interlobar arteries, renal function, and urinary albumin excretion, measured before and at 3 and 6 months of follow-up after denervation. Renal resistive index decreased significantly from baseline to 3 and 6 months after denervation. Mean Cystatin C GFR and urinary albumin excretion remained unchanged; however, the number of patients with microalbuminuria or macroalbuminuria decreased. No renal vascular events were noted through the 6 months of follow-up [36].

Renal perfusion was assessed by magnetic resonance imaging with arterial spin labeling (MRI-ASL) in a study in 19 patients who underwent denervation, along with assessment of Cystatin C and serum creatinine before and at 1 day and 3 months after denervation. Central hemodynamics using pulse wave analysis were assessed before and at 6 months after denervation: there was significant reduction in peripheral and central blood pressures after denervation; renal perfusion and function did not change significantly. Additionally, renal vascular resistance (calculated as mean arterial pressure (mmHg) divided by renal perfusion measured by MRI-ASL (ml/min per 100 g kidney tissue) was significantly reduced 3 months after denervation [37].

Longer term follow-up is important to assess evolution of renal function post denervation, especially the effects of intensive diuretic or renin–angiotensin inhibitors, if any, in the setting of renal denervation.

Durability of Effects

In studies that did show benefit (SYMPLICITY HTN-1 and SYMPLICITY HTN-2), BP reduction was reported to be persistent through 36 months [28, 29]. Data from animal experiments suggests that renal re-innervation might occur; re-innervation has been reported to be complete and functional at 8 weeks post denervation in rats, and in 12–16 months in dogs [38, 39]. Human experience with renal transplantation indicates that although there is anatomic re-innervation of the efferent nerves, the functional significance of this is unclear [40, 41].

Cost-Effectiveness and Quality of Life

A study prior to results of SYMPLICITY HTN-3 used a state-transition Markov model to assess the cost-effectiveness of renal denervation. This model, based on effect size from SYMPLICITY HTN-2 results, concluded that renal denervation may be a cost-effective treatment strategy for treatment of resistant hypertension (to an order of magnitude below the recognized threshold of $50,000 per QALY) [42].

However, this conclusion may no longer be valid based on results of SYMPLICITY HTN-3 which did not indicate efficacy with renal denervation. Additionally, the model assumes that renal denervation will lower cardiovascular morbidity and mortality by lowering BP; morbidity and mortality data are not available for renal denervation in resistant hypertension.

Health related quality of life (QOL) measures were examined in a small study of 62 patients who underwent renal denervation, using the Outcomes Study 36-Item Short-Form Health Survey (SF-36) and the Beck Depression Inventory-II (BDI-II). Improvements in QOL measures (comparing before and 3 months after renal denervation) were reported, not associated with magnitude of BP reduction [43].

Renal Denervation in CKD

An eGFR lower than 45 ml/min/1.73 m^2 was arbitrarily chosen as a contraindication for renal denervation in the SYMPLICITY trials. Thus, little evidence exists on the effect of denervation in moderate-to-severe CKD patients. One small study in 15 patients with stage 3–4 CKD found that mean changes in office systolic and diastolic BP at 1, 3, 6, and 12 months were −34/−14, −25/−11, −32/−15, and −33/−19 mmHg, respectively. Night-time ambulatory BP significantly decreased, restoring a more physiologic dipping pattern. There were no significant changes in eGFR or microalbuminuria in 3–6 months of follow-up. Additional benefits included a trend towards increased hemoglobin concentration, decrease in brain natriuretic peptide, and a significant reduction in arterial stiffness [44]. Although beneficial effects on progression of CKD and albuminuria may be expected from a blood pressure-lowering effect and direct beneficial effect of less sympathetic activity with renal denervation, the evidence is currently limited. In patients on hemodialysis, only case reports and a small series have been published reporting safety and significant blood pressure decrease after denervation, although in the series only systolic BP, not diastolic BP, decreased [45]. In hemodialysis patients, suitability of the renal arteries (of the atrophic kidneys) for denervation would be of concern.

Other Uses

Small studies have reported other benefits of renal denervation beyond BP lowering in conditions associated with underlying enhanced sympathetic drive, including improved glucose metabolism, improved apnea–hypopnea index in obstructive sleep apnea, improved insulin sensitivity in polycystic ovarian syndrome, and reduced recurrences of atrial fibrillation [46–49]. Left ventricular mass regression and improvement in diastolic function has also been reported [50]. Thus, there is some evidence that there may be pleiotropic effects of renal denervation beyond BP reduction; these require further investigation to assess potential utility.

Summary

Although there is an attractive underlying rationale with strong pre-clinical data, renal denervation did not show significant benefit in the largest clinical trial to date. Interestingly, a randomized study published after SYMPLICITY HTN-3 showed that adjusted drug treatment (with emphasis on drug adherence) was superior to renal denervation in patients with "true" treatment resistant hypertension [51]. Other renal denervation devices, including those with multi-electrode catheters, and non-invasive ultrasound based technology, are also being studied [52]. It is possible that this procedure may still have a place in management of resistant hypertension, but not before there is better understanding of its effects, including identifying response predictors and appropriate selection of patients who may benefit from the procedure, ability to better assess degree of ablation, and long-term follow-up for durability of effects and safety.

Baroreceptor Activation Therapy

Pathophysiology

Arterial baroreceptors located in the carotid sinus (at the bifurcation of the external and internal carotid arteries) respond to increased BP (via stretch stimulation due to vascular distension) and send signals to the nucleus tractus solitarius (NTS) located in the medulla. Under normal physiological conditions, baroreceptor firing exerts a tonic inhibitory influence on sympathetic outflow; when activated, there is increase in efferent parasympathetic and decrease in efferent sympathetic activity from the medullary center, causing bradycardia and peripheral vasodilation which counteracts the increases in BP.

Experimental animal models have also evaluated the effect of long-term stimulation of baroreceptors using carotid sinus electrode implants in dogs; a significant reduction in mean arterial pressure and plasma catecholamines has been demonstrated in these models, without a concomitant increase in plasma renin activity. Studies have also shown that in animals with angiotensin-II induced hypertension, prolonged activation of the carotid baroreceptors results in decreased renal sympathetic nerve activity in those with an intact baroreflex mechanism, along with a resultant increase in natriuresis [53–56].

Technique

Modulation of the baroreflex mechanism is not a new concept; in the 1960s, case reports and case series with use of implantable electronic devices showed angina and blood pressure reduction [57–60], however, technical limitations precluded more widespread use. The devices were bulky, needed frequent recharging, and it was difficult to adjust the frequency and amplitude of stimulation. Adverse effects reported with these devices included dysphagia, coughing, gagging, and dyspnea [61].

Newer devices have been developed with changes in generator and lead technology. The Rheos Baroflex Activation Therapy System (CVRx Inc., Minneapolis, MN) works by electrically activating the carotid baroreflex. Increased signaling to the medullary brain centers results in changes in sympathetic and parasympathetic output to offset the perceived rise in blood pressure. This surgically implanted device consists of a battery-powered generator and 2 leads (with 5 electrodes), which run from the generator to the left and right carotid sinuses. The device is implanted in infraclavicular position, and is programmable by an external system linked telemetrically to the generator, and allows the physician to non-invasively adjust the stimulation parameters delivered to the leads. The implantation procedure requires surgical skill, and has been compared with carotid endarterectomy. The procedure is done under general anesthesia, and medications include anesthetic agents that blunt the baroreflex system should be avoided. Electrode placement in the area of the carotid sinus is done in a position that provides optimal hemodynamic response. The lead is connected to the generator and activated with impulses of 3 V, 100 Hz and a pulse width of 480 μ[mu]s; within 1 min, stimulation using these parameters at a correct location should reduce systolic blood pressure by at least 10–20 mmHg and heart rate by 5–10 beats/min. Once optimal location is confirmed, the electrode was sutured in place on the superficial aspect of the artery, avoiding direct suturing to the carotid sinus [62, 63].

Adverse events attributed to the Rheos device were mainly surgical (noted below), and although the side effect profile was felt to compare favorably with the results from endarterectomy trials involving intervention in the same anatomical region, a second-generation system of baroreflex activation therapy Barostim neo (CVRx Inc., Minneapolis, MN) has been designed to address shortcomings of the original Rheos device. A single electrode lead (compared to 5 electrodes with the Rheos device) is implanted at one carotid site (typically on the right), thus reducing the operating field and possible surgical complications. The battery is also smaller, with an extended life span ($\approx$3 years). Average implantation procedure time for the Barostim device is reported to be 107 ± 28 min [52, 64, 65]. Patient with carotid artery stenosis or orthostatic hypotension were not enrolled in the baroreflex activation therapy trials discussed below.

Therapeutic Effectiveness and Safety

The prospective nonrandomized DEBut-HT trial was a multicenter feasibility trial for the early generation Rheos device, performed in 45 patients with resistant hypertension. In this proof-of-concept study, there was a reduction of $21 \pm 4/12 \pm 2$ mmHg ($n = 37$) in office BP at 3 months, with further decreases of $30 \pm 6/20 \pm 4$ mmHg

($n = 26$) at 1 year and $33 \pm 48/22 \pm 26$ mmHg ($n = 17$) at 2 years (all $p = <0.005$), respectively. There was also a statistically significant reduction in 24 h ambulatory blood pressures at 1 year follow-up (no significant change was noted at 3 month follow-up). In contrast, no BP change was observed in 10 control patients who did not get device implantation. In total, 8 serious adverse events (7 procedure-related and 1 device-related) were reported. A sub-study of 12 patients from the DEBut-HT trial demonstrated that MSNA and BP were decreased after activation of baroreflex activation therapy (BAT) and increased without activation, providing evidence that reduction of sympathetic outflow is the primary mechanism for BP reduction with this therapy. The DEBut-HT trial did not report any carotid artery stenosis as assessed by ultrasound at 1 year. No evidence of orthostatic hypotension was found, and no events of collapse or syncope were reported in 32 patients after 3 months of device therapy in the DEBut-HT trial [66].

The double-blind, randomized, parallel-design Rheos Pivotal trial enrolled 256 patients with resistant hypertension. One month after Rheos device implantation, patients were randomized in a 2:1 manner to immediate BAT (device on) or delayed BAT (device remained off for 6 months). The pre-specified acute primary efficacy end point (proportion of patients achieving BP reduction of ≥ 10 mmHg after 6 months with a superiority margin of 20%) was not met, and the secondary efficacy end point (mean change in systolic BP after 6 months) failed statistical significance (group A [device on]: -16 ± 29 versus group B [device off]: -9 ± 29 mmHg; $p = 0.08$). The sustained primary efficacy end point, defined as BP reduction of ≥ 10 mmHg post-implant to 12 months, with $\geq 50\%$ of BP reduction seen at month 6 (primary end point) was reached. The procedural primary safety end point (30 day event free rate) was not met, mainly because of surgical complications (4.8%) and transient (4.8%) or residual (4.4%) nerve injuries, but the pre-specified criteria of both therapy (6 month event free rate) and device safety (12 month event free rate) were met [67]. After completion of the Rheos Pivotal Trial, participants continued in an open-label, nonrandomized follow-up for an average of 28 ± 9 months. A mean BP reduction of 36/16 mmHg ($p < 0.001$) was observed in the selected group of long-term responders ($n = 245$, 76%), defined by achieved systolic BP ≤ 140 mmHg (≤ 130 mmHg for patients with diabetes or CKD) or systolic BP reduction of ≥ 20 mmHg from device activation. ABPM results are not available from this study [68].

Using the newer Barostim neo device, a single-arm open-label study enrolling 30 patients with resistant hypertension showed a BP reduction of $26.0 \pm 4.4/12.4 \pm 2.5$ mmHg after 6 months. ABPM results are not available from this study. Three perioperative and 1 long-term procedure-related complication occurred [65]. The randomized Barostim Hypertension Pivotal trial is currently recruiting patients, and aims to study the safety and efficacy of the newer device, and includes assessment of change of 24-h ambulatory systolic blood pressure (SBP) between baseline and 12 months post-activation as a secondary outcome measure.

Renal Function

The Rheos pivotal trial and the Barostim study did not specify any exclusion based on renal function, whereas the DEBut-HT trial specified exclusion of patients on dialysis. In the Rheos pivotal trial, the estimated glomerular filtration rate (GFR) decreased from 92 to 87 ml/min/1.73 m^2 in group A (immediate activation/device on) at month 6—these values did not change any further after 12 months of therapy. Patients with highest GFR showed the greatest decrease in glomerular filtration. Group B (delayed activation/device off) showed the same trends as group A even before device activation at month 6. Systolic BP reduction seemed to be significantly related to the change in glomerular filtration rate in both groups. Albumin/creatinine ratio did not change in both groups during follow-up. Thus, baroreflex activation therapy was associated with an initial mild decrease in glomerular filtration rate, attributed to be a hemodynamic response to the drop in blood pressure, and long-term treatment (up to the time of 12 month follow-up) did not result in further decrease in renal function [67, 68].

Cost-Effectiveness and Quality of Life

A German study reported Barostim BAT to be cost-effective compared with optimal medical treatment with an incremental cost-effectiveness ratio of €7797 per QALY. In the model, Barostim reduced lifetime rates of myocardial infarction by 19%, stroke by 35%, heart failure by 12%, and end-stage renal disease by 23% [69]. It should be noted, however, that this model evaluated the cost-effectiveness of the second-generation Barostim System, whereas clinical effectiveness data are based on the first generation Rheos device. Additionally, the morbidity and mortality data are not available for BAT from current studies, and clinical effectiveness was extrapolated over a lifetime assuming durable effects. Additional considerations would include requirement for hospital stay after surgery, and need for surgical replacement of the implanted generator at least every 3 years (which is lifespan of the Barostim device).

Baroreflex Activation Therapy in CKD

The effect of BAT (using Barostim device) on renal function in 23 CKD patients with resistant hypertension (defined as systolic BP > 130 mmHg despite the use of at least 3 antihypertensive medications including a diuretic) was reported in a small pilot study. After 6 months of BAT, the office systolic and diastolic BP decreased significantly. Mean systolic BP decreased from 161 ± 31.9 to 144 ± 32.3 mmHg and mean diastolic BP decreased from 87.4 ± 15.2 to 77.7 ± 17.1 mmHg) ($p < 0.01$). The mean decrease of systolic ABPM was -5.7 ± 15.4 mmHg which was not statistically significant. Proteinuria decreased after 6 months of BAT by a median of -29.2% ($-67.6 \pm 42.1\%$) ($p=0.01$) and albuminuria by a median of -19.0% ($-60.9 \pm 5.1\%$) ($p=0.01$), with more pronounced effects in those with higher stages of CKD. Serum creatinine ($p=0.66$), eGFR-MDRD ($p=0.82$), and CKD-EPI creatinine equation ($p=0.98$) did not differ in the follow-up compared to baseline. Renin and aldosterone levels did not change before and after BAT, and a non-statistically significant trend for increase in fractional excretion of sodium and 24 h urinary sodium was noted [70].

Other Uses

In a randomized trial of medical therapy vs. Barostim BAT in addition to medical therapy for NYHA III heart failure and ejection fraction $\leq 30\%$, the group that received BAT had significantly improved functional status, quality of life, exercise capacity, N-terminal pro-brain natriuretic peptide, and a non-significant trend for lower heart failure hospitalizations at 6 months. No interactions with existing implantable cardiac rhythm management devices (pacemakers or ICDs) were seen [71]. An echocardiogram sub-study of the DeBUT-HT trial using the Rheos device in 34 patients indicated that after 1 year of BAT, there was reduced left atrial (LA) dimension, left ventricle (LV) wall thicknesses, LV mass, and LV stroke work ($p<0.001$). Significant reduction in mitral A-wave velocity, LA dimension, and LV mass index (LVMI) suggested reduced LV diastolic filling pressures with BAT. No signs of deteriorating LV systolic function were present (i.e., no reduced LV ejection fraction and no increased LV end-diastolic diameter) [72]. These cardioprotective effects of BAT need to be evaluated in larger trials.

Summary

As with renal denervation, more data on efficacy, safety, and durability of effects, especially with the newer generation Barostim devices, will be needed before widespread use of this technique. While there are no head-to-head comparisons of renal denervation vs. BAT in patients with resistant hypertension, the Barostim BAT study showed lower BP and heart rate in a subset of patients who had previously undergone renal denervation therapy that failed to adequately control their hypertension [65]. A pre-clinical study in dogs with complete bilateral renal denervation has also demonstrated that intact renal nerves were not required for BAT to provide BP and heart rate reductions [73]. Grassi and colleagues have summarized similarities and differences between renal denervation and baroreceptor stimulation [61].

Other Devices

Arteriovenous Fistula

The ROX coupler system (ROX Medical Inc., San Clemente, CA) attempts to lower blood pressure by targeting the mechanical characteristics of the arterial tree in hypertension, and involves the addition of a low-resistance, high compliance venous segment to the stiff central arterial tree (that occurs with chronic hypertension). The device creates a 4 mm arteriovenous fistula (AVF) between the iliac artery and vein, generating a sustained calibrated shunt volume ($\approx$800 ml/min) within a short period of time ($\approx$1 h). A reduction in total systemic vascular resistance, despite an increment in cardiac output, is considered to be the key mechanism by which blood pressure is lowered [52]. Adverse effects include induction of venous stenosis and thrombosis and potential worsening or development of right ventricular failure. The randomized ROX CONTROL HTN study showed that in the ROX coupler group ($n=44$), office BP decreased by 26.3/20.1 mmHg (control group ($n=39$) 3.7/2.44 mmHg) and ambulatory BP by 13.5/13.5 mmHg (control group 0.5/0.1 mmHg) after 6 months. Patients with eGFR of less than 30 ml/min/1.73 m^2 were excluded from this study [74]. There are no reports of this device being specifically tested in CKD patients.

Carotid Implant Device

A first-in-man study (CALM-FIM_US) of the MOBIUS HD device (Vascular Dynamics Inc., Mountain View, CA) is currently recruiting patients to evaluate efficacy and safety of a device implanted in the region of the carotid sinus, and designed to amplify baroreceptor signaling and lead to blood pressure lowering (NCT01831895).

References

1. Rao MV, Qiu Y, Wang C, Bakris G. Hypertension and CKD: Kidney Early Evaluation Program (KEEP) and National Health and Nutrition Examination Survey (NHANES), 1999–2004. Am J Kidney Dis. 2008;51(4 Suppl 2):S30–7.
2. Calhoun DA, Jones D, Textor S, Goff DC, Murphy TP, Toto RD, White A, Cushman WC, White W, Sica D, Ferdinand K, Giles TD, Falkner B, Carey RM, Resistant hypertension: diagnosis, evaluation, and treatment. A scientific statement from the American Heart Association Professional Education Committee of the Council for High Blood Pressure Research. Hypertension. 2008;51(6):1403–19.
3. De Nicola L, Gabbai FB, Agarwal R, Chiodini P, Borrelli S, Bellizzi V, Nappi F, Conte G, Minutolo R. Prevalence and prognostic role of resistant hypertension in chronic kidney disease patients. J Am Coll Cardiol. 2013;61(24):2461–7.

4. Bangalore S, Fayyad R, Laskey R, Demicco DA, Deedwania P, Kostis JB, Messerli FH, Treating to New Targets Steering Committee and Investigators. Prevalence, predictors, and outcomes in treatment-resistant hypertension in patients with coronary disease. Am J Med. 2014;127(1):71–81.
5. Muntner P, Davis BR, Cushman WC, Bangalore S, Calhoun DA, Pressel SL, Black HR, Kostis JB, Probstfield JL, Whelton PK, Rahman M, ALLHAT Collaborative Research Group. Treatment-resistant hypertension and the incidence of cardiovascular disease and end-stage renal disease: results from the Antihypertensive and Lipid-Lowering Treatment to Prevent Heart Attack Trial (ALLHAT). Hypertension. 2014;64(5):1012–21.
6. Kumbhani DJ, Steg PG, Cannon CP, Eagle KA, Smith SC Jr, Crowley K, Goto S, Ohman EM, Bakris GL, Perlstein TS, Kinlay S, Bhatt DL, REACH Registry Investigators. Resistant hypertension: a frequent and ominous finding among hypertensive patients with atherothrombosis. Eur Heart J. 2013;34(16):1204–14.
7. Tanner RM, Calhoun DA, Bell EK, Bowling CB, Gutiérrez OM, Irvin MR, Lackland DT, Oparil S, Warnock D, Muntner P. Prevalence of apparent treatment-resistant hypertension among individuals with CKD. Clin J Am Soc Nephrol. 2013;8(9):1583–90.
8. United States Renal Data System, 2014 Annual Data Report: Epidemiology of Kidney Disease in the United States. Bethesda: National Institutes of Health, National Institute of Diabetes and Digestive and Kidney Diseases. http://www.usrds.org/2014/view/v1_01.aspx. (2014) Accessed 28 May 2015.
9. Schlaich MP, Sobotka PA, Krum H, Whitbourn R, Walton A, Esler MD. Renal denervation as a therapeutic approach for hypertension: novel implications for an old concept. Hypertension. 2009;54:1195–201.
10. Zanchetti AS. Neural regulation of renin release: experimental evidence and clinical implications in arterial hypertension. Circulation. 1977;56:691–8.
11. Kon V. Neural control of renal circulation. Miner Elecrolyte Metab. 1989;15:33–43.
12. DiBona GF, Kopp UC. Neural control of renal function. Physiol Rev. 1997;77(1):75–197. Review.
13. Mancia G, Grassi G, Giannattasio C, Seravalle G. Sympathetic activation in the pathogenesis of hypertension and progression of organ damage. Hypertension. 1999;34:724–8.
14. Campese VM. Neurogenic factors and hypertension in renal disease. Kidney Int. 2000;57:S2–6.
15. Katholi RE. Renal nerves in the pathogenesis of hypertension in experimental animals and humans. Am J Physiol. 1983;245:F1–14.
16. Smithwick RH, Thompson JE. Splanchnicectomy for essential hypertension; results in 1,266 cases. J Am Med Assoc. 1953;152:1501–4.
17. Krum H, Schlaich M, Sobotka P, Scheffers I, Kroon AA, de Leeuw PW. Novel procedure- and device-based strategies in the management of systemic hypertension. Eur Heart J. 2011;32(5):537–44.
18. Judd EK, Oparil S. Novel strategies for treatment of resistant hypertension. Kidney Int Suppl (2011). 2013;3(4):357–63.
19. Krum H, Schlaich M, Whitbourn R, Sobotka PA, Sadowski J, Bartus K, Kapelak B, Walton A, Sievert H, Thambar S, Abraham WT, Esler M. Catheter-based renal sympathetic denervation for resistant hypertension: a multicentre safety and proof-of-principle cohort study. Lancet. 2009;373(9671):1275–81.
20. Symplicity HTN-2 Investigators, Esler MD, Krum H, Sobotka PA, Schlaich MP, Schmieder RE, Böhm M. Renal sympathetic denervation in patients with treatment-resistant hypertension (The Symplicity HTN-2 Trial): a randomised controlled trial. Lancet. 2010;376(9756):1903–9. doi:10.1016/S0140-6736(10)62039-9. Epub 2010 Nov 17.
21. Kandzari DE, Bhatt DL, Sobotka PA, O'Neill WW, Esler M, Flack JM, Katzen BT, Leon MB, Massaro JM, Negoita M, Oparil S, Rocha-Singh K, Straley C, Townsend RR, Bakris G. Catheter-based renal denervation for resistant hypertension: rationale and design of the SYMPLICITY HTN-3 Trial. Clin Cardiol. 2012;35(9):528–35.

22. Atherton DS, Deep NL, Mendelsohn FO. Micro-anatomy of the renal sympathetic nervous system: a human postmortem histologic study. Clin Anat. 2012;25(5):628–33.
23. Templin C, Jaguszewski M, Ghadri JR, Sudano I, Gaehwiler R, Hellermann JP, Schoenenberger-Berzins R, Landmesser U, Erne P, Noll G, Lüscher TF. Vascular lesions induced by renal nerve ablation as assessed by optical coherence tomography: pre- and post-procedural comparison with the simplicity catheter system and the EnligHTN multi-electrode renal denervation catheter. Eur Heart J. 2013;34(28):2141–8, 2148b.
24. Myat A, Redwood SR, Qureshi AC, Thackray S, Cleland JG, Bhatt DL, Williams B, Gersh BJ. Renal sympathetic denervation therapy for resistant hypertension: a contemporary synopsis and future implications. Circ Cardiovasc Interv. 2013;6(2):184–97.
25. Rippy MK, Zarins D, Barman NC, Wu A, Duncan KL, Zarins CK. Catheter-based renal sympathetic denervation: chronic preclinical evidence for renal artery safety. Clin Res Cardiol. 2011;100(12):1095–101.
26. Hering D, Lambert EA, Marusic P, Walton AS, Krum H, Lambert GW, Esler MD, Schlaich MP. Substantial reduction in single sympathetic nerve firing after renal denervation in patients with resistant hypertension. Hypertension. 2013;61(2):457–64.
27. Vink EE, Verloop WL, Siddiqi L, van Schelven LJ, Liam Oey P, Blankestijn PJ. The effect of percutaneous renal denervation on muscle sympathetic nerve activity in hypertensive patients. Int J Cardiol. 2014;176(1):8–12.
28. Krum H, Schlaich MP, Sobotka PA, Böhm M, Mahfoud F, Rocha-Singh K, Katholi R, Esler MD. Percutaneous renal denervation in patients with treatment-resistant hypertension: final 3-year report of the Simplicity HTN-1 study. Lancet. 2014;383(9917):622–9.
29. Esler MD, Böhm M, Sievert H, Rump CL, Schmieder RE, Krum H, Mahfoud F, Schlaich MP. Catheter-based renal denervation for treatment of patients with treatment-resistant hypertension: 36 month results from the SYMPLICITY HTN-2 randomized clinical trial. Eur Heart J. 2014;35(26):1752–9.
30. Bhatt DL, Kandzari DE, O'Neill WW, D'Agostino R, Flack JM, Katzen BT, Leon MB, Liu M, Mauri L, Negoita M, Cohen SA, Oparil S, Rocha-Singh K, Townsend RR, Bakris GL, SYMPLICITY HTN-3 Investigators. A controlled trial of renal denervation for resistant hypertension. N Engl J Med. 2014;370(15):1393–401.
31. Bakris GL, Townsend RR, Flack JM, Brar S, Cohen SA, D'Agostino R, Kandzari DE, Katzen BT, Leon MB, Mauri L, Negoita M, O'Neill WW, Oparil S, Rocha-Singh K, Bhatt DL, SYMPLICITY HTN-3 Investigators. 12-month blood pressure results of catheter-based renal artery denervation for resistant hypertension: the SYMPLICITY HTN-3 trial. J Am Coll Cardiol. 2015;65(13):1314–21.
32. Persu A, Jin Y, Fadl Elmula FE, Jacobs L, Renkin J, Kjeldsen S. Renal denervation after simplicity HTN-3: an update. Curr Hypertens Rep. 2014;16(8):460.
33. Pathak A, Ewen S, Fajadet J, Honton B, Mahfoud F, Marco J, Schlaich M, Schmieder R, Tsioufis K, Ukena C, Zeller T. From SYMPLICITY HTN-3 to the renal denervation global registry: where do we stand and where should we go? EuroIntervention. 2014;10(1):21–3.
34. Joyner MJ. Renal denervation: what next? Hypertension. 2014;64(1):19–20.
35. Kandzari DE, Bhatt DL, Brar S, Devireddy CM, Esler M, Fahy M, Flack JM, Katzen BT, Lea J, Lee DP, Leon MB, Ma A, Massaro J, Mauri L, Oparil S, O'Neill WW, Patel MR, Rocha-Singh K, Sobotka PA, Svetkey L, Townsend RR, Bakris GL. Predictors of blood pressure response in the SYMPLICITY HTN-3 trial. Eur Heart J. 2015;36(4):219–27.
36. Mahfoud F, Cremers B, Janker J, Link B, Vonend O, Ukena C, Linz D, Schmieder R, Rump LC, Kindermann I, Sobotka PA, Krum H, Scheller B, Schlaich M, Laufs U, Böhm M. Renal hemodynamics and renal function after catheter-based renal sympathetic denervation in patients with resistant hypertension. Hypertension. 2012;60(2):419–24.
37. Ott C, Janka R, Schmid A, Titze S, Ditting T, Sobotka PA, Veelken R, Uder M, Schmieder RE. Vascular and renal hemodynamic changes after renal denervation. Clin J Am Soc Nephrol. 2013;8(7):1195–201.
38. Kline RL, Mercer PF. Functional reinnervation and development of supersensitivity to NE after renal denervation in rats. Am J Physiol. 1980;238(5):R353–8.

39. Nomura G, Kurosaki M, Takabatake T, Kibe Y, Takeuchi J. Reinnervation and renin release after unilateral renal denervation in the dog. J Appl Physiol. 1972;33(5):649–55.
40. DiBona GF. Renal innervation and denervation: lessons from renal transplantation reconsidered. Artif Organs. 1987;11:457–62.
41. Hansen JM, Abildgaard U, Fogh-Andersen N, Kanstrup IL, Bratholm P, Plum I, Strandgaard S. The transplanted human kidney does not achieve functional reinnervation. Clin Sci (Lond). 1994;87(1):13–20.
42. Geisler BP, Egan BM, Cohen JT, Garner AM, Akehurst RL, Esler MD, Pietzsch JB. Cost-effectiveness and clinical effectiveness of catheter-based renal denervation for resistant hypertension. J Am Coll Cardiol. 2012;60(14):1271–7.
43. Lambert GW, Hering D, Esler MD, Marusic P, Lambert EA, Tanamas SK, Shaw J, Krum H, Dixon JB, Barton DA, Schlaich MP. Health-related quality of life after renal denervation in patients with treatment-resistant hypertension. Hypertension. 2012;60(6):1479–84.
44. Hering D, Mahfoud F, Walton AS, Krum H, Lambert GW, Lambert EA, Sobotka PA, Böhm M, Cremers B, Esler MD, Schlaich MP. Renal denervation in moderate to severe CKD. J Am Soc Nephrol. 2012;23(7):1250–7.
45. Schlaich MP, Bart B, Hering D, Walton A, Marusic P, Mahfoud F, Böhm M, Lambert EA, Krum H, Sobotka PA, Schmieder RE, Ika-Sari C, Eikelis N, Straznicky N, Lambert GW, Esler MD. Feasibility of catheter-based renal nerve ablation and effects on sympathetic nerve activity and blood pressure in patients with end-stage renal disease. Int J Cardiol. 2013;168(3):2214–20.
46. Mahfoud F, Schlaich M, Kindermann I, Ukena C, Cremers B, Brandt MC, Hoppe UC, Vonend O, Rump LC, Sobotka PA, Krum H, Esler M, Böhm M. Effect of renal sympathetic denervation on glucose metabolism in patients with resistant hypertension: a pilot study. Circulation. 2011;123(18):1940–6.
47. Schlaich MP, Straznicky N, Grima M, Ika-Sari C, Dawood T, Mahfoud F, Lambert E, Chopra R, Socratous F, Hennebry S, Eikelis N, Böhm M, Krum H, Lambert G, Esler MD, Sobotka PA. Renal denervation: a potential new treatment modality for polycystic ovary syndrome? J Hypertens. 2011;29(5):991–6.
48. Witkowski A, Prejbisz A, Florczak E, Kądziela J, Śliwiński P, Bieleń P, Michałowska I, Kabat M, Warchoł E, Januszewicz M, Narkiewicz K, Somers VK, Sobotka PA, Januszewicz A. Effects of renal sympathetic denervation on blood pressure, sleep apnea course, and glycemic control in patients with resistant hypertension and sleep apnea. Hypertension. 2011;58(4):559–65.
49. Pokushalov E, Romanov A, Corbucci G, Artyomenko S, Baranova V, Turov A, Shirokova N, Karaskov A, Mittal S, Steinberg JS. A randomized comparison of pulmonary vein isolation with versus without concomitant renal artery denervation in patients with refractory symptomatic atrial fibrillation and resistant hypertension. J Am Coll Cardiol. 2012;60(13):1163–70.
50. Brandt MC, Mahfoud F, Reda S, Schirmer SH, Erdmann E, Böhm M, Hoppe UC. Renal sympathetic denervation reduces left ventricular hypertrophy and improves cardiac function in patients with resistant hypertension. J Am Coll Cardiol. 2012;59(10):901–9.
51. Fadl Elmula FE, Hoffmann P, Larstorp AC, Fossum E, Brekke M, Kjeldsen SE, Gjønnæss E, Hjørnholm U, Kjaer VN, Rostrup M, Os I, Stenehjem A, Høieggen A. Adjusted drug treatment is superior to renal sympathetic denervation in patients with true treatment-resistant hypertension. Hypertension. 2014;63(5):991–9.
52. Oparil S, Schmieder RE. New approaches in the treatment of hypertension. Circ Res. 2015;116(6):1074–95.
53. Lohmeier TE, Lohmeier JR, Haque A, Hildebrandt DA. Baroreflexes prevent neurally induced sodium retention in angiotensin hypertension. Am J Physiol Regul Integr Comp Physiol. 2000;279(4):R1437–48.
54. Lohmeier TE, Irwin ED, Rossing MA, Serdar DJ, Kieval RS. Prolonged activation of the baroreflex produces sustained hypotension. Hypertension. 2004;43(2):306–11.
55. Barrett CJ, Guild SJ, Ramchandra R, Malpas SC. Baroreceptor denervation prevents sympathoinhibition during angiotensin II-induced hypertension. Hypertension. 2005;46(1):168–72.

56. Lohmeier TE, Dwyer TM, Irwin ED, Rossing MA, Kieval RS. Prolonged activation of the baroreflex abolishes obesity-induced hypertension. Hypertension. 2007;49(6):1307–14.

57. Schwartz SI, Griffith LS, Neistadt A, Hagfors N. Chronic carotid sinus nerve stimulation in the treatment of essential hypertension. Am J Surg. 1967;114:5–15.

58. Neistadt A, Schwartz SI. Effects of electrical stimulation of the carotid sinus nerve in reversal of experimentally induced hypertension. Surgery. 1967;61:923–31.

59. Brest AN, Wiener L, Bachrach B. Bilateral carotid sinus nerve stimulation in the treatment of hypertension. Am J Cardiol. 1972;29:821–5.

60. Braunwald E, Epstein SE, Glick G, Wechsler AS, Braunwald NS. Relief of angina pectoris by electrical stimulation of the carotid-sinus nerves. N Engl J Med. 1967;277(24):1278–83.

61. Grassi G, Seravalle G, Brambilla G, Cesana F, Giannattasio C, Mancia G. Similarities and differences between renal sympathetic denervation and carotid baroreceptor stimulation. Curr Vasc Pharmacol. 2014;12(1):63–8.

62. Scheffers IJ, Kroon AA, Tordoir JH, de Leeuw PW. Rheos Baroreflex hypertension therapy system to treat resistant hypertension. Expert Rev Med Devices. 2008;5(1):33–9.

63. Tordoir JH, Scheffers I, Schmidli J, Savolainen H, Liebeskind U, Hansky B, Herold U, Irwin E, Kroon AA, de Leeuw P, Peters TK, Kieval R, Cody R. An implantable carotid sinus baroreflex activating system: surgical technique and short-term outcome from a multi-center feasibility trial for the treatment of resistant hypertension. Eur J Vasc Endovasc Surg. 2007;33(4):414–21.

64. Alnima T, de Leeuw PW, Kroon AA. Baroreflex activation therapy for the treatment of drug-resistant hypertension: new developments. Cardiol Res Pract. 2012;2012:587194. Epub 2012 Jun 12.

65. Hoppe UC, Brandt MC, Wachter R, Beige J, Rump LC, Kroon AA, Cates AW, Lovett EG, Haller H. Minimally invasive system for baroreflex activation therapy chronically lowers blood pressure with pacemaker-like safety profile: results from the Barostim neo trial. J Am Soc Hypertens. 2012;6(4):270–6.

66. Scheffers IJ, Kroon AA, Schmidli J, Jordan J, Tordoir JJ, Mohaupt MG, Luft FC, Haller H, Menne J, Engeli S, Ceral J, Eckert S, Erglis A, Narkiewicz K, Philipp T, de Leeuw PW. Novel baroreflex activation therapy in resistant hypertension: results of a European multi-center feasibility study. J Am Coll Cardiol. 2010;56(15):1254–8.

67. Bisognano JD, Bakris G, Nadim MK, Sanchez L, Kroon AA, Schafer J, de Leeuw PW, Sica DA. Baroreflex activation therapy lowers blood pressure in patients with resistant hypertension: results from the double-blind, randomized, placebo-controlled rheos pivotal trial. J Am Coll Cardiol. 2011;58(7):765–73.

68. Bakris GL, Nadim MK, Haller H, Lovett EG, Schafer JE, Bisognano JD. Baroreflex activation therapy provides durable benefit in patients with resistant hypertension: results of long-term follow-up in the Rheos Pivotal Trial. J Am Soc Hypertens. 2012;6(2):152–8.

69. Borisenko O, Beige J, Lovett EG, Hoppe UC, Bjessmo S. Cost-effectiveness of Barostim therapy for the treatment of resistant hypertension in European settings. J Hypertens. 2014;32(3):681–92.

70. Wallbach M, Lehnig LY, Schroer C, Hasenfuss G, Müller GA, Wachter R, Koziolek MJ. Impact of baroreflex activation therapy on renal function—a pilot study. Am J Nephrol. 2014;40(4):371–80.

71. Abraham WT, Zile MR, Weaver FA, Butter C, Ducharme A, Halbach M, Klug D, Lovett EG, Müller-Ehmsen J, Schafer JE, Senni M, Swarup V, Wachter R, Little WC. Baroreflex activation therapy for the treatment of heart failure with reduced ejection fraction. JACC Heart Fail. 2015.

72. Bisognano JD, Kaufman CL, Bach DS, Lovett EG, de Leeuw P, DEBuT-HT and Rheos Feasibility Trial Investigators. Improved cardiac structure and function with chronic treatment using an implantable device in resistant hypertension: results from European and United States trials of the Rheos system. J Am Coll Cardiol. 2011;57(17):1787–8.

73. Lohmeier TE, Hildebrandt DA, Dwyer TM, Barrett AM, Irwin ED, Rossing MA, Kieval RS. Renal denervation does not abolish sustained baroreflex-mediated reductions in arterial pressure. Hypertension. 2007;49(2):373–9.
74. Lobo MD, Sobotka PA, Stanton A, Cockcroft JR, Sulke N, Dolan E, van der Giet M, Hoyer J, Furniss SS, Foran JP, Witkowski A, Januszewicz A, Schoors D, Tsioufis K, Rensing BJ, Scott B, Ng GA, Ott C, Schmieder RE; ROX CONTROL HTN Investigators. Central arteriovenous anastomosis for the treatment of patients with uncontrolled hypertension (the ROX CONTROL HTN study): a randomised controlled trial. Lancet. 2015;385(9978):1634–41.

Index

© Springer Science+Business Media New York 2016
A.K. Singh, R. Agarwal (eds.), *Core Concepts in Hypertension in Kidney Disease*, DOI 10.1007/978-1-4939-6436-9

Printed in the United States
By Bookmasters